T0255636

CONDENSE WISDOM

and

CONQUER CANCER

for the

BENEFIT OF MANKIND

HOW TO CONQUER CANCER? HOW TO PREVENT CANCER?

Part I

Xu Ze; Xu Jie; Bin Wu

authorHOUSE®

AuthorHouse™
1663 Liberty Drive
Bloomington, IN 47403
www.authorhouse.com
Phone: 1 (800) 839-8640

© 2018 Xu Ze; Xu Jie; Bin Wu. All rights reserved.

No part of this book may be reproduced, stored in a retrieval system, or transmitted by any means without the written permission of the author.

Published by AuthorHouse 02/15/2018

ISBN: 978-1-5462-1832-6 (sc)
ISBN: 978-1-5462-1833-3 (e)

Library of Congress Control Number: 2017917861

Print information available on the last page.

Any people depicted in stock imagery provided by Thinkstock are models, and such images are being used for illustrative purposes only. Certain stock imagery © Thinkstock.

This book is printed on acid-free paper.

Because of the dynamic nature of the Internet, any web addresses or links contained in this book may have changed since publication and may no longer be valid. The views expressed in this work are solely those of the author and do not necessarily reflect the views of the publisher, and the publisher hereby disclaims any responsibility for them.

Contents

A Brief Introduction To The First Author

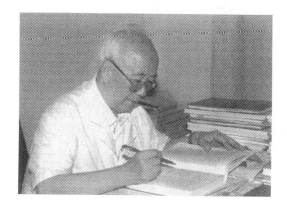

Xu Ze, male, born in Leping County of Jiangxi Province in Oct. 1933, gradated from Tongji Medical University in 1956, successively held the post of director of department of surgery of Affiliated Hospital of Hubei College of Traditional Chinese Medicine, professor, chief physician, tutor of postgraduate and doctoral student, President of Experimental Surgery Restitute Institute of Hubei College of Traditional Chinese Medicine, Director of Abdominal Tumor Surgery Research Room and Director of Anti Carcinomatous Metastasis and Reoccurrence Research Room. in addition, he held concurrent posts of Standing Director of China Medical Association Wuhan Branch, Vice President of Wuhan Micro-circulation Academy, Academic Member of International Liver Disease Research, Cooperation and Exchange Center, Member of International Surgeon Union, Standing Member of 1st, 2nd, 3rd and 4th Editorial Board of China Experimental Surgery Journal, Standing Member of 1st, 2dn and 3rd Editorial Board of Abdominal Surgery Journal. Enjoying Special Allowance of State Council.

He has been engaged in surgery work for 49 years and accumulated rich experience in radical operation of lung cancer, esophageal carcinoma, liver cancer, carcinoma of gallbladder, adenocarcinoma of pancreas, gastric carcinoma and intestinal cancer as well as in clinical therapy with Chinese Traditional Medicine combined with Western Medicine of prevention of reoccurrence and metastasis after operation.

He has been engaged in scientific research of surgery for 15 years and obtained many fruits, among which the task of Experimental Study and Clinical Application of Self-made Type Z-C1 Abdominal Cavity—Vein Flow Turning Unit in Therapy of Chronic Ascites of Hepatic Cirrhosis issued by Science Commission of Hubei Province was awarded Second Prize of Scientific Fruit by People's Government of Hubei Province and was popularized and applied in 38 hospitals in 12 provinces all over the country in 1982. The task "Experimental Study on Physiological Mechanism and Pathogenesis of Schistosome with Method of Experimental Surgery", issued by National Natural Fund Commission was awarded Second Prize of Scientific Fruit by People's Government of Hubei Province in 1986.

He began to study the tumor experience, established the tumor animal model and metastasis and reoccurrence animal model and probed into the mechanism and rules of carcinomatous metastasis and reoccurrence to find out the method to inhibit the metastasis. 48 kinds of Chinese traditional herbs that could counteract the intrusion, metastasis and reoccurrence were found and selected from a large number of natural herbs. Based on this, he invented and developed China Xu Ze (Z-C) Medicine Treating Malignancy, which had remarkable curative effects through over 10 years' clinical validation of many cases.

He has been engaged in teaching for 40 years and has cultivated many young doctors, 10 masters and 2 doctors. He has released 126 papers, published New Understanding and New Mode of Therapy of Cancer as the editor in charge, participate in writing 8 medical exclusive books including Therapeutics of Liver Disease, Surgery of Liver, Gallbladder and Pancreas and Surgical Operation of Abdomen.

A Brief Introduction To The Second Author

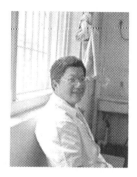

Xu Jie, male, graduated from Hubei College of Traditional Chinese Medicine in 1992, graduated from Hubei Medical University in 1996, Department of Clinical Medicine. Now He is chief physician in Hubei University of Traditional Chinese Medicine Hospital and Hubei Provincial Hospital of Surgery, engaged in experimental surgical tumor research and general surgery, urology clinical work.

Since 1992, he has been involved in the experimental tumor research of the Institute of Experimental Surgery of Hubei College of Traditional Chinese Medicine. He has carried out cancer cell transplantation and established a tumor animal model. He has carried out a series of experimental tumor research: exploring the mechanism of recurrence and metastasis of cancer and in vivo screening experiment of more than 200 kinds of Chinese herbal medicine in vivo tumor model of tumor inhibition s from a large number of natural medicine to find out, screening out of 48 kinds of anti-cancer invasion, metastasis, relapse traditional Chinese medicine

He participates in clinical validation and followed up for XZ - C immunoregulatory Chinese herbal medicine and completes the experimental research and clinical verification, data collection, collection and summary of this book.

A Brief Introduction To The Third Author And The Main Translator And One Of The Editors

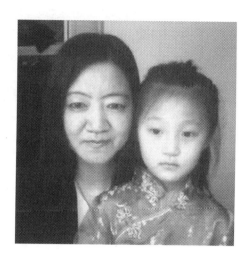

Bin Wu, MD, Ph.D., graduated from College of Yunyang of Tongji University of Medical Sciences for her MD degree; Studied her Master degree and her Ph. D degree in Sun Yat-Sen University of Medical Sciences. After she received her Ph.D., she worked as a Post-doctoral Follews in the Johns Hopkins Medical School and University of Maryland Medical School. She passed her USMLE tests and is going to do her residency training in America. She dedicated herself to oncology clinical and research. Her goal is to conquer cancer, which she believes this great contribution to our health. She has a daughter, named Lily Xu who drew all of the pictures in this book.

A Brief Introduction To The Illustrator And The Advisor

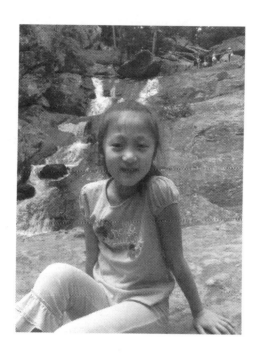

Lily Xu was born on November 17th 2006 and had an art presented in the Walter Art Museum in Baltimore at the age of 6; she got the fourth place trophy in the ES Double Digits or 24 and 24 games in the Baltimore County in Maryland; she got the first trophy in the BCPS STEM FAIR PHYSICS in Baltimore County; when she was in the sixth grade, she passed the advanced Math for 7th grade(which means the 8th grade math) test and moved the 8th grade math class; she loves the reading and the writing and she finished many seires of books. She got $3000 scholarship award for the Peabody music program in the Johns Hopkins University. She edits all of my books for the publication. She is a very smart advisor on the computer and on some medical-related topics.

XU ZE think of conquering cancer, where is the road? The road is in the scientific research – the road is on the prevention and treatment of cancer scientific research and the road is the study under the guidance of the concept of the scientific development.

Science is an endless frontier, our scientific work has followed the scientific concept of development, based on the known medical, future-oriented medicine, the new disciplines,interdisciplinary, cross-disciplinary,basedon the known material science, to explore the future of science and unknown knowledge, look forward, through the static mind, a long-term hard work and practice the scientific concept of development, in scientific, difficult journey, a scientific step by step and step, to the forefront of science, for innovative and forward, to overcome cancer research hall brick by Tim watts.

Preface

This book is to help with conquering cancer and with launching a total attack and with building the scientific city of conquering cancer.

The overall design and the planning and the blueprint of XZ-C's conquering cancer are the scientific thinking and the theoretical innovation and the experimental basis of conquering cancer are the reform and development of the overall strategy of cancer treatment and the crystallization of my 60 years of experience in medical work and 30 years of the scientific research results and achievement and the scientific and technological innovation and the scientific thinking and the scientific research wisdom which the direction of the research is to conquering cancer. It is proposed that to set up a test area sitting in Wuhan City, Huang Jiahu University City; the implementation of this research program will be done by my research team experts, professors ... ... and so.

The scientific research plan of conquering cancer is put into the focused on scientific research in the international and is the forefront of science.

In January 12th, 2016 the US President Barack Obama in the State of the Union addressed the national cancer program of "to conquer cancer" and named the new moon plan (Cancer moon shot) which is responsible by the vice president Joe Biden for the implementation which its specific plan is unknown.

Cancer is a disaster of the mankind. It must struggle with cancer all over the world and people of the world struggle together and gather wisdom and move forward together to overcome cancer.

Cancer disaster is covered by the world. The people worldwide are eager to overcome the cancer one day. It is the urgent hope that the states and the governments and the experts and the scholars and the scientists can find anti-cancer measures to keep people from cancer.

Acknowledgements

This book is for all of people who concern human being health. We are deep grateful to all of people who like our new ways to improve our human being health.

My daughter Lily Xu gives me many smart and creative ideas while we were finishing this book. Lily Xu drew all of the pictures such as the Thymus etc.

I would like to express our sincere gratitude to the following:

1. All of Authorhouse staffs
2. Dr. Xu Ze's family and Dr. Xu Jie's family
3. Mrs. Bo Wu's family and Mrs. Tao Wu's famly: espeicaly their daughters Chongshu Luo and Xunyue Wang
4. Medchi CEO: Gene Ransom III gives us great help

Bin Wu, M.D., Ph.D

In October, 2017 in Baltimore, Maryland in USA

The Guidance Information

Condense Wisdom and Conquer Cancer
— for the benefit of mankind

How to conquer cancer? how to prevent cancer by my opinions?how to treat cancer by my opinions

Table of Contents

1, the guidance to read
2, the guidance words
3, the guidance to act

1, the guidance to read

1), In this medical monograph the book is divided into the next two parts, a total of 10 volumes, which wisdom are condensed to be used to conquer cancer?

Part I (Volume 1-4) condense how to conquer cancer and how to prevent cancer by my opinions

Part II (5-10 volumes) condense how to conquer cancer and how to treat cancer by my opinions?

Prevention cancer and anti-cancer, and the prevention is as the main are the health work policy, especially the prevention cancer for the top priority so that people can be away from cancer to reduce cancer incidence.

This is a medical monograph with the more complete and more systematic and more comprehensive design and more specific planning of how to conquer cancer which can be used as the reference for the various countries and the provinces and the states to carry out the implementation of how to overcome cancer? how to prevent cancer? how to control cancer? how to treat cancer?

2), the agglutination of the following wisdom which can be used to overcome cancer:

Part One

Condense How To Conquer Cancer?
How To Prevent Cancer I See.

Volume I

(A), How to overcome cancer? XZ-C proposed three targets

After analysis: XZ-C proposed that the target or the goal of conquering cancer should be:

A target: it should be directed against the gene mutations and the abnormal expression or the deletion.

B target: it should be for environmental factors:
The external environment — air, water, soil, physical, chemical, biological factors, clothing, food, shelter.
The internal environment — immune, endocrine, neurohumoral
It should create "the environmental protection research institute" and carry out the prevention cancer system engineering research.

C target: it should be to adjust the normal immune system and to restore the immune system to identify cancer cells, thereby remove tumor cells, and conduct the immunotherapy and the immunoprophylaxis.

(B), How to overcome cancer? XZ-C presents: two wheels

The details of the situation analysis (a), (b), (c), (d)
The basic situation is:
The United States:

life sciences, biomedicine, genetic engineering, targeted therapy, drugs, minimally invasive techniques, instruments, and precision medicine are far ahead.

China:

It has the rich resources of the immune regulation and control traditional Chinese medication and the immune regulation traditional Chinese medications, the traditional Chinese medications with activating blood and removing stasis and anti-microvascular thrombosis and anti-micrometastasis as well as the traditional Chinese medication which controls precancerous nodules by soften the firm and scatter the knot.

It should cooperate complement each other and move forward together.

(C). Why is the cooperation between China and the United States?

Because:

(1) in 1971 the US Congress passed a "national cancer regulations", and President Nixon issued "anti-cancer declaration" in order to overcome cancer in one fell swoop.

(2) In January 12, 2016 US President Barack Obama announced **"the national plan to conquer cancer"** and the plan is responsible by Vice President Joe Biden.

The Plan name: **"Cancer moon shot"**
The Goal: to overcome cancer

(3) In 2011 Chinese doctor Xu Ze put forward in his published monographs: "the strategic thinking and suggestions of conquering cancer."

In August 2013 at the International Cancer Conference it was put forward " the XZ-C research program of conquering cancer and launch a total attack"

In July 2015 it proposed" the dawn of the C-type plan of conquering cancer and launch a total attack"

In December 2016 in the English version of the monograph it was put forward " the initiative of conquering cancer and launch the general attack."

Therefore: China and the United States both are conducting the scientific research of conquering cancer and it should be co-operation and move forward toward the scientific hall of conquering cancer.

Volume II

What wisdom is condensed which can be used to overcome cancer?

Its focus is:

- How to prevent cancer I see and how to carry out conquering cancer and launching a total attack?
- How to create the scientific research bases and the Science city with a multidisciplinary and cancer research group?
- it must create an "Innovative Oncology School" and a graduate school in order to o overcome cancer.
- it must set up To overcome the cancer, it must create " the prevention and treatment hospital with innovative tumor integrated traditional Chinese and Western medications during tumor whole process and the prevention, control and treatment of cancer are at the same attention in order to conquer cancer.
- it must create an "Innovative Molecular Cancer Institute" in order to overcome cancer.
- it must create "Innovative Environmental Protection Cancer Research Institute" and prevention cancer system engineering.

Volume III

What wisdom is condensed which can be used to conquer cancer?

Its focus is:

How to prevent cancer I see: how to prevent cancer from the big environment and the small environment?

- How to prevent cancer from clothing, food, shelter, and walking?
- it should be carried out prevention cancer from improving carcinogenic factors in external causes (external environment) and internal causes (internal environment).
- Environmental and cancer research groups should be set up to study the relationship between environment and cancer.
- To study what the carcinogenic factors are in the environment and how should they be prevented?
- XZ-C proposes to create the "Innovative Environmental Protection Institute" and the prevention cancer system project
- How can we prevent cancer from "two types of society"?
- The catastrophe of cancer is the global and the people of the world must struggle with it and struggle together.

Volume IV

What wisdom is condensed which can be used to conquer cancer?

Its focus is:

- the proposals was put forward "cancer treatment reform, innovation and development."
- XZ-C proposes a plan to tackle the total attack on cancer.
- it was put forward the necessity and feasibility of proposing a total attack on cancer.
- it was proposed "the general design and imagine of conquer cancer and the basic design of the Science City" and the feasibility report.
- it was put forward the suggestions that at the same time when a well-off society is constructed, the ride research is built and the scientific research on prevention cancer and anti-cancer is conducted.

Part II

The agglomeration of how to overcome cancer? Each opinion I see of how to treat cancer is this part.

Volume V

What wisdom is condensed which can be used to conquer cancer?

Its focus is: "walked out of a new way to overcome cancer"

- From the experimental results it was found that: the thymus has the acute progressive atrophy in the host with inoculated cancer cells and the cell proliferation was blocked and the volume was significantly reduced.

- From the above experimental study it was found that thymic atrophy and the immune dysfunction may be one of the etiology and pathogenesis of the tumor, it must try to prevent from the thymic atrophy and to promote thymocyte proliferation and to increase immune function.

- In order to try to prevent thymic atrophy and to promote thymocyte hyperplasia and to increase immune function, it was to find from both the traditional Chinese medication and Western medication. In western medication there is rare medication which can improve immunity and promote the proliferation of thymocytes so that it was changed from the Chinese medication to find because in the traditional Chinese medication the increasing tonic drugs generally have immune regulation.

- After 7 years of laboratory scientific research, XZ-C1-10 immune regulation and control anti-cancer and anti-transfer medications were screened out from the natural and traditional Chinese medication and composed of which can protect the thymus and the hematopiene in bone marrow . On the basis of the success of the animal experiment The clinical validation work was performed, after 20 years of more than 12,000 cases of cancer specialist clinical application it achieved good results.

- After the experimental study and the anti-cancer research of Chinese medicine immunopharmacology and the combination of Chinese and Western medications on the molecular level, it walked out of a new path of conquering cancer with XZ-C immune regulation and control which regulates immune activity, prevents thymus atrophy, promotes thymocyte proliferation, protects bone marrow hematopoietic function, improves immune surveillance and with the Combination of Chinese and Western medication—the "Chinese - style anti - cancer" new road.

Volume VI

What wisdom is condensed which can be used to conquer cancer?

Its focus is:

- During more than 20 years it has been walked out of a new path to overcome the cancer and has formed the theoretical system of XZ-C immune regulation and control and has undergone the clinical application, observation and verification.

- The new model that it is considered cancer treatment is that **healing should be done through immunoregulation rather than a single killer**, and the last step in curing cancer is to regain the control of the host's immune regulation and control function rather than destroy the last cancer cells.

- From the experimental results to analyze thinking, the new revelation is that: thymus atrophy are immune dysfunction are one of the factors of the cause and pathogenesis of cancer so that in the international academic conference Xu Ze Professor proposed that one of the cause and the pathogenesis of cancer may be thymus atrophy, central immune organ motility damage, immune dysfunction, immune surveillance capacity decline and immune escape.

- Based on the findings of the laboratory above experimental results, the treatment principle must be to prevent thymus atrophy, promote thymic hyperplasia, protect bone marrow hematopoietic function, improve immune surveillance, control malignant cells immune escape.

- XZ-C (XU-ZE-China) immunoregulation therapy was first presented by Professor Xu Ze in his book "New Concepts and Methods for Cancer Transfer

Treatment" in 2006, and he believes **that under the normal circumstances, both cancer and body defense are in a dynamic balance ; the occurrence of cancer is caused by this dynamic imbalance. If the state has been adjusted to the normal level, you can control the growth of cancer and make it subside.**

- **It is well known that the occurrence, progression and prognosis of cancer is determined by a combination of two factors, namely, the biological characteristics of cancer cells and the host body itself; if the balance between the two can be controlled, the cancer cells can be controlled; if the two are imbalance, the cancer will occur and develop.**

- Cancer treatment should be changed to observe and establish **a comprehensive treatment concept.**

The goal of treatment only kill cancer cells which is only one aspect and it is one-sided treatment concept and it can not overcome cancer. **The goal of treatment should be in both the areas of the host and cancer cells and not only kill cancer cells, but also protect the host, enhance immune function and protect thymus and increase immune functions and protect the hematopiene of the bone marrow and enhance the host anti-cancer ability; this is a comprehensive treatment concept, it is possible to overcome cancer.**

Therefore, the principle of cancer treatment should change the concept and it should establish a comprehensive treatment concept.

Volume VII

What wisdom is condensed which can be used to conquer cancer?

To challenge the status quo of cancer treatment and to reform can develop.

Its focus is:

- the review and the analysis and the questioning of the three major treatments for cancer

- Through the review and the analysis and the reflection it is found the traditional problems and shortcomings of traditional therapy.

- The analysis and the evaluation and the questioning of systemic intravenous chemotherapy for solid tumors:

- The analysis and questioning of whether the method and the route of the systemic intravenous administration for the solid tumors are scientific and reasonable or not?

- The analysis and questioning of whether the method of calculating the dose of the systemic intravenous chemotherapy for the solid tumors is reasonable or not?

- The analysis and query on the evaluation standard of Intravenous Chemotherapy and Curative Effect of Solid Tumor.

- the century review, analysis and comment of the three major treatments for cancer.

Respectively, the problems existing in the surgery and the radiotherapy and the chemotherapy are analyzed and commented:

The Surgical treatment:

Comments:

It is the main technology and the main treatment method in the future of conquering cancer. The surgical treatment of cancer is the exact and effective method.

The Radiation Therapy:

Comments:

The radiotherapy is for local treatment and the transfer is the entire body and the systemic problems which is a major contradiction. The reason for its failure is not for the transfer and is not for controlling the transfer because the main problem of cancer treatment is to anti-transfer and how to play its role during anti-transfer therapy which must be carefully considered and in-depth study.

The Chemotherapy:

Comment 1:

Comment on the route of administration of systemic intravenous chemotherapy

This route of administration is not the real point of targeted administration, but through the heart pump to the blood spray to the body and has the whole body cytotoxic distribution and the whole body target so that the whole body organs obtain the cytotoxic. It is very unreasonable and is very unscientific . The result is:

① very few foci cancer, only about 0.4%, the effect is minimal (because the foci accounts for a small body surface area and is very small proportion).
② 99.6% of the cytotoxic kill to the body of normal cells, causing the adverse reaction to the brain, heart, liver, lung, kidney, gastrointestinal system, hematopoietic system, the immune system, endocrine system.

The toxic side effects of these chemotherapy is irrational route of administration, which should be avoided.

Therefore, this route of intravenous chemotherapy is unreasonable, unscientific, easily lead to iatrogenic toxic side effects.

How to do? Should it be reformed? should it be changed the route of administration into target organ intravascular chemotherapy pathways? the drug can directly go the "target" organs so that the dose is very small, effective, no side effects, and is conducive to patients.

Comment 2:

The assessment of the dose calculation of the solid body tumor intravenous chemotherapy is applied according to the experience and methods of leukemia treatment; the guiding ideology is calculated by the body surface area, which is unwise, unreasonable, easy to lead Iatrogenic toxic side effects.

Why?

It is because solid tumors are confined to an organ, it should not be calculated with whole body surface area, which is unreasonable and unscientific.

Comment 3:

The evaluation of the efficacy evaluation criteria for the solid tumor systemic intravenous chemotherapy:

The current assessment criteria for the efficacy of solid tumors are:

a, the size of the tumor; b, remission periods, remission (CR, PR) - as the name suggests, to be ease is not cured and it is only the improvement in a few short weeks; after this short-term improvement, it will progress, increase, transfer, so that to be ease is not the purpose of treatment, it can not be cured and it can only alleviate and it is only the short-term relief, so that this is not the desired purpose of the patients and should not be the goal of treatment.

Comment 4:

Why did the abdomen solid tumor after adjuvant chemotherapy fail to prevent the recurrence and metastasis of cancer? In the abdominal solid tumor (gastric cancer, cardiac cancer, colorectal cancer, liver cancer, gallbladder cancer, pancreatic cancer, abdominal tumor) the postoperative adjuvant chemotherapy is the systemic intravenous chemotherapy, this way from the vena cava can not directly reach the portal vein.

Abdominal solid tumor cancer cells are mainly in the portal vein system; the vena cava system and the portal vein system is generally not connected; the medications administered by the superior vena cava can not reach the portal vein so that this route of administration is unreasonable, does not meet the anatomy, not scientific.

Comment 5:

There are some important errors and shortcomings in current chemotherapy.

Chemotherapy can suppress immune function and inhibit the bone marrow hematopoietic function so that the overall immune function decreased. In cancer patients thymus is inhibited and chemotherapy can inhibit bone marrow, as "snow adds frog or worse" so that the entire central immune organs are damaged and it promotes the further decline in immune surveillance and it may cause that while chemotherapy, cancer metastasis ; the more treatment, the more chemotherapy.

Volume VIII

What wisdom is condensed which can be used to conquer cancer?

The Study on Anti - cancer Traditional Chinese Medication of XZ - C Immunomodulation

Its focus is:

(1) In our laboratory the experimental study of finding and screening anti-cancer and anti-transfer medications was conducted from the Chinese medications:

1) **The in vitro culture method of cancer cells was used to study the anti-tumor rate of Chinese herbal medication.**

   a, in vitro screening test: the cancer cells were used in vitro culture to observe the direct damage to cancer cells.

   b, the test in the tube screening test: in the tubes which the cancer cells were cultured, the biological crude products (500ug / m) were placed to observe whether it could inhibit the cancer cells.

2) To make the animal models and to do the experimental study on the tumor inhibition rate of Chinese herbal medications:

Each group of mice were divided into 8 groups, each group of 30, the group 7 for the blank control group, the group 8 with 5-F or CTX as the control group. The whole mice groups were inoculated with EAC or S180 or H22 cancer cells. After 24 hours of inoculation, each mouse was orally fed with the crude drug powder, and then the selected Chinese herbal medication was fed for a long period of time. The survival time and the medication toxicity and side effects were observed, and the survival rate was calculated and the tumor inhibition rate was calculated.

In this way, we conducted four consecutive years of experimental study, each year with more than 1,000 animals models, during 4 years there were the total of nearly 6000 cancer-bearing animal models; after each mouse died the pathological sections and the slides were made for the liver, spleen, kidney, lung, thymus, which a total has more than 20,000 slices.

The experimental results:

In our laboratory 200 kinds of Chinese herbal medications were screened through animal experiments and then screened out 48 kinds with the certain, even excellent tumor inhibition rate which is 75% -90% or more. During the experimental screening tests 152 kinds of Chinese herbal medication with no obvious anti-cancer effects were gotten rid of .

(2) The clinical validation:

On the basis of the success of the animal experiments the clinical validation was conducted and it was established the cancer specialist outpatient and it was retained outpatient medical records and each outpatient record was recorded. It established the regular follow-up observation system to observe long-term efficacy. The standard of the Observation of the efficacy of the standard is: the patients have the long survival time and the good quality of life.

After 30 years of the clinical application and verification in the cancer specialist outpatient service in more than 12000 cases of advanced patients XZ-C immunoregulation anti-cancer traditional Chinese medication preparation has achieved significant effect. XZ-C immunomodulatory medications can improve the quality of life of patients with advanced cancer and enhance immune function and increase the body's anti-cancer ability and enhance appetite and significantly extend the survival period.

Volume IX

What wisdom is condensed which can be used to conquer cancer?

The focus is:

(1) how to carry out clinical research data summary and collation and expression?

1. China is a large country with 1.3 billion population and thus it is a large resource for cancer cases. China has a large number of cancer cases for the clinical observation and the analysis.

   In the daily clinical work the clinicians conduct the subtle observation of cancer and the careful thinking and the analysis and the actively exploring study. After the long-term accumulation of the practice medical experience it will also have some discovery and the development and the continuous progress; the medical research is to improve clinical diagnosis and treatment work. The medical research is to Improve the quality of medical care and medical level so that the clinical research work is also an important part of clinical work.

2. **it creates a table form to explain the scientific research materials which can be achieve to be both concise and comprehensive and to be easy to read and easy to understand.** Through a few decades of the bitter and meticulous clinical research work it received a lot of scientific research data and experimental data and the summary and the collation and the collection. Through the table form for the narrative expression it is concise

and structured and the readers can understand their core content in ten minutes.

3 to retain the outpatient medical records and the information accumulation about the outpatient visits, treatment, rehabilitation and follow-up; to fill in a complete detailed table outpatient medical records so as to obtain clinical validation of complete information and it is easy analysis, statistics and in order to facilitate follow-up treatment of patients.

If there is no preservation of the outpatient medical records, the analysis and the statistics of the outpatient efficacy of scientific research work can not be carried out.

4 **to stay outpatient medical records is to observe the long-term efficacy, is conducive to clinical research outpatient to improve the quality of medical care.**

Volume X

What wisdom is condensed which can be used to conquer cancer?

Its focus is:

- How to overcome the cancer? I see one: the road to scientific research is the experimental basic research to explore the cause of cancer, pathogenesis, pathophysiology.

- **the experimental surgery is extremely important in the development of medication. It is a key to open the medical closed area, many diseases prevention and control methods were applied to the clinical practice after many animal experimental research to achieve a stable effect and promote the development of medical career.**

- We conducted a series of animal experiments to explore the etiology, pathogenesis and pathophysiology of cancer. We have obtained new findings from the experimental results. The new findings: thymus atrophy and the immune dysfunction are one of the the cause and pathogenesis of cancer.

- As a result of our laboratory study, we found that thymus has atrophy, and the central immune sensory has dysfunction, and the immune function decreases, and the immune surveillance decreases in the cancer-bearing mice. Therefore, the principle of treatment must be to prevent thymic atrophy and promote thymus Cell proliferation and protect bone marrow hematopoietic function and improve immune servillence . For the immune regulation of cancer, it provides a theoretical basis and experimental basis.

- **XZ-C believes that under normal circumstances the cancer and the body defense arc in a dynamic balance . The occurrence of cancer is caused by** dynamic imbalance. **If the state has been adjusted to the normal level, you can control the growth of cancer and may make it subside.**

- **No matter how complex the mechanism behind cancer, immunosuppression is the key to cancer progression**. Removal of immunosuppressive factors and restoring the immune system to cancer cell recognition can effectively inhibit cancer. More and more evidence shows that by regulating the body's immune system, it is possible to achieve the purpose of cancer control. Through the activation of the body's anti-tumor immune system to treat tumors is currently the majority of researchers excited areas.

Second, the guidance words

1, It outlined the research process of anti-cancer research:

(A) a brief description of the research process of anti-cancer research

In 1985 I have done the petition for more than 3,000 cases of thoracic and abdominal cancer patients whose surgeries were operated by my own. The results were found that most patients had the recurrence and the metastasis and died within 2-3 years, and some were even after a few months, or 1 year. So that I realized that surgery was successful and the long-term efficacy was not satisfied and the postoperative recurrence and metastasis are a key factor affecting the long-term efficacy of surgery. And therefore it also raised a question: to study the prevention and treatment of postoperative recurrence and metastasis is the key to improve the survival. Therefore, it is the need for clinical basic research. If there is no breakthrough in basic research, the clinical efficacy is difficult to improve.

So we established the Institute of Experimental Surgery, from the following three aspects it took 30years to carry out a series of experimental research and clinical validation work:

(1) The experimental study of exploring the pathogenesis of cancer, invasion mechanism and recurrence and metastasis mechanism and of finding the effective control of invasion and the effective methods of cancer recurrence and metastasis.

I and my colleagues in our laboratory did the experimental tumor research work for a full four years; the research project topics are from the clinical problems and it attempted to explain or to solve some clinical problems through the experimental stud. All of them are the clinical basic research.

(2) The new drug experimental study of finding the new anti-cancer, anti-metastasis ad anti-recurrence from the natural herbal medication.

The existing anti-cancer drugs are that kill both cancer cells and the normal cells and have the toxic side effects . In our laboratory through the tumor-bearing mice in vivo tumor inhibition test, it was to find the new drugs that it only inhibited cancer cells without affecting the normal cells from the natural Chinese medication. We spent a total of three years in the laboratory testing 200 kinds of Chinese herbal medications which were the traditional commonly used anti-cancer prescription and reported anti-cancer prescriptions in the cancer-bearing animals in vivo tumor inhibition experiments to find the new drugs which only inhibit cancer cells without affecting the normal cells. The results: 48 kinds of Chinese medication with good tumor inhibition rate were screened out and at the same time with the better effect of increasing immune function and it was also found the traditional Chinese medication TG which could inhibit neovascularization.

(3) the clinical validation work: through the above four years of the basic experimental study to explore the recurrence and metastasis mechanism, and after three years of the basic experimental study screening the natural herbal medication it was found a group of XZ-C1-10 anti-cancer immune regulation traditional Chinese medications, and then through 30 years of clinical validation in more than 12,000 cases of patients with advanced or postoperative metastatic cancer the application of XZ-C immunomodulation of traditional Chinese

medication had achieved the good results, improved the quality of life, improved the symptoms and significantly prolonged survival period.

After the review, analysis, reflection of nearly 60 years of clinical practice cases and their own experience and more than 30 years of experimental results and discovery in the animal experiments, from the experimental to clinical, also from the clinical to the experiments and the data sorting and ummary of the collection from the experimental researches and clinical validation, it was published three monographs:1).In 67-year-old sixtieth year it was published the first monograph "new understanding and new model of cancer treatment " by Hubei Science and Technology Press in January 2001; 2).In 73 years old seventy years it was published the second monograph " new concepts and new methods of cancer metastasis treatment " by Beijing People's Medical Publishing House in January 2006;In April 2007 the People's Republic of China Publishing House issued a "three hundred" original book certificate.3).In 78 years old seventy years it was published the third monograph "new concept and new methods of cancer treatment " by Beijing People's Medical Publishing House in October 2011; followed by American medical doctor Dr. Bin Wu who translated it into English, the English version on March 26, 2013 was published in Washington, the international distribution; 4).The New Concept and the New Way Of Treatment of Cancer, published in Washington, DC in March 2013, in English, the international distribution of the third edition. 5).In 82-year-old it was published the fifth monograph "On Innovation of Treatment of Cancer" - "cancer treatment innovation" published in full English, worldwide in December 2015 in Washington, 6). At the age of 83 it was published the sixth monograph "New Concept and New Way of Treatment of Cancer Metastais" in August 2016 in Washington in the full English version, the global release;7).In 83 years old the seventh monograph "The Road To Over come Cancer" - to overcome the road of cancer in December 2016 in Washington, published in full English, the global release.

(B). The Cognition and Scientific Thinking of Our Scientific Research journey

Our 30 years of cancer research work research journey of ideological awareness and scientific research thinking can be divided into four stages:

(A) The first phase of 1985—1999

- Find problems from follow-up results → Ask questions → Research questions;
- From the review, analysis, reflection to find the questions existing in the current cancer traditional therapies and it needs to be further studied and improved;
- Recognize the existence of problems and it should change thinking and change ideas;
- summarized and organized and collected the information, it was publish the first monograph "new understanding and new model of cancer treatment " in January 2001 by Hubei Science and Technology Publishing House.

(B) The second phase after 2001 –

- The "target" and key of cancer research and treatment is anti-metastatic cancer therapy;
- Conducted a series of basic and clinical validation studies of anti-cancer metastasis, recurrence and rised to the theory of innovation, put forward new ideas, new methods of anti-metastasis;
- Summarized information, sorted into collection, published "new concepts and new methods of cancer metastasis treatment" second monograph January 2006 by People's Medical Publishing House, Xinhua Bookstore issued in April 2007 won the People's Republic of China and Publication issued by the department "Three hundred" original book award.

(C) The third phase after 2006 -

A. Study the whole process of development of cancer prevention and treatment;
B. Reform and innovation of cancer research and development ;
C. "three early" is the strategies of cancer prevention and treatment
D. I have been 60 years in the tumor surgery, more and more patients, the incidence of cancer is also on the rise, the mortality rate remains high, so I deeply appreciate, not only pay attention to the treatment of cancer, but also to focus on prevention from cancer source. There is a series of related studies, summary data, sorting and collection which was published in the third of my monograph "The new concept and a new approach to cancer treatment," in October 2011 by People's Medical Publishing House, Xinhua Bookstore. Later it was published in English on March 26, 2013 in Washington publication, international distribution.

(4) the fourth stage after 2011 -

- It is now the fourth stage of our research work, which is being carried out and developed ; the research work is conducted with step by step; the research goal or "target" is positioned to reduce the incidence of cancer, to improve the cure rate and to prolong the survival period.
- Our 30 years of cancer research work: the first three stages of experimental research and clinical research work were mainly in the treatment to study the new drugs, new methods of diagnosis, new technologies, new concepts of treatment, new methods.

But today in the 21ˢᵗ century, the second 10 years cancer is still rampant, the more treatment and the more patients, the incidence of cancer continues to rise, it has the high mortality rate so that I deeply appreciate that the cancer is not only to pay attention to treatment, but also to pay attention to prevention in order to stop at the source.

The current tumor hospital or oncology mode to go all out is to focus on treatment and aimed for patients with advanced disease and it had poor efficacy and it exhausted human and financial resources, and failed to achieve lower morbidity, the more treatment and the more patients. The status quo is: through a century the road which was walked on was to focus on treatment and ignore the prevention, or only treatment. Over the years we have just been working on cancer. But the prevention of cancer was done very little, almost did not do so that the incidence of cancer continues to rise.

The Review, reflection, cliché anti-cancer of the prevention of cancer and anti-cancer work: for a century, what have we done in the prevention of cancer research or work? What has it been done?

Medical school textbooks teaching content does not attach importance to the knowledge of the prevention of cancer ;

Hospital hospital mode does not attach importance to the prevention of cancer science setting up work;

Medical school or hospital research projects do not attach importance to the prevention of cancer research projects;

Journal of Cancer Medical Science does not attach importance to the cancer prevention work papers .

In short, the cancer prevention is not attached importance and the prevention is not paid attention. Cliché the cancer prevention is as the main and was not paid attention to and is not implemented.

How to do? How to reduce the incidence of cancer? How to improve cancer cure rate? How to reduce cancer mortality? How to extend life? How to improve the quality of life?

It should be launched the total attack to conquer cancer and the prevention and treatment are at the same attention and the level.

The goal of conquering cancer should be: reduce morbidity, improve the cure rate, reduce mortality, prolong survival, improve quality of life, reduce complications.

The current global hospitals and the hospitals in China are going all out to engage in treatment and focus on treatment and ignore the defense, or only treatment .

XZ-C thinks of that this hospital model or cancer treatment model can not overcome the cancer, can not reduce the incidence. Global hospitals and the hospitals in China must change the overall strategy of cancer treatment from focusing on treatment into focusing on prevention and treatment.

Therefore, we propose the general idea and design of launching the attack to conquer cancer and XZ-C (Xu Ze-China) proposed to launch the general attack, that is, the prevention of cancer and cancer control and the treatment of cancer three-phase work are carried out simultaneously .

It is put forward the " the necessity and feasibility report of conquering cancer to start the general attack ."

It is put forward " the XZ-C research program to conquer cancer and launch a total attack"

(C) why do I study cancer and propose to launch a total attack and to build "the science city to overcome cancer"? it is because:

① In 1985, I have done the petition for more than 3,000 cases of thoracic and abdominal cancer patients whose surgeries were operated by my own, the results were found that within 2-3 years most patients had the recurrence or metastasis. Therefore, we must study the prevention methods of the postoperative recurrence and metastasis to improve postoperative long-term efficacy.

② I suddenly had acute myocardial infarction in 1991. After treatment it was mproved; after recovery I should not be on the operating table and I was to calm down and to hide in the small building to concentrate on scientific research.

③ through experimental studies it was found that thymus atrophy and immune dysfunction are one of the etiology and pathogenesis of cancer and it should be to be expanded in-depth study.

④ through experimental research and clinical validation, after 30 years of more than 12,000 cases of clinical validation observation, I found the new path of the combination of chinese medication and western medication in the molecular level with the modernization of this "Chinese-style anti-cancer" and walked out this innovation new path of Chinese medicine immunoregulation which prevent thymus atrophy, promote thymic hyperplasia, protect bone marrow hematopoietic function, improve immune surveillance, at the molecular level of the combination of chinese medication and Western medication to overcome cancer, so that it is to be perseverance and persistence to stuy. Therefore, it is proposed to overcome the cancer and launch the total attack, to build the "Science City" of conquering cancer in an attempt to achieve: reduce the incidence of cancer; improve cancer cure rate; extend cancer survival; to be "three early" (early detection, early diagnosis, early Treatment), early can be cured; to achieve cancer prevention and treatment at the same attention and level; Both of prevention and treatment at the same attention and level can overcome the cancer, reduce the incidence of cancer.

All basic research must be for clinical to improve patient efficacy so that patients benefit. The evaluation criteria for the efficacy of cancer patients should be: prolong survival, good quality of life, less complications.

In 1951 I come to Wuhan and attended the Zhongnan Tongji Medical College, in 1956 graduated from Tongji Medical College, assigned to the Hubei College of

Traditional Chinese Medicine Hospital, has served as director of surgery, Professor, Hubei College of Experimental Surgery, director of the Institute.

In 1991 due to sudden acute myocardial infarction, I was to have emergency rescue and rehabilitation after six months hospitalization . It was because I can not go to power surgery, I was quiet to hide into the small building to do the basis of cancer and clinical research. As a result of that my experimental laboratory equipment conditions were better, it made a large number of the experimental research about the cancer etiology, pathology, pathogenesis, cancer metastasis mechanism and the experimental screening study for anti-cancer Chinese herbal medicine suppression rate in cancer-bearing animal model mice.

I was 63 years old in 1996 and applied for retirement. After the retirement I was to continue to do the scientific research; the science (science) journey is non-stop. (No one to ask, no one support), go it alone, self-reliance, from the years over sixty, to the seventy years of the year, to more than eighty ripe old age, it still perseveres and is to be perseverance, continues to carry out a series of experimental research and clinical validation observation. And it finally made a series of scientific research and scientific and technological innovation series. All of these experimental and clinical data, data conclusions, summary collection were written into more than 100 research papers, published by the new book monographs. It was to be published a series of monographs about these cancer study, of which 3 for the Chinese version, 4 for the English version. The English version is published in Washington, USA. **In the books it was put forward a series of new concepts and new methods to overcome cancer, put forward the theory of cancer treatment innovation, put forward the road to overcome the cancer and it formed the theoretical system of the immune regulation and control which is the experimental basis of cancer immunotherapy and the observation and verification of clinical application; it walked out of a new way to overcome cancer. Why is the English version? It is because cancer is a disaster of all mankind, the people of the world must work together. I contribute the scientific thinking, scientific research, experience, lessons, wisdom of my 60 years of clinical work and 30 years engaging in** cancer research experimental research and clinical validation to the people for the benefit of mankind.

I am 83 years old this year, I was the total designer of XZ-C research program "to capture the cancer and to attack the total attack and to build the cancer research base science city", I will participate in this practice of the preparation of "the science city to overcome the Cancer " with my academic, knowledge, wisdom and strength, to build "global demonstration of cancer prevention and treatment hospital", the cancer prevention and treatment and control of cancer at the same attention to build a good laboratory and multidisciplinary and cancer research group.

Change the mode of hospital from the focusing treatment with light defense into prevention and control and treatment of cancer at the same level! Change the treatment mode from the treatment of serious illness in the late stage to focus on the "three early" (early detection, early diagnosis, early treatment) precancerous lesions and early in situ cancer! This will benefit the human race and will open up a new era of anti-cancer research so that our prevention and treatment of cancer medical care go into the forefront of the world.

(D) I experienced 30 years to overcome the cancer as the direction of cancer research and clinical research, deeply appreciate: to achieve the purpose of cancer prevention and control:

① It must start the total attack. The prevention of cancer and cancer control and cancer treatment three stages of work should be the same attention; three carriages go hand in hand in order to achieve lower incidence of cancer, improve cancer cure rate, reduce cancer mortality and prolong cancer survival. If it is only treatment, or the focusing treatment with light defense, it will never be able to overcome the cancer, because it can not reduce the incidence, the more treatment and the more patients.

How to launch a total attack and to implement the cancer prevention + control cancer + cancer treatment? It is necessary to establish the hospital with the prevention and treatment of cancer during the whole process of the occurrence and the development of cancer and to change the current only treatment mode. Change the current treatment model for the middle and advanced cancer patients.

② It must be the government-led, the masses to participate, the mobilization of all the people, the work of thousands of households involved in order to conquering cancer ; in preset our country is building the new country, which it is the government-led, the masses involved; Time is good; if it can do the medical science research of cancer prevention and treatment and cancer control, it will be able to improve the awareness of the whole people prevent cancer to achieve the effects of the prevention cancer and control cancer to significantly reduce the incidence of cancer in our city and province and country.

③ **Why should it launch the total attack? It is because the status quo is:**
   a, the current hospital mode is to pay attention to treatment with light defense, or only treatment, the more treatment the more patients.
   b, the current treatment model is mainly cancer patients in the middle and late stage and late transfer, the effect is very poor.
   c, the current radiotherapy and chemotherapy can not be cured, can only alleviate, slow interval of 4 weeks which can still progress, the effect is very poor, there are still problems and drawbacks.

It must emphasize early diagnosis, early treatment, early rehabilitation and adhere to the main prevention:

   a, To change the hospital mode for the prevention, control, treatment at the same attention.
   b, To change the treatment model for the "three early", precancerous lesions.
   c, the anti-cancer way-out is the prevention and the research and the cancer prevention research.

(5) I have been working on experimental research and clinical validation for the study of cancer for 30 years both in the laboratory and in the hospital. Why now is it to apply for government support?

It is because 90% of the cancer is related to the environment. The occurrence of cancer is closely related people's clothing, food, shelter, line and living habits so that I think deeply about prevention cancer and cancer control work are not just to rely on medical staff, experts, scholars to do it. It must rely on the government's major policy ; the current serious environmental pollution and ecosystem degradation may be closely related to the rising incidence of cancer.

Cancer treatment is dependent on medical staff and researchers to study new drugs, new treatment techniques.

However, the prevention and control of cancer, how to reduce the incidence of cancer and the cancer prevention work must rely on the government's major policy and rely on government-led and leadership, experts, scholars efforts to participate in the masses to make true.

The current status quo is:

1, the more treatment and the more patients ; the incidence is on the rise, which 90% are related to the environment. **We deeply appreciate not only to pay attention to cancer treatment, but also to pay attention to prevention; in order to stop at the source,** it must be prevention and treatment at the same attention and level.

2, the current diagnostic methods, B ultrasound, CT, MRI are currently the most advanced diagnostic methods, but once diagnosed, it mostly in in the late, the effect is very poor. **We must try to do the research and find new methods, new reagents and new technologies that can be diagnosed early.** If the early and precancerous lesions can be diagnosed, the early cancer can be cured. Therefore, the way out of cancer treatment is the "three early". (Early detection, early diagnosis, early treatment).

What should I do next? Now it is proposed to overcome cancer and to launch a total attack. Hope to get leadership support at all levels. I know that to achieve the purpose of cancer prevention and control cancer and treatment of cancer must be government leadership, government-led, experts, scholars efforts, the masses involved, thousands of households to participate in order to do.

In China daily about 8550 people were diagnosed with cancer, 6 people per minute was diagnosed with cancer. Therefore, the study of launching a total offensive research work can not walk slowly and it should run forward, save the dying.

We should avoid empty talking about and conduct the hard work and start to go. No matter how far the way to overcome cancer it is, it should always start to go.

(6) In 2013 → 2014 → 2015, I have been studying and formulating the basic idea and design of how to overcome cancer; formulate the theoretical basis and experimental basis for how to overcome cancer; formulate the planning and blueprint and guideline and method of how to overcome cancer.

It came up with:

① " the XZ-C research program of capturing the cancer and launch a total attack"

② " the necessity report to build a comprehensive cancer prevention and treatment of hospital necessity report"

③ " the the necessity and feasibility report of the proposed" ride research in building a moderately society at the same time " —conducting the medical science research of cancer prevention and cancer control and cancer prevention and treatment work."

④ "The planning and the total design to build a science city of conquering cancer and launching the total attack."

These four research projects were put forward in the international community for the first time, opened up a new field of anti-cancer research. Professor Xu Ze proposed to capture the total attack of cancer, which is unprecedented work. To July 2015, it was developed as "dawn of the C-type plan." That dawn is the morning sun and the sunrise, C type = China, the "Chinese model" to overcome the cancer plan. This "4" reports " is "tackling cancer and launching a total attack" and "establishing a science city to overcome cancer".

How to implement the specific plan to overcome the cancer? I detailed the overall design, the overall planning, the specific program research team talent ... ... and other planning, blueprint.

It was put forward the "the total blueprint and design of the science city of launching the total attack of cancer"

The total design and preparation work of the Science City; to establish a pilot area for cancer prevention work (station)

To set up the following:

1, the Cancer Academic Committee of overcoming cancer
2, the working group to build Science City (of the medical, teaching, research, science schoo to attack the cancer and launch a total attack)

(7) This work is ongoing, we have taken three to four years in the cancer research, but step by step to move slowly forward.

In January 12, 2016 US President Barack Obama in the State of the Union made a national cancer plan: to overcome cancer.

The program name: "Cancer moon shot"

Goal: to overcome cancer

Nature: A national plan to overcome cancer

The program leader: Vice President Joe Biden

We have been walking in the cancer on the road to this research for 3-4 years, but only the individual living alone building alone, step by step to move forward, just slow forward.

Now the US President Barack Obama in the State of the Union issued a national cancer plan: to overcome cancer which the vice president I responsible for the implementation. Vice President Biden is actively pursuing. He goes to the cancer centers in the United States every month to preach: "Cancer moon shot".

On June 29, 2016 in the White House to the United States live "national cancer lunar landing plan". It was called the nation scientists to gather wisdom and to overcome cancer.

This international scientific research situation is gratifying, but also the situation is pressing, inspiring. In this case, the government has to be asked to support, ask the government to lead and to guide and to support this unprecedented work for the benefit of mankind.

This is a big deal and it is an unprecedented event for the benefit of mankind.

Therefore, XZ-C proposed: common progress, toward the scientific temple to overcome cancer.

Third, the guidance to act

XZ-C proposed the scientific research plan to build a science city of conquering cancer and launching the total attack. How to implement? How to do it? How to achieve? Now the brief explanation is as the following:

(1), the goal of conquering cancer: reduce the incidence of cancer, improve cancer cure rate, extend the survival time of cancer patients

To achieve:

1/3 can be prevented

1/3 can be cured

1/3 can be treated to relieve pain, is a chronic disease; is the survival with tumor; is to prolong survival

The evaluation criteria for the efficacy of cancer patients should be:

1. live a long time, prolong survival time
2 good quality of life
3 no complications, or less complications

(2) the road of conquer cancer

The way:

1. capture cancer and launch a total attack
   What is the total attack?

That is, cancer prevention + control cancer + treatment cancer, at the same time it is to launch the total attach and to go hand in hand.

2 to build science and technology city to overcome the cancer:
   a, how to overcome cancer? It must be the founder of "innovative molecular cancer medical school" and graduate school

   - and modern high-tech experimental talents

   b, how to overcome cancer? It must be founded " Chinese and Western combined hospital with the full process of the preventation and treatment of cancer on the innovative molecular tumor level."
   c, how to overcome cancer? It must be the founder of "Innovative Molecular Cancer Institute" and multidisciplinary and cancer research group.

d, how to overcome cancer? It must be the founder of "innovative molecular tumor nano-pharmaceutical factory"

e, how to overcome cancer? It must create "innovative environmental protection anti-cancer research institute" and carry out the cancer prevention system engineering.

f, how to overcome cancer? It must be the founder of "Cancer Animal Experimental Center." This is the only way to overcome cancer.

(3) how to prevent? How to control?How to treat cancer? It have developed specific measures, feasibility programs, planning, blueprint seeing (I) (II) (III) (IV) (Part I) in this book.

(4) how to start?

1. first to build the hospital with the cancer prevention, control, treatment → the establishment of various disciplines (departments) → the establishment of the school group (study group)

2 first to run, teach, research (Section, group) the prevention and control and treatment as a whole dragon and one-stop; the prevention and treatment at the same attention ; there are clinical basis and there are "three early", precancerous lesions.

3 first to build the graduate school, personnel training methods and ways;

To overcome the cancer, the cultivation of multidisciplinary senior personnel is the key; it is to train the personnel through experimental research, clinical practice.

a, first to run graduate tutor course, seminar, training personnel, the above content of how to overcome the cancer to start the total attack is to be discussed and to be studied by the division of the sub-topics for special, special study

b, Talent training program:

Graduate School Recruit graduate students (Ph.D, Master); while working, learning, 100 people, after graduation, all stay in the Science City, so generation of training, it requires results and achievements, patents (not just papers), three years and five years later, it will be talented and the scientific research results will acculated.

- **In order to overcome cancer and to launch a total attack, the policy of the prevention cancer + control cancer + treatment cancer at the same attention and same level are is the right way.**

- **To Create a scientific base to conquer cancer and to launch the total attack—the Science City, is the necessity way to set up agglutination wisdom and capture cancer. This approach is the right way to overcome cancer.**

How to implement?

- **It is necessary to establish a pilot area for the Cancer Working Group (station) to explore the experience in prevention, control and treatment.**

- **This set of cancer planning, program, the total design is applicable to a country, a province, a city reference implementation.**

- **Because cancer is a disaster for the people of the world, the people of the world, people of all countries, people of all provinces and cities must struggle with them.**

- **To apply for the International Conference on Oncology in Wuhan, China, November 16-18, 2018, the world's first "Challenging Cancer Summit". To be organized, the United States ... ... global cooperation research organization, once a year to promote the development of Summit Forum.**

The Conference Theme:

1, **to look forward to the promising prospects of 21st century cancer metastasis, recurrence prevention and treatment;**

2, to gather wisdom, capture cancer, launch a total attack, for the benefit of mankind.

To overcome the cancer and launch a total attack is an unprecedented human event, is the forefront of science

- **to emphasize on the cancer prevention and cancer control and cancer treatment at the same lever. The way-out of Cancer treatment is in the "three early".**
- **the emphasis on anti-cancer out of the way is in the prevention, the establishment of the department of the prevention cancer and the department of cancer control and the cancer prevention research institute,** because 90% of the cancer is related to the environment and it must be from the big environment, small environment to prevent cancer and from air, water to prevent and from the clothing, food, live to prevent cancer and from changing the living habits, and changing the life to prevent cancer.

(5) XZ-C proposed that it must establish the prevention cancer research institute and the prevention of cancer system engineering in order to conquer cancer and to launch a total attack.

The most prominent of the discovery is that more than 90% of the cancer is caused by environmental factors during the process of that Human beings is in the search for cancer etiology and conditions.

How to implement the creation of the cancer prevention research institute?

Professor Xu Ze XZ-C proposed anti-cancer design, proposed anti-cancer system engineering:

To study the prevention measures of how to reduce or prevent from these carcinogens?

It is because cancer patients cover the world, industrial and agricultural waste water, waste residue, waste gas pollution is also covered the world, therefore, it must be the whole world to conquer cancer and launch a total attack.

Professor Xu Ze suggested:

① each country, each province, each state should establish the prevention of cancer research institute (or organization), carry out the prevention of cancer system engineering, for their own country, the province, the city to carry out anti-cancer work.

② to establish the prevention of cancer regulations, to carry out (some should be legislation)

③ I will recommend this project to the World Health Organization to launch anti-cancer operations, the goal is to try to reduce the incidence of cancer. Capture cancer is the forefront of science, is a worldwide problem; cancer is a human disaster, covering the whole world, people around the world are eager to one day to overcome cancer, for the benefit of mankind.

④ to promote scientific research ethics; medicine is benevolence and the legislation is the first

Scientific research ethics: the products should have moral standards.

The standard: it should not harm human health as the standard and as the bottom line.

It should pay attention to the prevention of cancer regulations

The basic ethics: all products should be harmless to people and do not harm people's health, especially for children. (To be beautiful, the flower of the living environment, living environment)

3   health administrative departments is to defend life, to protect health, should lead and guide and support to guide the prevention of cancer measures,

the prevention of cancer engineering, the prevention of cancer testing, the prevention of cancer monitoring.

The summary after guidance

"Condense Wisdom and Conquer Cancer - for the benefit of mankind"

This is a medical monographs with the more complete, more systematic, more comprehensive design and more specific planning of how to overcome the cancer. The whole book content is divided into two parts: ①how to overcome cancer? how to prevent cancer by I see. ②how to overcome cancer? How to treat cancer I see?

1.the book to the length of 40% on the specific programs and planning sand the blueprints of how to prevent cancer. It raised how to overcome cancer? how to prevent cancer by I see .

The target of the study or "target" is located in how to reduce the incidence of cancer.

The current status quo is: the more treatment and the more cancer patients, and the incidence of cancer is continuing rising and the mortality rate is high. The road which walked through for a century is to focus on treatment and to ignore the defense or only treatment and no defense. It was done very little in the prevention work and it almost did not do. The cancer prevention did not attach importance; the prevention did not pay attention so that the incidence of cancer is rising.

How to prevent cancer? Where is the target or goal of the cancer prevention?

It must have a specific prevention cancer object and a clear goal so that it can have operational.

Professor Xu Ze proposed how to prevent cancer I see (a), (b), (c), (d) proposed that it should analyze what causes or which factors lead to an increase in cancer incidence. Currently the more number of patients and the more treatment; the incidence is on the rise and 90% is related to its environment. It should study and explore for the environmental carcinogenic factors (the external environment and the internal environment).

The causes of cancer are related to the carcinogenic factors of the external and internal environment.

If we have a better understanding of the causes of cancer, then in the future it will be able to put forward:

How to prevent which carcinogenic factors? how to monitor which carcinogenic factors? how to clean which carcinogenic factors? so that we can stay away from cancer and prevent cancer.

Therefore, Professor Xu Ze proposed: it should prevent cancer from the big environment and the small environment and it should be from the clothing, food, live and walking to prevent cancer.

2. 60% of the length in this book is the disscussion of how to treat cancer. The study of the target or "target" is located in how to improve cancer cure rate, extends the survival of cancer patients, improve the quality of life and put forward how to cure cancer by I see.

We are taking the new road of cancer treatment in the molecular level of the combination of Western medication and Chinese medication and it is the new road of finding the immune regulation methods and drugs on the basis of new discoveries in animal experiments in our laboratory. After years of animal experiment screening and clinical validation it finally found out this new road of immune regulation of cancer with XZ-C1-10 immune regulation of anti-cancer Chinese medication series.

- From our laboratory experiments it was found that: thymus of the host was acute progressive atrophy and the volume was significantly reduced after the host was inoculated with cancer cells.

- From the above experimental results it was found that thymus atrophy, immune dysfunction may be one of the etiology and pathogenesis of the tumor so the principle of treatment must try to prevent thymic atrophy, promote thymocyte proliferation, increased immune function.

- In order to prevent thymic atrophy and to promote thymocyte proliferation and to increase immune function, we look for from both the traditional Chinese medication and Western medication. Western medication which can improve immune function and promote the proliferation of thymocytes is very rare. So we changed to find from the Chinese medication because the traditional Chinese medication tonic drugs generally have immune regulation.

- After 7 years of laboratory scientific research, we selected XZ-C1-10 immune regulation anti-cancer, anti-transfer traditional Chinese medication with protecting thymus and increasing immune function and protecting bone marrow and hemotesise from the natural drug. on the basis of the success of the animal experiment the clinical validation work was conducted. After 20 years of more than 12,000 cases of clinical application in the cancer specialist outpatient center it achieved the good results.

- After the experimental study, with anti-cancer research of Chinese medication immunopharmacology and the combination of Chinese and Western medication on the molecular level, it walked out of the new path of conquering cancer with XZ-C immune regulation, regulating immune activity, preventing thymus atrophy, promoting thymocyte proliferation, protecting bone marrow hematopoietic function, improve immune surveillance.

3. This medical monograph is the outline of the practical and the applied and the research and the implementation of how to overcome cancer.

This set of scientific research programs and scientific research and design and scientific research planning and blueprint can be used for each country and each province and each of the state as the reference to implement the ambitious of conquering cancer for the benefit of mankind.

The main project of this medical monograph is:

The Main Project

1. To conquer cancer and to launch cancer the total attack: the prevention and the control and the treatment at the same level of the attraction and moving together

2 To create the cancer - related research base with a multi - disciplinary — Science City

Two wing works:

A wing - how to prevent cancer - to reduce the incidence of cancer

B wing - how to cure cancer - to improve cancer cure rate

The goals and the aims:

A: to reduce the incidence of cancer

B: to improve cancer cure rate and to extend the survival of patients and to improve the quality of life

If it is implemented and it achieves this total design and planning blue of conquering cancer, it is possible to overcome cancer.

4. The next step is how to implement the work, how to achieve this total design and the programs and the planning and the blueprint.

It should set up the research team of conquering cancer and launching the total attack".

In order to capture cancer and to launch the total attack, the talent is the key and the first thing is to set up research team

The conditions of the research team and the academic members:

Genuine talent; in the cancer research, basic research or clinical work it has academic achievements, academic achievements, monographs, editor, special issue, international papers; has the practical clinical experience and the experimental research results, its direction of the research and academic is to capture cancer.

The leadership leaders who leads and organizes to conquer cancer should support anti-cancer research and support cancer research; the scientists and the entrepreneurs and the leaders and the volunteers of conquering cancer must have both ability and political integrity and medicine is benevolence and the legislation is for the first.

Part I: How to prevent cancer in order to conquer cancer

Volume 1

Table of Contents

14 The situation analysis

(c) how to overcome cancer? Can traditional therapy (surgery, chemotherapy, radiotherapy) be relied on to overcome cancer

15 The situation analysis

(d) moving forward together toward the scientific hall to conquer the cancer.

1. The historical records of putting forward the "to conquer cancer" program internationally within a hundred years

(1) In 1971 the US Congress passed a "National Cancer Regulations", which the "anti-cancer declaration" was issued by President Nixon, therefore it was put the considerable human and financial resources in order to conquer cancer in one fell swoop.

In December 1971, President Richard Nixon presented the anti-cancer slogan in the United Nations.

(2) On January 12th, 2016, US President Barack Obama announced a national plan to "to conquer cancer" in his annual State of the Union address, which was run by Vice President Joe Biden.

The name of the program: "Cancer moon Shot"

Objective: To overcome cancer

In June 29th, 2016 Vice President Biden convened a summit in the White House from 9 am to 6 pm to broadcast the United States "national cancer lunar landing program" lively and the dozens of cancer centers and the doctors, nurses, scientists, volunteers, patients, family members, cancer survivors, rehabilitation in the communities organizations .. .... participating in this publicity activity to prevent cancer, encouraging the scientists to focus on the wisdom of cancer.

The White House calls on Americans to join them to host the community activities.

Immunotherapy opens a new era of cancer treatment and it announced that $ 1 billion per year will be used for the cancer research.

(3) In 2011 Chinese physician Xu Ze put forward "to overcome the cancer of the strategic ideas and suggestions" in his published monographs; in August 2013 at

the International Conference on Cancer for the first time it is put forward: " XZ-C Research plans of conquering cancer and launching a total attack ".

In July 2015 it was proposed "the dawn of the C-type plan to overcome the cancer and to launch a total attack."

- In the 38 chapters in the third monograph "new concepts and new methods of cancer treatment" with the length of a chapter Xu Ze addressed "the strategic ideas and the suggestions to overcome the cancer"

1. How to overcome the cancer by I see one: the road to scientific research is the experimental basic research of exploring cancer Etiology, pathogenesis, pathophysiology.
2. How to overcome the cancer by I see two: the road to scientific research is the scientific research of studying the prevention and treatment during the whole process of cancer occurrence and development.
3. How to overcome the cancer by I see three: the road to scientific research is to carry out multidisciplinary research and to set up the formation of cancer-related research group and to specialize in clinical basis and clinical scientific research in-depth.

The book was translated into English in 2013, entitled "New Concept and New Way of Treatment of Cancer". The English text was published in Washington, DC in March 2013 and is released worldwide.

- Xu Ze's fourth monograph "On Innovation of Treatment of Cancer"
  --------(the theory of cancer treatment innovation)

The English edition is published in Washington, DC in December 2015 and is electronically distributed worldwide

The Introduction of this book: the experimental study and the anti-cancer research of Chinese medication immunopharmacology and of the combination

of Chinese and Western medications on the molecular level; XZ-C immune regulation of anti-cancer has formed the theoretical system.

Walking out of the new path of an immune regulation of traditional Chinese medication with regulating immune activity, preventing thymic atrophy, promoting thymic hyperplasia, protecting bone marrow hematopoietic function, improving immune surveillance at the molecular level of the combination of Chinese and Western medications to overcome cancer.

- Xu Ze's fifth monograph "The Road To Overcome Cancer" (to overcome the road of cancer)

The English edition was published in Washington, DC, on December 6, 2016, and is available electronically and worldwide.

In this book:

Chapter 11 the initiative of conquering cancer and launching a total attack

------The overall strategic reform of cancer treatment

Section I: the necessity to launch a total attack

Section II: the feasibility of launching the overall attack

Section III: the XZ-C plan of conquering cancer and launching the total attack

Chapter 12 to strengthen the anti - cancer prevention and treatment research, to change the status of light defense and the attention of treatment

The first section: It must be aware of the existing problems and the clear research direction

Section II: In order to overcome cancer it must pay attention to the prevention and the treatment effect is in the "three early"

Chapter 13: the suggestions on the Cultivation of Scientific and Technological Talented Personals and the Transformation of Scientific Research Achievements

The first section: In order to overcome cancer the science and technology talented persons are the key

Section II: To build a good laboratory

Chapter 14 Adhering to the new path of anti-cancer with Chinese characteristics

This book is a full English version and has been published in all of the global for more than six months. Therefore, China, Hubei, Wuhan should catch up to capture cancer research work. Because conquering cancer and launching the total attack is in China; it is put forward by Wuhan professor in China and the monographs have been published. It should be carried out in the country to catch up to conquer cancer and to launch a total attack and should be applied to the provincial and municipal.

In the contemporary era and now chinese physicians do the research work of conquering cancer the most and the earliest and published the monographs and there are the experimental research and the theory and the clinical practice.

<u>The original hope was that our leadership can report to the United Nations about conquering cancer and launching a general attack, but the US president has announced the conquering cancer national plan, called the United States and the global scientists condense wisdom to capture cancer.</u>

<u>It should remember the story of smallpox and Vaccinia in the Ming Dynasty Cattle! Putting Vaccinia was invented by a Chinese physician, but after this research result was spread to France; however it was reported by the French physician.</u>

<u>How to do? To apply to hold an international tumor academic conference in November 16- 18th, 2018 in Wuhan: " the peak of the academic forum to overcome the cancer and to launch a total make the international announcement</u>

of which China has made the first series of scientific research of conquering cancer and launching a total attack.

2. Why is it said as moving forward together? What is inside in common?

(1) It was put forward: "conquer cancer" in Chapter 38 in Xu Z e's third monograph "new concepts and new methods of cancer treatment" which was published in Beijing in 2011 (Chinese version), and then published in Washington, 2013 (in English)

In " the strategic thinking and suggestions of conquering cancer " it was put forward "conquering cancer"

1. How to overcome the cancer by I see one: the road to scientific research is the experimental basic research of exploring cancer Etiology, pathogenesis, pathophysiology.
2. How to overcome the cancer by I see two: the road to scientific research is the scientific research of studying the prevention and treatment during the whole process of cancer occurrence and development.
3. How to overcome the cancer by I see three: the road to scientific research is to carry out multidisciplinary research and to set up the formation of cancer-related research group and to specialize in clinical basis and clinical scientific research in-depth.

The book was published by the American medical scientist Dr. Bin Wu in English and published in Washington, DC, in June 2013, published in Europe and America.

This book focuses on: to conquer cancer and to launch a total attack

(2) Xu Ze's fourth monograph "On Innovation of Treatment of Cancer" ---- (Cancer Treatment Innovation) The English edition was published in Washington, DC in December 2015, with electronic and global distribution

This book focuses on: immune regulation of anti-cancer

The experimental study: the anti-cancer research of Chinese medication immunopharmacology and of the combination of Chinese and Western medications on the molecular level; XZ-C immune regulation of anti-cancer has formed the theoretical system.

Walking out of the new path of an immune regulation of traditional Chinese medication with regulating immune activity, preventing thymic atrophy, promoting thymic hyperplasia, protecting bone marrow hematopoietic function, improving immune surveillance at the molecular level of the combination of Chinese and Western medications to overcome cancer.The above two books:

The former focuses on: to overcome cancer

The latter focuses on: immune regulation cancer treatment

(3) In January 12, 2016 US President Barack Obama in the State of the Union address put forward the national cancer plan: to overcome cancer.

The program name is: "Cancer moon shot", by that Vice President Joe Biden is responsible for the implementation. Biden proposed the focusing on the study of immunotherapy and the immunization prevention; the immunotherapy opens a new era of cancer treatment.

On June 29th, 2016, Vice President Biden convened a summit to broadcast to the United States from 9:00 am to 6:00 pm at the White House. The National Cancer Monthing Program encourages the scientists to focus on intelligence to conquer cancer and announced $ 100 million per year for the research on cancer.

The above goal: to overcome cancer

Methods and pathways: the immune anti-cancer treatment and immune prevention

In short, in Chapter 39 of Xu Ze's third monograph it was proposed: to overcome cancer and how to overcome cancer; in the fourth book there was the whole Chapter which was discussed: the immune regulation treatment of cancer and walking out of a new way to overcome cancer.

In the United States the goal of the "new moon program (Cancer moom Shot)" is to conquer cancer and its method and way are immunotherapy.

The above two goals are to overcome cancer, its methods and pathways are the immune therapy and the immune regulation and the immune prevention; the two goals and methods are the same way.

Therefore, it is put forward to going forward together. Rush toward the science hall to overcome cancer.

3. To do an unprecedented event for the benefit of mankind

Cancer is a disaster of all mankind and it must be struggling with cancer in the whole world. People all over the world work together.

How to implement this unprecedented human event?

- To report the government and to apply for the instructions
- To report the provincial and municipal and to request instructions
- To provide recommendations to the city and to build in Wuhan City:

"The first Science City of overcoming the Cancer in the country ";

"The world's first Science City of overcoming the Cancer"

Location: to be in the University City Huangjia Lake

Referred to as: "Huangjia Lake Science City" Cancer Medical Research Center

Leadership support:

To overcome the cancer and to launch the total attack is unprecedented in human work; it must personally create experience; it must practice in person; this is a new cement road and every step will leave the eternal footprints.

(1) it needs the leadership support
(2) to apply for an international conference on tumor

China-US cooperation and AACR cooperation, to be held in November 16-19th, 2018 in Wuhan, China, the world's first summit forum of the "conquering cancer and launching a total attack." To be organized cooperation research for China and the United States … …the global cooperation research organizations, once a year to promote the development of Summit Forum.

- To put forward the "race", it should invite the United States to have the common progress and to have their own strengths and the co-operation and the complementary advantages and the common progress toward the scientific hall of overcoming cancer.

4. (1) how to overcome cancer? XZ- C proposed that it needs two wheels: A wheel and B wheel

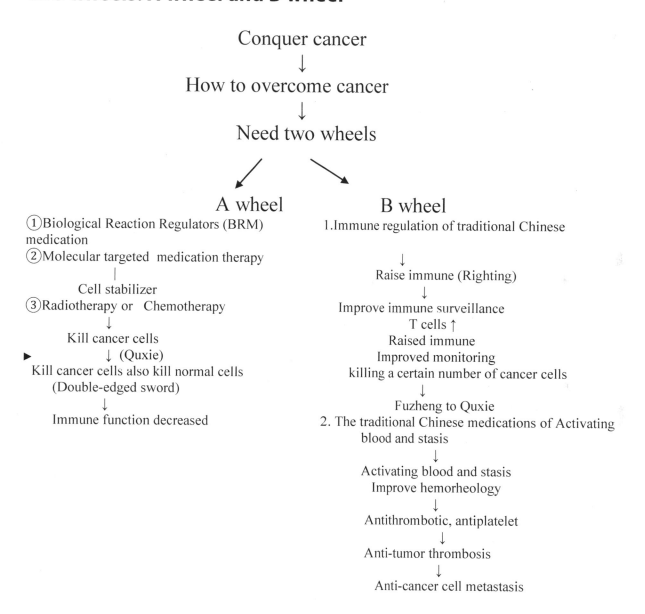

Conquer cancer
↓
How to overcome cancer
↓
Need two wheels

A wheel

①Biological Reaction Regulators (BRM) medication
②Molecular targeted medication therapy
|
Cell stabilizer
③Radiotherapy or   Chemotherapy
↓
Kill cancer cells
► ↓ (Quxie)
Kill cancer cells also kill normal cells
(Double-edged sword)
↓
Immune function decreased

B wheel

1.Immune regulation of traditional Chinese

↓
Raise immune (Righting)
↓
Improve immune surveillance
T cells ↑
Raised immune
Improved monitoring
killing a certain number of cancer cells
↓
Fuzheng to Quxie
2. The traditional Chinese medications of Activating blood and stasis
↓
Activating blood and stasis
Improve hemorheology
↓
Antithrombotic, antiplatelet
↓
Anti-tumor thrombosis
↓
Anti-cancer cell metastasis

A + B
↓
The Combination of Chinese and Western Medications

4. (2) how to overcome cancer? XZ-C put forward to require A wheel and A runway, and B wheel and B runway

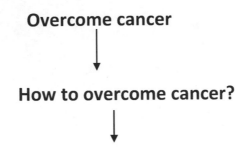

Overcome cancer

↓

How to overcome cancer?

↓

Need two wheels and two runways

A	B
one wheel	one wheel
A runway	**B** runway (clinical basis)
(Life Sciences and Biomedical)	Etiology, pathogenesis, pathophysiology, related factors

The A wheel is:

a. the DNA found

Under a variety of internal and external factors the body occurs the mutation or error, causing DNA structure and function changes, resulting in cancer.

b. the gene mutation

1928 it was considered that gene mutation is the root cause of cancer and tumor occurrence and the development is involved in genes and the basic life activities such as the cell proliferation, differentiation, apoptosis and other etc, therefore, it is now recognized as a disease of the tumor.

c. the Philadelphia chromosome opens targeted therapy

In 1960, the researchers in Philadelphia found that there was a chromosomal abnormality in patients with chronic myeloid leukemia (CML), and that years later it was found to be the result of chromosomes of chromosome 9 and chromosome 22. The chromosome became the target of CML targeted therapy for 40 years. In 2001 it was the first time confirmed to the drug of being against Philadelphia chromosome molecular defects - imatinib.

The B wheel is:

a. The virus

- 1951 it was found that virus can transmit the mice leukemia.
- In 1960 the African sub-Saharan region reported that Hodgkin's lymphoma was thought to be caused by a virus and later confirmed as an AIDS virus.
- 1983 human papillomavirus infection is one of the factors of cervical cancer.
- Preventive vaccines for cervical cancer in 2006 were approved by the US FDA.

b. the immune

- in 2001 in the Animal experiments it was found that removal of thymus can produce a mouse model of mice.

    Mouse thymus had the acute progressive atrophy after inoculated with cancer cells and cell proliferation was blocked and the immune function was low, the volume was significantly reduced, thymus atrophy, immune function was slow and it could promote cancer metastasis.

c. the hormones

- in 1916 it was found that removal of ovaries can reduce the incidence of breast cancer, suggesting that ovarian can promote the occurrence of breast cancer.
- in 1941 the hormone dependence of the prostate cancer was confirmed and the injection of androgen could promote metastasis.

d. the environmental pollution

- In 1907, the sun exposure was associated with skin cancer
- in 1978 the nitrosamines in tobacco leaves were confirmed to be carcinogens in cigarettes and were found to be carcinogenic in animal models

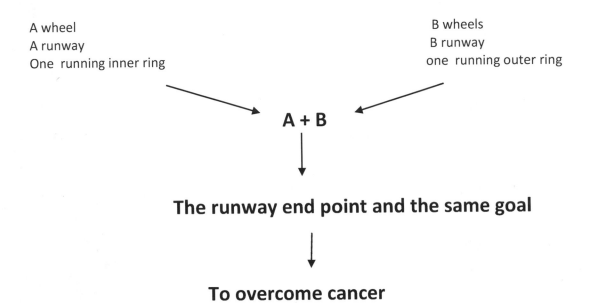

A wheel
A runway
One running inner ring

B wheels
B runway
one running outer ring

A + B

The runway end point and the same goal

To overcome cancer

4. (3) how to overcome cancer? XZ-C proposed the need to aim for A, B, C three targets in order to conquer cancer

The treatment of the diseases must aim on the cause, pathogenesis, pathophysiology for the prevention and the treatment.

The prevention of cancer and cancer treatment must also aim on the mechanism of the cause, pathogenesis, cancer metastasis for prevention and treatment

How did the tumor happen?

The research and attack should be performed by each goal or each target in the process of tumor generation.

Tumorigenesis is the result of the occurrence of the gene mutations and the abnormal expression or deletion under genetic and environmental factors

leading to tumor cells which all have a common characteristics - out of the control infinite reproduction.

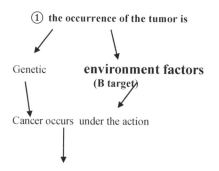

① the occurrence of the tumor is

Genetic   **environment factors**
(B target)

Cancer occurs under the action

Gene mutation and the abnormal expression or deletion

(A target)

Eventually leading to the abnormal cell proliferation results

 ② **the body's normal immune system**

it can identify, recognize, and remove tumor cells
(C target)
(it should adjust the immune system, thus identify and remove the tumor cells)

③ but the process of interaction between tumor cells and immune system

is regulated by a large number of immune activation / or inhibition of molecular regulation
(C target)
(C target) (in the application of up-regulated immune activating molecules; thereby inhibiting immune escape and inhibiting tumor growth)

④ tumor cells through
Either the up-regulation of immunosuppressive molecules or the down-regulation of immune activating molecules

Inhibiting the body's anti-tumor immune response

To achieve immune escape and excessive growth

According to the above brief description of the process of the occurrence of the tumor, XZ-C proposed: the goal or target to overcome the cancer should be:

A target: it should be directed against gene mutations and the abnormal expression or deletion

However: are the gene mutation and the abnormal expression or deletion the cause of cancer? Or is it the result of cancer?

Why does the mutation occur? What is the cause of its mutation? What are the consequences of the mutation?

It is the environmental factor that causes genetic mutation.

B target: it should aim on environmental factors.

B target is the goal of anti-cancer.

The environmental factors:

The external environment - air, water, soil, physical, chemical, biological factors, clothing, food, shelter and travel

The Internal environment - microscopic, ultramicro, immune, endocrine, neurohumoral

It is the environment (inside and outside) → lead to gene mutation

Therefore, we must create "anti-cancer research institute" to carry out anti-cancer system engineering.

C target: it should adjust the normal immune system, thereby remove the tumor cells.

- the Large amounts of immune activation and the up-regulation activation make the balance between the tumor and immune system interact with each other.

- the Immune activators should be up-regulated to inhibit immune escape and inhibit tumor growth.

- **the Immunization and immunotherapy and vaccination are human expectations.**

5. (1) why is it put forward "the race" (the scientific and technology race)

(1) **Because I have been done the research work of conquering cancer for 3-4 years and made a series of ideas and design and published in 2011 monograph "the new concepts and new methods of cancer treatment". In Chapter 38 with the whole chapter it wasput forward "the strategic thinking and suggestions of conquering cancer " and put forward "to overcome cancer and to launch a total attack."**

And then in 2013, it was put forward "the total design of building a city of conquering cancer." In August 2013 the first time in the international community it was put forward: " XZ-C research program of attacking the cancer and launching a total attack." In July 2015 it was put forward the "dawn of the C-type plan" and put forward "to attack the cancer and to launch a total attack" and "to build a science city to overcome cancer." This work is being reported to the provincial office with step by step to move forward.

On January 12, 2016, US President Barack Obama in the Unite State issued a national cancer plan: to overcome cancer.

The plan was run by Vice President Joe Biden, and Vice President Biden went to the Cancer Research Center in person and was in a row meeting and held a live broadcast at the White House on June 29, 2016, preaching "Cancer moon Shot " and called on scientists across the United States to gather wisdom and o overcome cancer.

We are on the research work of conquering cancer along the way which is a step by step and is slow forward. The review and the reflection is like the race between the tortoise and the rabbit race. I still propose the "race" word for encouraging myself to move forward with a view to self-reliance forward

(2) Can you race? Can! because the technology races can motivate yourself and encourage yourself to move forward. With the race it will has the power.

Because we have made a set of basic plans and the design and the planning and blueprint to capture cancer, in July 2015 it was known as the "dawn of the C-type plan." It was Put forward "to attack the cancer and to launch a total attack" and "to build the science city to overcome the cancer", pending reporting and asking for the implementation.

(3) How to race? Is it a runway, or two runways?

A. after 28 years of the experimental research and clinical validation which to conquer cancer is as the research direction and the review and the reflection and the analysis and self-evaluation and the decades of the failure lessons and successful experience clinical treatment, we took the clinical basic research. Why has the basic and clinical research been done and walked on? Because the results of follow-up were found that the postoperative recurrence and the metastasis are the key to impact the long-term effect → and thus it must study the relapse and metastasis factors → how to prevent recurrence and metastasis → → it must study the clinical basis → → how to carry out clinical basic research? The human being is the most valuable and many experiments and observations do not allow the researchers to be directly tested on the human body and the need to use simulation methods and the establishment of animal models to do the experimental study → → so we first set up experimental laboratory; after the establishment of experimental surgery Research institute, the animal experiments were done → the animal model experiment new discovery →after the animal inlocation or vaccination of cancer cells, the host thymus was acute progressive atrophy, cell proliferation was blocked, the immune function decreased, the volume was significantly reduced and had atrophy → and thus it must try to prevent thymic atrophy and to promote cell proliferation and to increase the immune regulation → → how to carry out immune regulation?→ → we searched the drug of the immune regulation of from two aspects of both the Western medication and Chinese medication; however Western medication is very small, so turned to find from the Chinese medication and to find with animal models Experimental screening method → → it was found the immunomodulating drugs with much better effect inside the herbal medication →→ After three years of screening 200 kinds of Chinese herbal medication in the experiments in animal models, it was found that there are 48 kinds of Chinese herbal medications which have the good inhibition rate and can increase the immune function . 152 kinds of Chinese herbal medication were gotten rid of and were invalid → the final combination of the formation of optimal combination of XZ-C1-10, and then after 20 years of the clinical validation they achieve the good results.

Our research is carried out by following the following scientific research routes:

1. **Find the problem:** →2. **ask questions:** →3. **research questions:** →4. **solve the problem:**

1. Through the large number of patients follow-up, it was found that the key factors of the impact of postoperative long-term efficacy are postoperative recurrence, metastasis.

2. In order to improve long-term efficacy it must be researched of solving the recurrence, transfer problems and it is put forward that the anti-cancer target is how to anti-transfer.

3. Set up a research institute, a series of experimental studies, looking for anti-recurrence, transfer of technology and new drugs, screening 200 kinds of traditional Chinese medicine, to find 48 kinds of anti-cancer, anti-metastasis effect.

4. Clinical validation and clinical research were done to explore the law of cancer metastasis, and to explore the new model of anti-metastatic treatment and new programs.

From the follow-up to find the problem → the new findings of the experimental study → the experimental study of traditional Chinese medication → the clinical application

This kind of the clinical basic research runway is a B wheel.

B, from the basic research of the life sciences and the biomedical medication:

(A) **DNA discovery**: the body has the mutation or error in a variety of the internal and external factors, causing DNA structure and function changes, resulting in cancer;

(B) **Gene mutation**: that gene mutation is the root cause of cancer and it is now recognized that the tumor is a genetic disease;

(C) **Philadelphia chromosome opens targeted therapy** due to the discovery of chromosomal abnormalities in chronic myeloid leukemia (CML), chromosome 9 and 22 of the long arm ectopic. As the target study 40 years later developed the drug against Philadelphia chromosome defects - imatinib.

From the life sciences, molecular biology, DNA, gene mutations, chromosomal abnormalities → conducting biomedical basic research → molecular biology, genetic engineering, targeted therapy, this is the fundamental treatment of cancer treatment runway, an A wheel.

This is the life science and is high, fine, sharp theory and technology and is precision medicine.

If it is racing, it should be a running inner ring and a running outer ring and is two wheels and is the car with the two wheels.

The end point of the runway and the same goals: to overcome cancer.

So on the academic it should move forward together, rush toward the science temple of conquering cancer, what is the end of the runway? What is the goal of tackling cancer?

It should be:

① **The long survival time and the good quality of life and the fewer complications;**
② **To reduce morbidity and to improve the cure rate and to prolong survival.**

To achieve:

1/3 can be cured;

1/3 can be prevented;

1/3 can extend life with tumor survival.

5. (2) Cancer is a disaster of the mankind, it must struggle with cancer all over the world and the people all over the world struggle with cancer together and China and US cooperate together and joint research

(a). "Cancer moon shot"

The foundation and the peak of the study precise oncology

↓

Life sciences, bioscience,molecular biology, genetic engineering, proteome

$\downarrow$

Targeted drugs, Precision medicine, diagnosis and treatment

$\downarrow$

High, fine, sharp equipment and instrument, high level of diagnosis and treatment technology

(b). Dawn of the C-type plan

The direction of research is clinical basic research

$\downarrow$

Immunity, virus, fungi, chemistry, hormones ...

$\downarrow$

And cancer-related group study ... to find relevant effective control measures

$\downarrow$

Experimental study of etiology, pathology, physiology, pathogenesis
------Seeking effective measures to prevent and control

$\downarrow$

Study on Immunopharmacology of Chinese Herbal Medicine

$\downarrow$

Molecular Biology of Chinese Herbal Medicine

$\downarrow$

Study on Anti - tumor Effect of Immuno - regulation of Traditional Chinese Medicine

$\downarrow$

Chinese and Western medicine combined with anti - cancer research, clinical research

↓

Analysis of Effective Components of Anti - cancer of Chinese Herbal Medicine

↓

Study on Immunomodulation of anti - cancer and Traditional Chinese Medicine by

↓

Objective: to prolong survival time, living with cancer survival
"Three early" study, pre- cancerous and cancer change research

↓

Objective: To reduce the incidence and improve the cure rate

6. (1) how to overcome cancer? XZ-C proposed the four major dedications

Cancer is a disaster of mankind and people should be aroused to move forward together to struggle with cancer all over the world.

Four great dedications

(the Historic and the global for the benefit of mankind)

(1). The first time in the international community it is put forward

"to Capture cancer and to launch a total attack"

---- Change the hospital model
----Change the treatment model

It proposed the total attack design and the blueprint and the implementation details and the program

(See the additional information)

(2) The first time in the international community it is put forward

"To build science city of overcoming cancer"

-----to establish a holistic framework for tackling cancer

This is the only way to overcome cancer.

It proposed the overall design and the blueprint and the implementation details and the programs of the science city

(See the additional information)

(3) The first time in the international community it is put forward

"Walking out of a new way to overcome cancer"
The experimental study of Chinese medication immunopharmacology and anti - cancer research of the molecular level of the combination of Chinese and Western medication

----Walk out of the new path of a XZ-C immune regulation and the combination of Chinese medication and Western medication on the molecular level to capture cancer.

---Walk out of the new path of conquering cancer of an immune regulation with traditional Chinese medicine, regulate immune activity, prevent thymus atrophy, promote thymic hyperplasia, protect bone marrow hematopoietic function, improve immune surveillance and the combination of Chinese medications and Western medication at the molecular level.

---- we have walked out of the new road of conquering cancer of XZ-C immune regulation and the combination of Chinese medications and Western medication at the molecular level – the "Chinese-style anti-cancer" path .

(See additional information)

(4) The exclusive research and the development of XZ-C immunosuppressive anti-cancer traditional Chinese medication products series

----the experimental study + the clinical application + the typical cases + the case lists

----Self-developed XZ-C (XU ZE-China) (Xuze - China) immunoregulation anti-cancer series of traditional Chinese medication preparation, from the experimental research to the clinical validation, on the basis of successful animal experiments and then it was applied th clinical practice. In the more than 20 years after more than 12000 cases of clinical validation it has the significant effect and is Innovation and is independent intellectual property rights

--- XZ-C immunoregulation anti-cancer traditional Chinese medication is from more than 200 kinds of traditional Chinese herbal medications in the tumor-bearing mice in vivo tumor inhibition test in our country to select 48 kinds of Chinese herbal medications with the good anti-tumor Inhibition rate, then after composed of the compound, which was tested for the tumor inhibition rate in the cancer-bearing mice which is much greater than the single herbicide inhibition rate and XZ-C1 inhibition rate of cancer cells is 100% and 100% does not kill normal cells with Fuzheng Guben and with the effect of improving the human immune function.

From our experiments on XZ-C pharmacodynamics study it showed that: on the Ehrlich ascites cancer, S_{180}, H_{22} hepatocellular carcinoma they have a better tumor inhibition rates.

There were no obvious side effects on acute toxicity test in mice. In the clinical long-term oral years (2-6 years), it also has no obvious the side effects.

In the middle and advanced cancer patients there is mostly weak in righting and weak, fatigue, loss of appetite; however, after XZ-C immune regulation of anti-cancer Chinese medicines were used 4-8-12 weeks later, the patients can have significantly improvement on appetite, sleep, relieve pain, gradually restore physical levels.

6. (2) the readme file – 4 of why?

(1) why do I study cancer?

I am a clinical surgeon doing chest and general surgical work. Why do I do research on cancer?

This is due to the results of the mail survey after a number of cancer patients were followed up after their cancer surgery:

Since 1985, I have done the petition for more than 3,000 cases of thoracic and abdominal cancer patients whose surgeries were operated by my own. The results were found that most patients had the recurrence and the metastasis and died within 2-3 years, and some were even after a few months, or 1 year . From the results of follow-up it was found: the postoperative recurrence and metastasis are the key to the long-term effect of surgery. And therefore an important question is put forward that clinicians must pay attention to and study the prevention and the treatment measures of the postoperative recurrence and the metastasis to improve the long-term efficacy after surgery.

So we established a laboratory surgery laboratory and did the experimental tumor research and had the implementation of cancer cell transplantation and established the tumor animal models and carried out a series of experimental tumor research: to explore the recurrence and the metastasis mechanism and regularity of cancer;

to seek the effective measures of the regulation of metastasis and recurrence; to do the experimental study from the natural drug to find the new drugs of anti-cancer and anti-metastasis and anti-recurrence.

(2) Why do I study Chinese herbal medication against cancer?

I am a clinical surgeon and have a lot of patients, usually in the morning have the surgery and the rounds and come to the laboratory four- afternoon every week.

We conducted a full four years of laboratory experiments in the laboratory, is the research of the clinical basis.

From the experimental results it was found that: the hosts' the thymus after inoculated cancer cells were acute progressive atrophy, the cell proliferation was blocked and the volume was significantly reduced. From the above experimental study it was found that thymus atrophy, immune dysfunction may be one of the etiology and pathogenesis of the tumor, it must try to prevent thymic atrophy and to promote thymocyte proliferation and to increase immune function.

In order to try to prevent thymic atrophy, to promote thymocyte hyperplasia, to increase immune function, we searched from both the traditional Chinese medication and Western medication. **In Western medication which can improve the immune function and promote thymus hyperplasia it is rarely**. So we changed from the Chinese herbal medication to find.

Why were the medications which can promote thymus hyperplasia, prevent thymus atrophy, enhance immune functions searched from Chinese medication?

Because the traditional Chinese medication with tonic drugs generally contains the immunomodulatory effects.

The traditional Chinese medication and the polysaccharides medication and the tonic medication may have the regulation of immune function.

Anti-cancer immune research of chinese medication polysaccharide progresses quickly. There are a large number of immunopharmacological studies from the molecular level; THE polysaccharides can improve the body immune surveillance system. The traditional Chinese medications have the rich source and are the clinical effective and good medications in the long-term clinical treatment. After extraction the active ingredients can be gotten and have obvious pharmacological effects (including immunomodulatory effects) and the study process saves people and saves time with the high efficiency.

We experimented with a series of experimental studies to find the new medications of anti-cancer, anti-metastatic, anti-thymic atrophy, and no immune-resistant anti-cancer Chinese medication from the natural medication.

After 7 years of the laboratory scientific research, we selected the natural drug XZ-C1-10 immune regulation of anti-cancer, anti-transfer of Chinese medication with the prevention of thymus and the increase of immune function and the protection of bone marrow and the production of blood. Based on in the successful animal experiment, the clinical validation work was carried out. After the application for 20 years in more than 12,000 cases of the clinical specialist outpatient clinics the good results are achieved.

(3) why do I continue to do the cancer research after my rehabilitation of myocardial infarction?

In December 1991 I suddenly had acute myocardial infarction and was hospitalized after six months after the restoration of health. I can no longer come to the power surgery and keep my heart calm down to hide in a small building to do the basis and clinical cancer research.

In 1996 I was 63 years old and was retired. After I retired I has been staying in the building for 18 years and was the sola army and fought alone; the Science journey is non-stop and continuously carried out a series of the experimental research and the clinical validation observation, then a series of scientific research was made.

(4) why did I put "racing"?

- --moving forward together toward the scientific temple of overcoming cancer

Because in October 2011 I published the third monograph "new concepts and new methods of cancer treatment," and in Chapter 38 it was put forward "the strategic ideas and suggestions to capture cancer ":

1, how to overcome the cancer I see 1: the road to scientific research is to explore the cause of cancer, pathogenesis, pathophysiology of experimental basic research

2, how to overcome the cancer I see 2: the road of scientific research is to study the occurrence of cancer, the development of the whole process of prevention and treatment of scientific research

3, how to overcome the cancer I see 3: the road to scientific research is to carry out the multidisciplinary research, to form the relevant specialist group and specialize in the basis and clinical research in-depth

After 2011 it is the fourth stage of our research work. We carried out and conducted the research work with step by step. The research goal or "target" **was located to reduce the incidence of cancer, to improve the cure rate and to prolong the survival period.**

From 2013 onwards, we proceeded the design work of conquering cancer and launching a total attack and building the science city of conquering cancer.

From 2013 → 2014 → 2015 the "Science City" basic assumptions and design, as well as preparation, planning work were proceeded.

In May 2015 Volume (I), (II), (III), (IV) have been the basic manuscript order and have been prepared to "the report outline", and it seems that current is time which welcomes the flourishing and the scientific spring and the

country is creating an innovative country the prosperity and technological innovation. It coincides with the "new moon program" proposed, although other people have favorable conditions, we have as early as 2-3 years of the thinking and the design and the planning; also it shows that the designs, planning and the direction of overcoming cancer are right and are for the people to seek health benefits in the past few years so that it is proposed the "race" to make self-motivated forward.

Because cancer is a disaster of all mankind, we must struggle with cancer all over the whole world and all the people of the whole world.

7. The exclusive research and development products: a series of products of Z-C immune regulation of anti-cancer Chinese medication (Introduction)

The Self-developed ZC (Xu Ze China) immunoregulation anti-cancer series of traditional Chinese medication products, from the experimental research to the clinical validation, on the basis of the successful animal experiments it was applied to the clinical practice, after years of clinical practice in a large number of clinical Validation, they have the significant effects. It is the independent invention of the results, the independent innovation and independent intellectual property rights.

The research of which was done from the research traditional Chinese medication to find and to screen the new drugs of anti-cancer, anti-metastasis:

The purpose is to screen out the intelligent drugs of the anti-cancer and the anti-metastasis and the anti-recurrence with no the drug-resistant and the non-toxic side effects and the high selectivity which can be used by the long-term oral route.

To this end, our laboratory conducted the following experimental study screening the new anti-cancer, anti-transfer drug from the Chinese medications:

(A). The screening experimental study with the cancer cells in vitro culture method screening anti-cancer and anti-metastasis medication from of Chinese herbal medications:

In vitro screening test: the use of cancer cells in vitro culture to observe the direct damage to cancer cells.

In vitro tube screening test: in the culture of cancer cells in the tube the raw and crude drugs (500ug / ml) were placed to observe whether it inhibits the cancer cells. 200 kinds of traditional Chinese medicine herbs having anticancer function were screened one by one in vitro screening tests. And under the same conditions with a normal fiber cell culture the toxicity of these cells was tested and compared.

(B) Built cancer-bearing animal model for the screening of anticancer Chinese herbs

In vivo screening test: in cancer-bearing animal model screening Chinese anti cancer herbs, 240 mice were divided into eight experimental groups, each group 30 mice, Group 7 was the blank control group, Group 8 with 5-Fu or CTX was the control group. The whole groups were inoculated with EAC or S180 or H22 cancer cells. After 24 hours of inoculation, each mouse was orally fed with crude bio-powder, and the traditional Chinese medicine was screened for a long time. The survival time and the toxicity were observed. The survival rate was calculated and the tumor inhibition rate was calculated

We conducted experimental studies for seven consecutive years in more than 1000 rats each year. A total of nearly 6,000 tumor-bearing animal models were made and autopsy each mice after died to observe liver, spleen, sheets, pituitary gland, kidney and to get pathological anatomy with a total of 20,000 slices to explore to find out whether There may be slight carcinogenic pathogens and the establishment of tumor micro-vessels beds and microcirculation was observed with the microscope in 100 tumor-bearing mice.

Through experimental study we first found that Chinese medication TG had a significant effect on inhibiting tumor angiogenesis. Now it has been used as anti metastasis in more than hundreds of patients in clinic treatment.

Experimental results: In our laboratory animal experiments after screening 200 kinds of Chinese herbal medicine, 48 kinds of medications with certain and excellent inhibitory effect on cancer cells and inhibition rate of more than 75-90% were selected. 152 kinds with no significant anti-cancer effects were screened-out.

Screening out of 48 kinds of traditional Chinese medications with having good tumor suppression rates, and then optimized the combination and repeated tumor suppression rate experiments in vivo, and finally developed XU ZE China1-10(XZ-C1-10) immunomodulatory anticancer Chinese medication with Chinese characteristics.

$Z-C_1$ could inhibit cancer cells, but does not affect normal cells; $Z-C_4$ specially can increase thymus function, can promote proliferation, increased immunity; $Z-C_1$ can protect bone marrow function and to product more blood.

Clinical validation: Based on the success of animal experiments, clinical validation was conducted. Namely the oncology clinics and the Research Group of combined Chinese with Western medicine for anti-cancer and anti-metastasis and recurrence were established. The patient medical records were retained and the regular follow-up observation system were established to observe the long-term effects. From experimental research to clinical evidence, the new questions were discovered during the new clinical validation process, then went back to the laboratory for the basic research, then applied the results of a new experiment for clinical validation. Thus, the experiment→ →the clinics→ the experiment again →the clinical again, all experimental studies must be clinically proven in a large number of patients observed many years, or even clinical observation of many years. According to evidence-based medicine, the long-term follow-up assessment information had gained and

they have been verified indeed to have a good long-term efficacy. The efficacy of the standard is: a good quality of life, longer survival. XZ-C sectional immune regulation anti-cancer medicine was made after a lot of applications in advanced cancer patients verification and achieved remarkable results and can improve the quality of life of patients with advanced cancer, enhance immune function, increase the body's anticancer abilities, increased appetite and significantly prolong survival.

In the chinese herbal medications many of them are the immune enhancer and the biological reaction regulator and the tonic medications; many can strengthen the body immune and have anti-cancer function. The two major global diseases that threaten human life are cancer and AIDS. The former is immunocompromised, the latter is immune deficiency. **At present, the world scientists agree that tumor formation is summarized as three processes: the first step, carcinogenic factors act on the body, interfere with cell metabolism; the second step, disrupting the genetic information within the nucleus, causing cell cancer; the third step, cancer cells escape the body Immune alert defense system; the body's immune defense capability is internal causes and the external causes have the action and the function through the internal factors. Cancer cells must be escaped from the alarm system monitoring in the body, breaking the body's immune line, to develop into a tumor. Therefore, trying to improve the body immune function is the key of the measures of the anti-cancer and the prevention of cancer. How to improve immune function? Chinese herbal medication has the extremely important advantage; there are many immune herbal preparations and there are a lot of drug sources and it should be an important anti-cancer and prevention cancer resources and it organizes the research and performs the development.**

The prevention and treatment of malignant tumors in the world are in progress. Each country focuses on a large number of experts and scholars with the experimental research and clinical experience to study and try to overcome cancer.

We should have advantages in our country areas to play the advantages of our country and to catch up with the international advanced level.

In the field of cancer research, the traditional Chinese medication is the advantage of our country. To play this advantage in the function of the field of cancer research and to explore and to develop the prevention of the cancer and anti - cancer Chinese herbal medications and to play this advantage of the study should be a strategic significance of the international significance.

On the road of human conquest cancer the research and the excavation and the development of effective and reproducible anti-cancer anti-cancer new Chinese herbal medication preparations must be promising and can be excavated into effective treasure and must be carried out the strict and objective and realistic and scientific and repetitive research with the strict scientific methods and the modern experimental surgical methods. All experimental studies must be rigorously and clinically proven in a large number of patients who demonstrate that there is a good curative effect and that the standard of efficacy is good quality of life and prolonged survival.

A series of products of XZ-C immunoregulation anti-cancer traditional Chinese medicine

1. **XZ-C1+4: for all kinds of cancer**
2. **XZ-C1: has the stable and significant anti-cancer effects, the inhibition rate up to 98%, no harmful to normal cells.**
3. **XZ-C4: protection of thymus and increase of immune function, promote the thymus proliferation, increase the immune function**
   XZ-C8: protection of bone marrow and production of blood, increase T cells, and anti-metastasis
4. **Lung cancer: XZ-C1+XZ-C4+XZ-C7**
5. **Breast cancer: XZ-C+XZ-C+XZ-C+ mushroom**
6. **Esphogus cancer: XZ-C1+XZ-C4+XZ-C2**

7 Stomach cancer: XZ-C1+XZ-C4 or +XZ-C5

8 Liver Ca: XZ-C1+XZ-C4+XZ-C5 + Mushroom+ Red ginseng

9 Bile cancer: XZ-C1+XZ-C4+XZ-C5 + Capillaris

10 Pancrease cancer: XZ-C1+XZ-C4+XZ-C5+XZ-C9

11 Colon and rectal cancer: XZ-C1+XZ-C4+XZ-C5

12 Kidney and bladder cancer: XZ-C1+XZ-C4+XZ-C6

13 Cervical and ovary cancer: XZ-C1+XZ-C4+XZ-C5+ Lms+ MDS

14 Lymphma: XZ-C1+XZ-C4+XZ-C2+ Dai Dai

15 Leukemia: XZ-C1+XZ-C4+XZ-C2+XZ-C8+ barge pole

16 Prostate cancer:XZ-C1+XZ-C4+XZ-C6

Comments: A series of XZ-C immune regulation anti-cancer traditional medications have been verified and tested for 20 years in Shuguang tumor special out-patient center on 12,000 of middle or later stage cancer patients. On clinical application they can change the symptoms, the patients have the good spirit and appetites are good, the life quality is improved, and they significantly prolong the survival time.

The scope of Clinical application of XZ-C immunoregulation anti-cancer traditional Chinese medicine XZ-C1-10 anticancer metastasis, recurrence

(1) **For a variety of distant metastatic cancer, such as liver metastases, lung metastases, bone metastases, brain metastases, abdominal lymph node metastasis, mediastinal lymph node metastasis, malignant pleural effusion, cancerous ascites, XZ-C Immune regulation of anti - metastatic therapy can be applied according to the transfer step, to intervene, block the transfer of cancer cells, to extend life.**

(2) **For the patients who completed a variety of radiotherapy and chemotherapy treatment course, XZ-C1-4 immune regulation of traditional Chinese medicine can be used to consolidate long-term efficacy and prevent recurrence.**

(3) For the patients who have chemotherapy, the reaction is serious and can not continue, XZ-C immunoregulation treatment to anti-metastasis, recurrence can continue to be applied.

(4) In the elderly or frail with other diseases who can not put, chemotherapy, XZ-C immune regulation of anti-metastasis, relapse treatment can be applied.

(5) On the patients who surgical exploration can not cut down the tumor XZ-C immune regulation treatment can be used.

(6) For the palliative surgery XZ-C immunoregulation anti-transfer therapy can be applied.

(7) After a variety of radical mastectomy, XZ-C immunoregulation treatment of traditional Chinese medicine anti-recurrence, metastasis should continue to serve to improve the long-term effect after radical operation.

8. how to overcome cancer? XZ-C put forward to the scientific research achievement and the scientific and technological innovation series

The anti-cancer and anti-cancer metastasis research and the scientific research achievement and the scientific and technological innovation series

The following arguments in the monographs of XZ-C (XU ZE - China)series are put forward the first time in the international and are the original papers and the first in the international and the international leader:

(1) In the international first it was proposed: "thymus atrophy and the immune dysfunction are one of the causes of cancer and pathogenesis"

- the wew findings of experimental studies on the etiology and pathogenesis of cancer

- This is the leading international independent intellectual property results. After investigation this is put forward the first time in the international.

- see the monograph "new concept and new method of cancer treatment" P.13

.... [Scientific research results] [Science and technology innovation] A

(2) In the international it was first proposed: " the theoretical basis and experimental basis of the " increase immune function and the prevention of thymus of XZ-C immunomodulation treatment ""

- put forward the theoretical basis and experimental basis of immunoregulation therapy for cancer

- Because of the above experimental study it was found that the new revelation so that the treatment principle must be to prevent thymus atrophy, promote thymic hyperplasia, protect bone marrow hematopoietic function, improve immune surveillance, control malignant cells immune escape.

- see the monograph "new concept and new method of cancer treatment" P.17

.... [Scientific research results] [Science and technology innovation A]

(3) The first international initiative: "Cancer treatment should change the concept of the establishment of a comprehensive treatment concept"

- put forward the new concept of cancer treatment principles

- the goal or target of cancer treatment must be for both the tumor and the host to establish a comprehensive treatment view.

- it should overcome of killing the cancer cells simply in the one - sided treatment view

- see the monograph "new concept and new method of cancer treatment" P.28

.... [Scientific research results] [Science and technology innovation B]

4) The international first initiative: " the new model of combination of Cancer multidisciplinary comprehensive treatment"

- Proposing a new concept of cancer treatment portfolio model

The new model of multidisciplinary comprehensive treatment is:

The long-term treatment: surgery + biotherapy + immunotherapy + Chinese medication+ the combination of Chinese and Western therapy

The short-term treatment as the supplemented: radiology therapy + chemotherapy, not long-term, not excessive

- see the monograph "new concept and new method of cancer treatment" P33

.... [Scientific research results] [Science and technology innovation B]

(5) In the international it was first pointed out: "the analysis and the evaluation and the questioning and the four comment of the solid tumor systemic intravenous chemotherapy"

----the discussion on the Problems and Disadvantages of the whole Body Venous Chemotherapy

--- questioned and commented on the route and the dose calculation and the curative effect evaluation of systemic intravenous chemotherapy

- see the monograph "new concept and new method of cancer treatment" P.57

.... [Scientific research results] [Science and technology innovation A]

(6) In the international it was first proposed: "the abdominal solid tumor systemic intravenous chemotherapy should be changed into the target organ of the intravascular chemotherapy and reform the traditional cancer chemotherapy"

- because the systemic intravenous chemotherapy cytotoxic from the superior vena cava route can not directly reach the portal vein system and the vena cava system and the portal vein system are generally not connected by the superior vena cava so that it is difficult to reach the portal vein.

- where are the cancer cells in the abdominal solid tumors (stomach, colorectal, liver, gallbladder, pancreas, spleen, abdominal and other malignant tumors)? It is mainly in the portal vein system. The postoperative adjuvant chemotherapy is injected by the elbow vein → vena cava route of administration. It is unreasonable and does not meet the anatomy and the physiological pathology because it can not directly into the portal vein system.

- therefore, it should change the route of administration into the administration of the target intravascular therapy

- see the monograph "new concept and new method of cancer treatment" P.63

.... [Scientific research results] [Science and technology innovation A]

(7) In the International it was first proposed: "cancer in the human body there are three main forms of expression"

---proposed the new concept of cancer metastasis therapy

- proposed that this third form of expression is the transit of the cancer cell population and the goals of cancer treatment should be based on the above three forms of existence, in particular, it should be on the transfer of cancer cells.

- see the monograph "new concept and new method of cancer treatment" P.38

.... [Scientific research results] [Science and technology innovation A]

(8) In the international it was first proposed: "the whole process of cancer development" two points and one line"

--proposed the theory of cancer metastasis therapy

- One of the purposes of cancer treatment is to prevent metastasis

Cancer metastasis of the whole process can be summed up as "two points and one line"

- the traditional cancer treatment only pay attention to "two points" while ignoring the "first line"

The new concept that should pay attention to both "two", but also to cut off "line"

- see the monograph "new concept and new method of cancer treatment" P.43

.... [Scientific research results] [Science and technology innovation A]

(9) In the international it was first proposed: "anti-cancer treatment of three steps"

---proposed the theory of cancer metastasis therapy

- The "eight steps" of the transfer of cancer cells are grouped into "three stages" and attempts to break each step

- see the monograph "new concept and new method of cancer treatment" P.47

.... [Scientific research results] [Science and technology innovation A]

(10) In the international it was first proposed: "open up the third area of anti-cancer metastasis"

- put forward the theory innovation of the new concept of cancer metastasis therapy and it was found and put forward the third field of human anti-cancer metastasis.

- The circulatory system has a large number of immune surveillance cells. The "main battlefield" which is annihilating the transit of cancer cells is in the blood circulation.

.... [Scientific research results] [Science and technology innovation B]

9. How to overcome cancer? XZ-C proposed: to attack the cancer and to launch a total attack which is unprecedented work

(11) In the international it was first proposed: "the XZ-C research program of capturing cancer and launching a total attack"

- The Overall Strategy Reform and Development of Cancer Treatment in China
- To avoid empty talk and to pay attention to the hard work and to start to go No matter how far away the cancer path is, it always should go.
- Proposed to conquer cancer and to launch a total attack, which is unprecedented work

(12) In the international it was the first time to put forward: " the necessity and feasibility report of conquering cancer and launching the total attack"

- The overall strategic reform of China's cancer treatment should change from focusing on treatment into pay attention to both the prevention and the treatment at the same attention
- XZ-C proposed the general idea and design of conquering cancer
- What is the target of the total attack against cancer and the total attack?
- XU ZE proposed the general offensive ideas and the strategies and the planning and the blueprint of conquering cancer and of launching the total attack

(13) In the international it was first proposed: "to build the prevention and treatment hospital during the whole process of cancer occurrence and cancer development"

(The global demonstration hospital of the prevention and treatment cancer)

- Current existing problems in the model of setting up hospital
- The road of how to overcome cancer is to study the establishment of the prevention and treatment hospital during the whole process of cancer

occurrence and development and reform the current mode of setting up the hospital which focuses treatment and ignores the prevention

- XU ZE proposed the strategic thinking of fighting cancer and the planning map and the cancer prevention and treatment for whole process of cancer occurrence and development

(14) In the international it was first proposed: "to build the general envisage of conquering cancer and launching the attack and the basic design of the science city"

- It is equivalent to the design of a Chinese charecteric framework for conquering cancer
- How to set up the basic idea and design of conquering cancer and launching the general attack?
- How to overcome cancer? It must set up

  "cancer animal experimental center"

  "Innovative Molecular Oncology School of Medicine"

  "Cancer and Multidisciplinary Research Institute"

- How to overcome cancer? It must be "to build the science base of the medicine, the teaching, the research and the development of conquering cancer and launching a cancer attack--- the Science City"

10. How to overcome cancer? XZ-C proposed that: to condense wisdom and to move forward together to overcome cancer

"Cancer moon shot" (US) and "the dawn of the C-type plan" (China)

---- move forward together toward the scientific temple of conquering cancer

(1) "Cancer moon shot" (Cancer moon shot) "profile

On January 12, 2016, US President Barack Obama announced a national plan to tackle cancer in his last State of the Union address during his term

of office, namely Vice President Joe Biden's "New Moon Plan" Shot ", which will be headed by Biden. In May 2015, the son of Biden died of brain cancer, only 46 years old. Since then, Biden announced not to participate in the 2016 presidential election and will remain in the remaining vice president of anti-cancer career.

Biden will visit the University of Pennsylvania School of Medicine at Abramson Cancer Center next week and discuss the plan. He said the "new moon program" is a commitment to the world to overcome cancer, will inspire a new generation of scientists to explore the scientific world.

Obama did not mention the specific plan for the plan in his speech, but he mentioned that the bill and tax bill passed by Congress in December 2015 had raised the financial budget of the National Institutes of Health (NIH).

The United States has recently set up a National Immunotherapy Consortium comprised of the pharmaceutical companies and the biotech companies and the academic medical organizations who have tried to develop a vaccine immunotherapy by 2020 to overcome cancer and complete "cancer Moon plan".

The American Society of Clinical Oncology (ASCO) issued a statement on its website that welcomed Obama's "the new moon program" and supported Biden's leadership that the "the new moon program" would reduce the pain of which cancer Cancer causes death. The "big data" technology application, such as ASCO's "CancerLinQ" fast learning system, can speed up the pace of cancer, but also improve the quality of cancer so that physicians better develop the treatment program for each patient's individual and understand what aspects of the urgent need to put more research work (Liu Quan).

(January 21, 2016, China Medical Tribune)

(2) Introduction to the dawn of the C-type plan

① **Before January 12, 2016, it was put forward to the progress situation of scientific research program "to overcome cancer and to launch the total attack of cancer."**

② **before January 12, 2016, we took " conquering cancer" as the research direction and had carried out the scientific research and the scientific and technological innovation series.**

③ **The dawn of the C-type plan**

(A).Cancer Moon Shot

The United States

Project Name: "New Moon Plan"
Objective: To overcome cancer
Nature: A national plan to overcome cancer
Announcement: The President's State of the Union statement
Announcer: President Obama
Announced on January 12, 2016
The head of the program: Vice President Biden
The program specific program: unknown
National Institutes of Health: Increased financial budget
(NIH)
Recently formed:
 pharmaceutical companies
Biotechnology companies ⟶ the national immunotherapy alliance
Academic medical organizations

The alliance is trying to develop a vaccine therapy by 2020 to tackle the cancer's new cancer landing program.

(B). The Dawn of the C-type plan

China

Project name: "dawn of the C-type plan"

Objective: To overcome cancer

Nature:

Advocates and

The total designer: Professor Xu Ze in 2011 proposed "to overcome the cancer and to launch the total attack" and in 2013 put forward " the total design of building the science city of conquering cancer and launching the total attack" and in 2013 put forward " the scientific and research plan of conquering cancer and launching the total attack XZ-C attack cancer launched a total offensive research project" ; In July 2015 put forward the "dawn of the C-type plan" ; in July 2015 put forward the application report of the feasibility report with four major items of conquering cancer and launching cancer; in August 2015 set up the Preliminary Design and Design of the establishment in Hubei, Wuhan of the Experimental Area of Cancer Working Group which will be used to apply for the government.

Racing with Cancer moon shot

In the January 12, 2016, we put forward the "to capture of cancer and to launch a total attack" has been carried out the research work. To put forward "conquering cancer and launch the total attack is the unprecedented work. XZ-C (Xu Ze-China) has been running in front of 3-4 years.

(1) Xu Ze published the monograph "the new concept of cancer treatment and new methods" . Chapter 38 with a chapter of the length it was put forward " the strategic thinking and suggestions of overcoming cancer" in October 2011

(2) In June 2013 Xu Ze also proposed " the general idea and design to overcome the cancer ", in an attempt to reduce the incidence of cancer, reduce cancer mortality, improve the cure rate, prolong survival, the total attack is anti- Cancer, three carriages go hand in hand

(3) Xu Ze in August 2013 for the first time in the international community proposed: " the XZ-C research program to overcome the cancer and launch a total attack " - the overall strategy and development of cancer treatment in China

(4) Professor Xu Ze in July 2015 to the Government made the following four to tackle the total attack on the feasibility report of cancer report

"XZ-C proposed the scientific and research program to attack the cancer and launcha total offensive"

The Overall Strategy Reform and Development of Cancer Treatment in China

① in the international first proposed:

"The need to capture the total attack of cancer and the feasibility of the report"

② in the international community for the first time:

"To build the whole anti-rule hospital of the prevention and treatment of cancer during the whole process of the development and occurance of cancer"

(Global Demonstration Prevention and Treatment Hospital)

"the imagination and feasibility report of building the hospital of anti-cancer throughout the prevention and treatment."

- Describe the necessity and feasibility of establishing a complete prevention and cure hospital

③ in the international first proposed:

"To build the general idea of conquering cancer and science city's basic vision and feasibility report"

- is equivalent to the design of a Chinese framework for cancer design

④ in the international first proposed:

> "In building a moderately society at the same time, the proposed" ride research "- for cancer prevention, cancer control of medical science and cancer prevention and control of the necessity and feasibility report" - adhere to the Chinese characteristics of anti-cancer,

Our dreams are tackling cancer, building a well-off society and everyone's health away from cancer.

The four scientific research programs in the international community for the first time was put forward and are the first in the international and the international leader and opened up the new areas of anti-cancer research and will open up a new era of anti-cancer research

It is unprecedented work to raise the total attack on cancer.

(5) Xu Ze in August 2015 proposed the initial design and imagination for the establishment of Wuhan in Wuhan to overcome the Cancer Working Group (station) pilot area which is apply to the Hubei Provincial Government.

(6) In July 2015, it was reported to the Provincial Science and Technology Department about the scientific research achievements, the series of scientific and technological innovation and put forward the scientific research plan and outline of launch the general attack of cancer (report outline) and the promotion of cancer treatment reform, innovation and development Four of the filings of the application

(7) in July 2015 it was reported to the Provincial Department of Education about capture the cancer as the research direction of scientific research and the scientific and technological innovation series

(8) Professor Xu Ze's fourth book "Monograph": "On Innovation Of Treatment Of Cancer" - (Cancer Treatment Innovation) was published in Washington, DC in December 2015, published in the world with electric Version.

Introduction to the new book: the experimental study of Chinese medicine immunopharmacology and the anti-cancer research of the combination of the traditional Chinese and Western medication on the molecular lever and it has formed XZ-C immune regulation of the theoretical system of cancer.

Walking Out of a traditional Chinese medication with immune regulation, regulate immune activity, prevent thymus atrophy, promote thymic hyperplasia, protect bone marrow hematopoietic function, improve immune surveillance, at the molecular level of combining Chinese medications and Western medication to overcome the new path of cancer.

Before January 12, 2016, we took the cancer as the research direction, has carried out the scientific research achievements of scientific and technological innovation series.

(1) The new discovery of experimental research:

Xu Ze published in January 2001 in its monograph "new understanding of cancer treatment and new model" published from the laboratory experimental tumor research new discovery:

①　Thymus (Thymus) removal can be made to produce animal model, injection of immunosuppressive drugs can help the establishment of animal model.

②　the thymus of the host inoculated with cancer cells, was acute atrophy, cell proliferation blocked, the volume was significantly reduced, the laboratory by 7 years more than 6,000 production of animal models of animal experiments observed, the experimental results show that: the progress of the tumor, even if the thymus Progressive atrophy.

(2) Xu Ze published in October 2011, "new concept of cancer treatment and new methods," Chapter 2 of the cancer etiology, pathogenesis, pathophysiology of the experimental study of the new discovery:

"Thymus atrophy, immune dysfunction is one of the causes and pathogenesis of cancer", and in Chapter 3, based on animal experiments inspiration, the principle of treatment, should protect, regulate and activate the body's anti-cancer immune system, Proposed: "XZ-C immunomodulation therapy" chest rhythm "theoretical basis and experimental basis.

(3) Reported at the American Society for International Oncology Cancer Research Paper:

① it received the American Cancer Research Society AACR for the meeting in September 2013 at the International Conference on International Oncology in Washington, "XZ-C immunomodulation anti-cancer therapy", has aroused widespread attention in the international tumor medical community And highly valued.

② It was Participated in the 12th International Conference on Cancer Research in the American Society of Cancer Research (AACR) in Washington, USA, from 27 to 30 October 2013, and it was reported that "thymic atrophy and immunocompromised are one of the causes and pathogenesis of cancer" The theoretical basis and experimental basis of the treatment of the principle of "protecting the thymus, improving the immune system", "protecting the bone marrow" (the protection of bone marrow stem cells) is warmly welcomed by the participants and attaches great importance.

(4) published monographs

In the above study of cancer to study the direction of the experimental study, basic research, clinical validation, wc have gone through 28 years, made a series of anti-cancer, anti-cancer metastasis, relapse research research, scientific and technological innovation series, which hundreds of original Innovative or independent innovation of scientific research papers, are published in my series of "monograph" in.

① published in January 2001 the first monograph "new understanding of cancer treatment and new model"

Hubei Science and Technology Press, Xu Ze with

② published in January 2006 the second monograph "cancer metastasis treatment of new concepts and new methods"

Beijing People's Medical Publishing House, Xu Ze with

In April 2007 issued by the People's Republic of China issued a "three hundred" original book publishing project certificate

③ published in October 2011 third book "new concept of cancer treatment and new methods"

Beijing People's Medical Publishing House, Xu Ze, Xu Jie / with

④ published in December 2015 the fourth monograph, for the English version of the English version of "On Innovation Of Treatment Of Cancer" - (Cancer Treatment Innovation Theory - Volume 1) published in Washington, the world, and issue electronic version, Xu Ze, Xu Jie with the

⑤ December 6, 2016 published the fifth monograph, the English version, published in Washington, the United States, "The ROAD To OVER Come Cancer" - "capture the road of cancer", the global distribution, and issue electronic version, three sites.

This five monographs are our difficult trek, hard climbing, step by step in four different scientific research stages of scientific research, four different levels of achievement. (The first monograph at the age of 67, published the second monograph at the age of 73, the third monograph at the age of 78, the English version of the third monograph at the age of 80, the English edition, the Washington publication, the international distribution, At the age of 82, he published the fourth monograph, the full English edition, published

in Washington, published worldwide, and published the fifth monograph at the age of 83 in December 2016.) Full English edition, published in Washington, USA.

(5) Visited the Stoutin Cancer Institute in Houston, USA

In order to strengthen the exchange and cooperation of international scientific and technological organizations, on 10 December 2009, we were invited to visit the Stoutin Cancer Institute in the United States. We were warmly welcomed and warmly received by the Institute. Many professors, researchers, nude mice animal model laboratory and anti-cancer drug analysis laboratory responsible person participated in the discussion, exchange, with a slides report the latest scientific research.

We presented to the United States Stoutin Cancer Institute of my Institute of "cancer metastasis, recurrence of experimental research" color Atlas, introduced the experimental study of radical surgery in the tumor-free technology and removal of thymus to produce animal model of animal experiments Research, and the exclusive development of the ZC immune regulation of anti-cancer, anti-transfer of traditional Chinese medicine products Z-C1-10 of the situation. And presented my published monograph "cancer transfer treatment of new concepts and new methods", the Department of the book award of three hundred original books, by the Institute of the warm welcome and appreciation.

(6) The innovation - plot 28 years of anti-cancer, anti-cancer metastasis of the basic and clinical research and walking out of a "Chinese-style anti-cancer" and the Chinese and Western medicine combined with immune regulation of cancer, we have accumulated 20 years more than 12000 cases Clinical experience, can be pushed to the country, you can go to the world, you can connect the "area along the way" to make Chinese medicine to the world, so that "Chinese-style anti-cancer", Chinese and Western medicine combined with immune regulation of cancer, both the development and enrich the immune Learn the content of cancer, but also the modernization of Chinese medicine and international standards, to the forefront of the world.

11. The dawn of C-type plan No. 1 -6

Why is the "dawn"?

Dawn is dawn light and is dawn sun and is sunrise;

Vibrant and Energetic Vibrant and the Original innovation and the Independent Innovation

C = China

Type C = Chinese model

In China daily 8550 people were diagnosed with cancer, 6 people per minute was diagnosed with cancer, therefore, the research to attack the cancer and to launch a total offensive research work cannot walk slowly and should run forward to save the dying.

Time is money, time is money = an inch of time is an inch of gold

Time is life

Time flies and it is like a light arrow

Empty talk is worsening the country and the hard work is flourishing the group.

To avoid empty talk and to pay attention to the hard work and to start to go.

No matter how far the way to overcome cancer it will be, it always should start to go.

This research program is the original innovation and it is put forward the "declaration of war to cancer" and it is the time and it should launch the total attack.

Our dreams are to overcome cancer, to build a well-off society, to keep everyone healthy, and far away from cancer

Xu Ze

In Wuhan, Hubei

July 2015

Dawn of the C-type plan
Developed in July 2015

(1) Dawn of the C-type plan No. 1: "capture cancer and launch a total attack"

-----The Overall Strategy Reform and Development of Cancer Treatment in China

It was proposed to the general designs and the ideas and the plannings and the blueprints and the rule of capturing cancer

To avoid empty talk and to pay attention to the hard work and to start to go.

No matter how far the road to overcome cancer it will be, it should always start to go

(See another article)

(2) Dawn of the C-type plan 2: "to build the hospital with the whole rules of prevention and treatment of cancer"

(Global Demonstration Prevention and Treatment Hospital)

----strategic reform and change of the mode of running hospitals

Reform and treatment model

(See another article)

(3) Dawn of the C-type plan on the 3rd: "to build the science and technology city to overcome the cancer"

- XZ-C proposed the Science City total design, planning, blueprint to conquer cancer and launch a total attack

This is the only way to overcome cancer

This is to overcome the cancer of the "high-speed rail", "high-speed" channel

(See another article)

(4) The Dawn of the C-type plan on the 4th "set up multi-disciplinary and cancer research group"

- for the cause of cancer, pathogenesis, pathophysiology, metastasis, recurrence mechanism ... ... to study anti-cancer, anti-recurrence, anti-transfer measures to improve the overall level of medical care to benefit patients.

- the efficacy evaluation criteria are: the patient survival time is long, good quality of life, complications or less, each school group are provincial key laboratories.

(See another article)

(5) dawn of type C plan on the 5th "vaccine is human hope and immunology prevention"

- today's immunology prevention and treatment have become a very important field in clinical medicine and preventive medicine

- $\triangle$ $\triangle$ school group + $\triangle$ $\triangle$ school group + $\triangle$ $\triangle$ school group $\rightarrow$ scientific alliance, the ally group

(See another article)

(6) Dawn of the C-type plan on the 6th: A "immunomodulatory drug prospects gratifying"

- no matter how complex the mechanism behind cancer, the body immunosuppression is the essential for cancer progression

- In our lab from the experimental results analysis the new discoveries and the new revelation were gotten:

Thymic atrophy and immune dysfunction and immune surveillance capacity decline and immune escape of cancer are one of the cancer etiology and pathogenesis so that the treatment principle should be to prevent thymus atrophy, promote thymic hyperplasia, improve immune surveillance.

- XZ-C immunomodulation traditional Chinese medications are 48 kinds of Chinese herbal medication with the good anti-cancer rate which 26 kinds are better Immune regulation screening out from more than 200 kinds of the traditional Chinese herbal medications on the animal model in vivo tumor inhibition experiments.

(See another article)

Dawn C type plan Number 6: B "XZ-C immunoregulation anti-cancer traditional Chinese medicine active ingredient, the research and scholar group and laboratory on the molecular level analysis and research"

- Further the development of XZ-C immunoregulation anti-cancer traditional Chinese medication active ingredients, molecular weight, structural formula, molecular level analysis

- the methods and the steps: animal experiments, molecular level experiments; gene level experiments, first active ingredients were isolated, so that our traditional medications of this valuable heritage can become modern and scientific.

(See another article)

Dawn C Shape Plan (China)

Hope: apply for the "dawn of the C-type plan" into the national cancer program

Expected results:

The modern science and technology and analysis and testing methods are used to do the traditional Chinese medicine research. Chinese medicine in clinics play a material basis because the chemical compositions are contained inside. The study of the traditional Chinese medicine anti-cancer and its mechanism must be in-depth study and analysis, of which active ingredients are inside, so that our traditional medicine is this valuable legacy, and more modern, scientific.

After 30 years of the experimental research, basic research and clinical validation it has been selected series of "protection of thymus and increase immune" immune regulation of anti-cancer Chinese medicine XZ-C1-10, after 30 years of clinical observation to verify more than 12,000 cases of cases, a list, Prolong life, improve symptoms, improve the quality of life, how to know, evaluation can extend the survival period? Some surgical exploration can not cut down (all confirmed by pathological biopsy), or has been widely transferred, estimated to survive only 3-6 months, or 6-12 months of the case, by XZ-C immunoregulation anti-cancer, Anti-metastasis, relapse treatment, some patients can still survive 4 years - 5 years - 8 years, are the original data and complete information and follow-up information.

By a retired professor, after the rehabilitation of heart, calm down, hide in the small building, self-reliance, hard work, adhering to the animal experiments and outpatient clinical research of anti-cancer, anti-cancer metastasis; from Sixty years (60 years old) → to the seventies (70 years old) → to the ripe old age (80 years old), still perseverance, perseverance to carry out scientific research to overcome cancer, because of retirement it cannot apply for projects and subjects so that there is no scientific research and sola fighting and no support with hard work for more than 20 years, it made a series of scientific and technological innovation, scientific research achievement .. Because the retirement has been 20 years, nobody cares and there is no support. As the retired professor, I do not know where the management is and where it can support and where the scientific research can be reported so that it just is to publish the "monographs" for the benefit of mankind and so that there are a series of monographs which are published, and then To report the Provincial Science and Technology Department, the Provincial Department of Education: ① hope to open an international high-end academic forum; ② report to the government to attack cancer, launched a total attack; ③ to the provincial,, The city to overcome the cancer test area (station), first try. Hope: to apply in Wuhan, Wuhan City, the establishment of "the first to overcome the cancer launched a total attack of the Science City", that "the world's first attack on cancer launched a total attack of Science City."

How to implement this unprecedented human event?

(1) report to the government, request instructions
(2) to the province, city report, request instructions
(3) to the city to make recommendations in Wuhan City to build:
    "the first Science City to overcome Cancer"
    "The world's first Science City to overcome Cancer"

Annex 2 Brief description of the scientific environment and the recent international research situation:

"Cancer moon shot" (US) and "the dawn of the C-type plan" (China)

---- move forward together toward the scientific temple of conquering cancer

(A). "new moon plan (Cancer moon shot)" (US) (Introduction)

Plan name: "Cancer moon shot"
Objective: To overcome cancer
Nature: A national plan to overcome cancer
Announcement: The President's State of the Union statement

Announcer: President Obama

Announced on January 12, 2016

The head of the program: Vice President Biden

The program specific program: unknown

National Institutes of Health: Increased financial budget

(NIH)

Recently formed:

pharmaceutical companies
Biotechnology company $\longrightarrow$ National immunization therapy union
Academic medical organization

The alliance is trying to develop a vaccine therapy by 2020 to tackle the cancer's new cancer landing program.

(1) In January 12, 2016, President Barack Obama announced in his State of the Union a national plan to tackle cancer, which was run by Vice President Joe Biden.

The name of the program: 'plant new moon program'

Objective: To overcome cancer

Nature: A national plan to overcome cancer

(2) In the second week of the plan, Vice President Joe Biden visited the Abrainson Cancer Center at the University of Pennsylvania School of Hearing and discussed the plan. He said the "new moon program" is a commitment to the world to overcome cancer, will inspire a new generation of scientists to explore the scientific world.

(3) In Feb 4th, 2016 American Society of Clinical Oncology (ASCO) in Washington State Capitol Hill: it was published the "2016 Annual Report: ASCO Clinical Oncology Progress" presented the progress of 2015, "Cancer Immunotherapy". Prof.

Julie MVose, the professor at ASCO, said that the most important progress in 2015 was the discovery of immunotherapy, which she said in the foreword: "We are not going to be treated only by tumor type and stage; in the accurate medicine Era, we choose or exclude treatment based on each patient and tumor gene data. No other significant progress like immunology can be transformed into clinical practice so that in 2015 the biggest progress is immunotherapy. "Immunotherapy opens the new era of the cancer treatment.

(4) On April 28, 2016: in US Congress Building it was held a policy luncheon and it was hosted by the former US Senator Tom Coburn. My fourth book (On innovation of Treatment of Cancer) third author and translator Bin Wu attended the meeting. (On Innovation of Treatment of Cancer), published in Washington, DC, February 25, 2015, published in English, published worldwide, and released an electronic version of the book.

Introduction to the new books:

The Experimental study of Chinese medicine immunopharmacology research and molecular level of Chinese and Western medicine combined with anti-cancer research has formed xz-C immune regulation of the theoretical system of cancer.

Walking Out of the new way of a traditional Chinese medicine with immune regulation and regulation of immune activity and preventing thymus atrophy, promoting thymic hyperplasia, protecting bone marrow hematopoietic function, improving immune surveillance in the molecular level combination of Chinese and Western medication to overcome cancer.

(5) In June 3, 2016 the American Society of Clinical Oncology Conference is held in Chicago which is the world's highest level of clinical oncology academic conference. The theme of the meeting focused on "focus on wisdom, to overcome cancer"; presidential presided over the meeting at the General Assembly reported the US anti-cancer "moon moon (moon Shot) division, the world a total of 50,000 participants, unprecedented, world attention.

(6) On May 25the 2016 Vice President Joe Biden visited Hopkins University and Cancer Research magazine, reported "New Moon Sword," said the future is mainly immunotherapy to conquer cancer, immunotherapy to control cancer, immunotherapy Is a new discovery by this, vigorously supporting immunotherapy, and knot Hopkins University 1-. $ 2 million in research funding. The magazine cover the photo of Vice President Joe Biden.

(7) On June 29, 2016 US Vice President Biden convenes a summit: broadcast from the National Palace from 9 am to 6 pm to the United States. National Children's Ten Cancer Centers and Societies organize physicians, nurses, scientists, volunteers, patients, families, cancer survivors, and those who have survived ... to participate in this missionary cancer leopard mission to encourage scientists to focus on cancer.

The American Cancer Society Cancer Action Network and the American Cancer Society [ACS] Chief Executive Officer and Chief Medical Officer and President attended the historic summit.

The white house called on the Americans to join them to host community activities.

Immunotherapy opens a new era of cancer treatment and it should be one billion dollars per year Yao Yu to overcome cancer research.

(B). "Dawn of the C-type plan" (China)(Introduction)

Project name: "dawn of the C-type plan"

Objective: To overcome cancer

Nature:

Advocate and Chief Designer:

(1) Xu Ze published in October 2011, "the new concept of cancer treatment and new methods" monograph of Chapter 38 with a chapter of the length of "to overcome the strategic thinking and suggestions of cancer"

(2) June 2013 Xu Ze also proposed "to overcome the cancer to start the general idea and design", in an attempt to reduce the incidence of cancer, reduce cancer mortality, improve the cure rate, prolong survival, the total attack is anti- Cancer, three carriages go hand in hand

(3) Xu Ze in August 2013 for the first time in the international community: "to overcome the cancer launched a total attack of the XZ-C research program" - the overall strategy and development of cancer treatment in China

(4) Professor Xu Ze in July 2015 to the Government made the following four to tackle the total attack on the feasibility report of cancer report

"XZ-C proposed to attack the cancer launched a total offensive research program"

The Overall Strategy Reform and Development of Cancer Treatment in China

① in the international first proposed:

"The need to capture the total attack of cancer and the feasibility of the report"

② in the international community for the first time:

"To build cancer, the development of the whole anti-rule hospital"

(Global Demonstration Prevention and Treatment Hospital)

"To build anti-cancer throughout the prevention and treatment of hospital vision and feasibility report"

- Describe the necessity and feasibility of establishing a complete prevention and cure hospital

③ in the international first proposed:

"To build the general idea of conquering cancer and science city's basic vision and feasibility report"

- is equivalent to the design of a Chinese framework for cancer design

④ in the international first proposed:
"In building a moderately society at the same time, the proposed" ride research "- for cancer prevention, cancer control of medical science and cancer prevention and control of the necessity and feasibility report" - adhere to the Chinese characteristics of anti-cancer,

⑤ before Januazry 12, 2016, we put forward the "capture of cancer launched a total attack" research work has been carried out 3-4 years. Put forward the "capture of cancer launched a total attack" research work, which is unprecedented.

In 2016 years before 01: 12 days: we attack the cancer as the research direction, has carried out the scientific research achievements of scientific and technological innovation series

(1) experimental study leopard new discovery:

Xu Ze published in January 2001 in its monograph "new understanding of cancer treatment and new touch type" published from the laboratory experimental tumor research new discovery:

1. Resecting Thymus can be used to make the animal model of the cancer-bearing mice and the injection of immunosuppressive agents can help the establishment of the animal model.

2 the host of the thymus inoculated with cancer cells was an acute progress and the inhibition of proliferation and the volume decrease and in the experimental observation in 6000 cancer-bearing mice model within seven

years it was found that while cancer pregresses, the thymus continues having atrophy.

(2) in October 2011 Xu Ze published "the new concept and new methods of cancer treatment" in which in Chapter 2 discussed the new discovery of the experimental study of cancer etiology and pathogenesis and pathophysiology:

<< one of the reasons of the cancar is thymus atropy and immune function reduction >>, in the chapter 3 it was put forward the revelation from the animal experiments which the rules of treatment are to protect, regulate, and activate the anti- Cancer immune function; also also put forward << the therapy and experimental basis of XZ-C immune regulation >>.

(3). Exchange the cancer research results at the American Society for International Oncology Cancer Research Paper:

1. reccived the American Cancer Research Society AACR in September 2013 in Washington, the United States International Cancer Society "XZ-C immunoregulation anti-cancer therapy", has great widespread attention in the international tumor medical community.

2. In October 27-30, 2013 in Washington to participate in the American Society for Cancer Research (AACR) academic conference, the 12th International Cancer Research Conference, it was reported: "one of the reasons of cancer is thymus atrophy and reduce of immune functions", and the theory basis of the treatment rules of protection of thymus and increase immune function (protecting thymus and increasing immune function and the protection of bone marrow and increase immune system "(prevention of the stem cells in bone marrow).

(4) published monographs

In the above research on the direction of cancer research, basic research, clinical validation, we have gone through 30 years and made a series of anti-cancer, anti-cancer metastasis, recurrence research research, scientific and technological innovation series, this hundred The original innovation or the main innovation of scientific research papers are published in my series "monograph".

1. in January 2000 the first book of new recognition and new model of cancer treatment was published by Hubei Science and Technology Press, the author is Prof. Xu Ze.

2   in January 2006 the second monograph "new concepts and new methods of cancer metastasis therapy" was published by Beijing People's Medical Publishing House, the author was Xu Ze

   in April 2007 the People's Republic of China issued the certificate of the original book publication of "Three of one hundred"

3   in October 2011 the third monograph "new concepts and new methods of cancer treatment was published by Beijing People's Military Publishing House and Xu Ze, Xu Jie are the authors.

(4) In 2015, the fourth monograph published the English version of "On Innovation Of Treatment Of Cancer") - (Cancer Treatment Innovation on the first volume) by Washington, the United States, the global distribution, and the issue of electronic Edition

(5)in 2016 the fifth monograph "the road to overcome cancer" is published.

(5) innovation ----- after 30 years of anti-cancer, anti-cancer metastasis of the basic and clinical research it has been walked out the new way with Chinese-style of anti-cancer and immune regulation and control of the combination of western and Chinese medication of cancer treatment; we have 30 years of the experience in more than 12000 cases of the application: it can be pushed to the country and to go on the world and it can connect the generation and the way and make Chinese medication to walk into all of the word and it is "Chinese anti-cancer Style and the combination of Chinese medication

and West Medication with immune regulation of cancer treatment and the development and enrichment of the content of the treatment of cancer, but also it makes the modernization of Chinese medication merge with the international so that it walks to the forefront world.

In Sept 9th, 2016 it was reported in China that American Specialists made the route of anti-cancer plans-------encourage to use the immunotherapy and gene therapy

12. The situation analysis (a)

Prevention of Cancer and Anti-cancer and Move Forward Together and Conquer Cancer

1. To analyze the respective technological advantages

The United States   China

Advantages: (+)   Advantage:(-)

1, life science   originated from   1, Life Sciences   learn from
                           the United States   the United States
Molecular biology   extremely high   Molecular biology
Genetic engineering   patent, invention   Genetic engineering
Proteomics Group   Precision medicine   Proteomics Group

2, cancer targeting   originated   2, cancer targeting   imports from
   Treatment, drug s   from the United States   Treatment   the United States
                           patent, invention   the drugs   it did not have
                                                                            (in 2015 had a selfroduced)

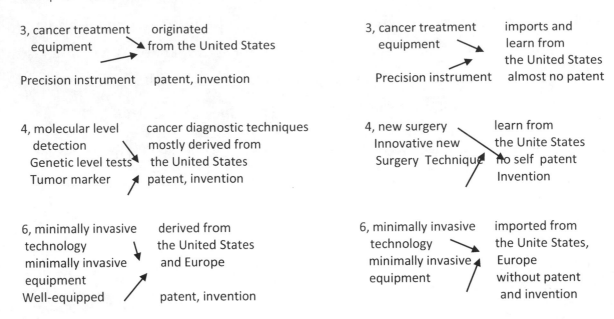

3, cancer treatment equipment → originated from the United States

Precision instrument patent, invention

3, cancer treatment equipment → imports and learn from the United States almost no patent

Precision instrument

4, molecular level detection
Genetic level tests
Tumor marker

cancer diagnostic techniques mostly derived from the United States
patent, invention

4, new surgery
Innovative new
Surgery Technique

learn from the Unite States
no self patent
Invention

6, minimally invasive technology
minimally invasive equipment
Well-equipped

derived from the United States and Europe

patent, invention

6, minimally invasive technology
minimally invasive equipment

imported from the Unite States, Europe without patent and invention

In short, the modern medicine was from Europe and the United States. The development and advance of American medicine nearly a hundred years has developed to micro → ultramicro → precision medicine, nanotechnology; and China's modern medicine is dependent on imported medicine and following behind by learning. The United States has 39 cancer research centers, Anderson Cancer Center is one of the earliest three comprehensive cancer treatment center designated by US "National Cancer Action" program in 1971, is also currently one of the 39 comprehensive cancer treatment center designated by Cancer Medical Association, Anderson Cancer Center is recognized as the world's best cancer hospital, and is ranked first in the United States in the field of cancer treatment and scientific research. The MD Anderson Cancer Center has more than 20,000 employees, including nearly 2,000 doctors, more than 500 beds, and more than 19,000 hospitalized patients in the United States and other countries each year, daily out-patient numbers is 1800 patients.

Since as the mentioned above, China's modern medicine is still far behind the United States, cancer treatment is more dependent on imported medicine; the self- invention and creation, patents, intellectual property rights are smaller.

Race with people, than what? Is it comparable? What's going to compare with?

Because the advantages of our country are:

1, Chinese medicine, anti-cancer Chinese medicine, immune regulation traditional Chinese medicine, anti-cancer Chinese medicine with increasing blood circulation and reducing stasis

2, Combination both Chinese and Western medicine, combination with innovation

The advantage of the United States is:

Modern medicine, advanced treatment technology, targeted drugs.

It should play our country's advantages, potential, and should increase efforts to develop, and to explore the advantages of Chinese herbal medicine.

Situation Analysis:

Western medicine: the United States>China

Chinese medicine: China > the United States

Surgery: the United States and China are the same (the United States can do the surgery, China can do and also has more cases)

Diagnostic technology equipment: The United States and China are the same (large hospitals have equipments)

Radiology therapy and chemotherapy: China and the United States are the same

Chinese medication: China >the United States [the majority can improve symptoms, improve physical fitness, prolong survival, increase immunity (lesions do not shrink, but can survive with tumors, live a long time), can be used as adjuvant therapy of surgery, can develop and dig.

Experimental research, innovation, patents, inventions, new drugs, targeted drugs: The United States>China

Second, analyze the current situation

1, the Current status: see today's status quo: (now is 20 years in the 21st century)

(1) the status of cancer incidence

The more treatment the more patients, China's new cases of cancer every year are for the 312 million cases, the average daily new cancer patients are 8550 cases, 6 people are diagnosed as cancer every minute in the country national.

(2) the status of cancer mortality:

Remains high and no decrease, and it has been the first cause of death in urban and rural areas in China, each year 2.7 million people are deaths due to cancer, an average of 7,500 people died of cancer every day.

(3) the status of treatment:

Although the application of the traditional three treatment for nearly a hundred years, tens of thousands of cancer patients bear radiotherapy and chemotherapy, but how are the results? So far the cancer is still the first cause of death, despite the postoperative formal, systemic radiotherapy and / or chemotherapy, or radiotherapy + chemotherapy, still failed to prevent cancer metastasis, recurrence, little effect.

(4) the status of the hospital model of the current tumor hospital or oncology department:

① go all out to focus on treatment, for the middle and late, poor efficacy, exhausted human and financial resources, and failed to achieve lower mortality, improve the cure rate, reduce morbidity.

② only cure and no prevention, or heavy treatment and light defense, the more the more patients.

③ ignored the "three early", ignoring the precancerous lesions.

④ many large-scale tumor hospital, university affiliated hospital oncology (or center) did not establish a laboratory, cannot carry out basic research or clinical basis of cancer research, because if there is no basic research breakthrough, the clinical efficacy is difficult to improve. "Oncology" is still the most backward in the current medical disciplines, why? Because the etiology, pathogenesis, pathophysiology of oncology have not yet clear, people on its pathogenesis, cancer cell metastasis mechanism is still lack of understanding of the complex biological behavior and cancer cells is still lack of sufficient understanding, and thus the current treatment program still is a considerable blindness, it is necessary to establish a laboratory for basic research and clinical basic research.

⑤ a century through the road is a focused treatment and light defense, or only cure. Prevention cancer, anti-cancer is the task of mankind, but over the years the cancer research is only on the cancer treatment, prevention cancer work is done very little, almost did not do.

2, how to do:

(1) To do cancer scientific research is an urgent need for current oncology disciplines.

    ① must understand the current problems of oncology
    ② must be aware of the problems of the current treatment

(2) how to reduce morbidity, improve the cure rate, reduce mortality

- **how to improve cancer cure rate, reduce mortality**

    ----**The out-way of cancer treatment is in the "three early"** (early detection, early diagnosis, early treatment), **early cancer treatment effect is good and cancer can be cured.**

Especially handling well in precancerous lesions can be cured. **1/3 of the cancer can be cured by early treatment.**

② **how to reduce the incidence of cancer**

- the way out of anti-cancer is in the prevention, 1/3 of the cancer can be prevented.

Third, the analysis of the next step of the study prospects

1, the analysis of we should play the advantages of our country in our advantage areas

However, our country also has our advantages, we should play the advantages of our country which our country already have advantages. In the field of cancer research, traditional Chinese medicine is the advantage of our country. To play this advantage in the field of cancer research, to explore, develop anti-cancer, anti-cancer Chinese herbal medicine, play this advantage of the study should be a strategic significance of international significance.

The combination of Chinese and Western medicine is Chinese medicine characteristics and advantages; the goal of the combination of Chinese and Western medicine should be combined innovation, the goals of combined with innovative should be to improve the treatment effect. The standard of efficacy of cancer patients should be: the patient survival time is long, good quality of life, fewer complications.

Combined Chinese and Western medicine comes from Chinese medicine, is higher than traditional Chinese medicine; it comes from Western medicine, higher than Western medicine, combined with the goal is to combine innovation, combined with innovative results should be innovative "Chinese medicine", innovation "Chinese anti-cancer".

At present, the world in addition to the study of synthetic drugs, but also the study of the region, the nation's herbs, scientists and return to nature to find anti-cancer drugs, the study of biological response regulator immunotherapy capacity. China in this field has many natural drugs, such as lentinan, ginseng polysaccharides, Ganoderma lucidum polysaccharides, Hericium polysaccharides and many other natural plant herbs which contain a variety of histones, polysaccharides, etc., have a better role in biological reaction regulator, and have immune regulation. All of them need to further be studied in experimental experiments with modern science and technology, strictly, scientifically, objectively, realistic and further study. And perform the traditional Chinese medicine immunopharmacology deep level, modern research.

Many of our Chinese herbal medicine are immune enhancer, biological response regulator, tonic, many can strengthen the body immune function and anti-cancer, and to try to improve the body immune is prevention cancer, anti-cancer important measures, how to improve immune function? Chinese herbal medicine is an extremely important advantage.

2, our research work of carrying out in 30 years:

(1) The new discovery of the anti-cancer and anti-cancer metastasis study

① **it was found from the results of follow-up**:

A, postoperative recurrence, metastasis is the key to long-term efficacy of surgery

B, suggesting that clinicians must pay attention to and study of postoperative recurrence, metastasis prevention and control measures

② **it was found from the experimental tumor study**

A, the experimental results suggest that: animal model can be made after the removal of thymus

B, the experimental results suggest that: the first low immunization, and then easy to occur the occurrence of cancer, development

C, the experimental results suggest that: metastasis is immune-related, and immune dysfunction may promote cancer metastasis

D, the experimental results suggest that: the host thymus immediately showed acute atrophy after inoculated cancer cells, cell proliferation was blocked, the volume was significantly reduced.

E, the experimental results suggest that some experimental mice are not vaccinated, or the tumor is very small, the thymus is not obvious atrophy, in order to study the relationship between tumor and thymus atrophy, cancer cells were inoculated in mice after the tumor grows to the thumb size and then removed them, after a month anatomical findings are that thymus is no longer atrophy.

F, the above experimental results show that: the progress of the tumor makes the thymus atrophy, then, we can use some ways to prevent the host thymus atrophy, so that the use of mice fetal liver, fetal spleen, fetal thymocyte transplantation to reconstruct immunization reconstruction The results showed that: S, T, L three groups of cells combined transplantation, the recent tumor complete regression rate was 40%, long-term tumor complete rate of regression was 46.6%, the group of complete regression of the tumor were long-term survival.

In short, from a series of experimental studies, it was found that thymus atrophy, immune dysfunction may be one of the causes and development of cancer.

③ XZ put forward to: "one of the cancer etiology, pathogenesis may be thymus atrophy and immune function" in the monograph and at the International Conference on Oncology. After investigation, it is the first time that it was reported in the international community.

④ XZ put forward to: "XZ-C immunomodulation therapy - the theory Basic and experimental basis of the principle of treatment" protect thymus and increase immune "(to protect the thymus, increase immune, protect marrow and produce blood (to protect bone blood stem cells)" in the monograph and at the International Conference on Oncology, which is the first time to be proposed in the international.

⑤ XZ proposed in the monograph: "the goals or targets of cancer treatment must be for both the tumor and the host, the establishment of a comprehensive treatment concept," the current domestic and foreign hospitals, chemotherapy is only to kill cancer cells, we think this is a one-sided treatment concept, not only did not protect the patient's immune system, but also a large number of killing the host immune cells and bone hematopoietic cells, resulting in the more chemotherapy the lower immune function; while chemotherapy is done, the metastasis is occurring.

⑥ XZ initiatives in the monograph: the establishment of a multi-disciplinary comprehensive treatment program

Whole course of treatment is as the main axis: to surgery-based + biological therapy, immunotherapy, integrated traditional Chinese and Western medicine treatment, XZ-C immunoregulation treatment … …

Short-term treatment for the auxiliary axis: to radiotherapy, chemotherapy-based, not a long course of treatment, cannot be excessive, and it should change the current treatment of over-treatment status quo in some hospitals.

⑥ XZ in t he book put forward the new concept of cancer anti-metastasis therapy, that: in the human body there are three manifestations of cancer: the first for the primary cancer; the second for the metastasis cancer cells; the third is the cells on the metastasis way

The annihilation, blocking or interference of the cancer cells on the metastasis way to cut off the new pathways of metastasis is the key to anti-cancer metastasis.

⑧ **It initially formed a theoretical system of XZ-C treatment cancer: immune regulation therapy.**

Laboratory animal ↘ 1.Resection of thymus can be made to produce animal model  found
experiments found ↗ 2.With the progress of cancer, thymus was progressive atrophy disease

Due to: thymus atrophy, immune dysfunction → put forward the theoretical basis of treatment: XZ-C immunoregulation "protect thymus and increase immune function" → exclusive development products: XZ-C1-10 → clinical validation: 20 years outpatient observation was followed up with advanced cancer patients more than 12,000 cases, can improve the quality of life, and extend the survival period.

(2) The research summary of XZ-C immunomodulation anti-cancer traditional Chinese medications

1. the experimental study of finding a new anti-cancer and the external anti-recurrence new drugs from the natural drug. The existing anti-cancer drugs kill both cancer cells and also the normal cells and have the adverse reactions. We searched the new drugs which only inhibit cancer cells without affecting the normal cells through the cancer-bearing mice in vivo tumor inhibition test from the natural drug.

    A, the use of cancer cells in vitro culture method, the screening experimental study of Chinese herbal medicine screening effect - in vitro screening test

    B, the manufacture of animal models, the experimental study of Chinese herbal medicine on the tumor in vivo tumor inhibition rate - in vivo tumor suppression screening test

    We spent a total of three years, the commonly used traditional anti-cancer prescription and reported anti-cancer prescription in the use of 200 kinds of Chinese herbal medicine, taste flavor of the tumor in vivo tumor inhibition test. A total of nearly 6,000 tumor-bearing animal models were obtained. After each mouse died, the anatomy of the liver, spleen, lung, thymus and kidney was performed. 48 kinds of them were screened out with having anti-tumor effect, meanwhile there are better immune regulation traditional Chinese medication.

2 clinical validation work

Through the above four years to explore the recurrence and metastasis of the basic experimental study, and after 3 years from the natural drug screening in the experimental study to find a group of XZ-C1-10 immune regulation of traditional Chinese medicine, and then through 30 years in more than 12,000 cases in the late or Postoperative metastatic cancer patients with clinical validation, the application of XZ-C immunomodulatory anti-cancer traditional Chinese medications have achieved good results and can improve the quality of life of patients, improve patient symptoms, significantly prolong the survival of patients.

(3) The experiment study and clinical observation of XZ-C immunoregulation anti-cancer traditional Chinese medicine in the treatment of malignant tumors

1. XZ-C immunoregulation anti-cancer traditional Chinese medication is the result of the modernization of traditional Chinese medication
2   XZ-C immunoregulation anti-cancer Chinese medication treatment of cancer cases and typical cases

(4) to study the traditional Chinese medication anti-cancer effect must carry out modern scientific research, analyze active ingredients, and purify and do modern immunopharmacology experiments and research.

Although we should play the advantages of our country with our country has the dvantage in our country, in the field of cancer research, Chinese drugs and Chinese medicine, the combination of Chinese and Western medicine is the advantage of our country, play this advantage in the field of cancer research, it should conduct scientific research, and conduct experimental research, active ingredient analysis, purification and modern pharmacological experiments to study the traditional Chinese medicine anti-cancer effect and its mechanism, we must study the active ingredients so as to Chinese medicine to become modern and scientific.

But it must be aware of the strengths of traditional Chinese medicine, what weaknesses are, and whether there is no toxicity or not, the application should be considered for the patient's "long", "short", "get", "lost", it must conduct modern scientific research, it should be scientific research, analysis, clinical validation, should be scientific, authenticity, safety, doctors in scientific research, clinical application must be both ability and political integrity, medical is benevolence, legislation and morals for the first.

(5) Analysis of the next step of the study prospects and the prospective assessment of cancer treatment:

- Molecular targeted drug therapy is eye-catching
- Immunomodulatory drugs are promising
- Immunotherapy opens a new era of cancer therapy
- Application of vaccine to cancer is a human hope
- The way out of cancer treatment is three early
- The way out of cancer is preventing

3, the initial work that we have been in the fight against cancer:

(1) Xu Ze published in October 2011, "the new concept of cancer treatment and new methods" monograph of Chapter 38 with a chapter of the length of "to overcome the strategic thinking and suggestions of cancer"

(2) In June 2013 Xu Ze also proposed "to overcome the cancer to start the general idea and design", in an attempt to reduce the incidence of cancer, reduce cancer mortality, improve the cure rate, prolong survival, the total attack is anti- Cancer, three carriages go hand in hand

(3) Xu Ze put forward in August 2013 for the first time in the international community that: "the XZ-C research program to overcome the cancer and

to launch a total attack" - the overall strategy and development of cancer treatment in China

(4) in July 2015 Xu Ze proposed the feasibility report from the following four aspects to attack the cancer and launch a total attack

"XZ-C proposed the research program to attack the cancer and launch a total offensive" - China's cancer treatment of the overall strategic reform and development

1. in the international it is the first time proposed:
   "the feasibility the need of the report to capture the total attack of cancer"

2. in the international community for the first time it was put forward:
   "To build the hospital with the prevention and the treatment of cancer during the development and occurrence of cancer of the whole process"

   (the Global Demonstration Prevention and Treatment Hospital)

   "the hospital vision and feasibility report of building anti-cancer and treatment of cancer throughout the prevention and treatment"

   - Describe the necessity and feasibility of establishing a complete prevention and cure hospital

3. in the international it was the first time proposed:
   "the basic vision and feasibility report To build the general idea of conquering cancer and the science city"

   - is equivalent to the framework of the design of conquering cancer with China characteristic.

4. in the international it was the first time proposed:
   "the necessity and feasibility report of building a moderately society at the same time, it was proposed" ride research "- perform ing the medicine

research and cancer prevention and cancer control and cancer prevention and treatment" ---- adhere to walk on the new way with the Chinese characteristics of anti-cancer and control cancer.

These four research projects in the international community were put forward for the first time and opened up a new field of anti-cancer research.

To propose to capture the total attack of cancer is unprecedented work.

(5) Xu Ze's fourth monograph book ": "On Innovation Of Treatment Of Cancer" - (Cancer Treatment Innovation Theory) was published in Washington, DC in December 2015, in English, published worldwide, and also released electronic version to Introduce the new book.

Introduction to the new book: the experimental study of Chinese medicine immunopharmacology of traditional Chinese and Western medicine combined with anti-cancer research at the molecular level has formed XZ-C immune regulation of the theoretical system of cancer.

Walking out the new path of an immune regulation with traditional Chinese medications which regulate immune activity, prevent thymus atrophy, promote thymic hyperplasia, protect bone hematopoietic function, improve immune surveillance at the molecular level of the combination of western and Chinese medications to overcome cancer.

How to overcome the cancer I see:

- To avoid empty talking, to focus on hard work, no matter how far away it is from the cancer, it should always start.
- To attack cancer should start to launch the total attack, what is the total attack against cancer?

The total attack is to conduct work and to develop in full swing simultaneously for three stages of cancer prevention, cancer control and cancer treatment during the whole process of the occurrence and development of cancer,.

That is:

To prevent cancer - before the formation of cancer

To control cancer - malignant transformation of precancerous lesions

To treat cancer - has formed a lesion or metastasis

The main target of launching the cancer attack: to reduce cancer lesions, reduce cancer mortality, improve the cure rate, prolong survival, improve quality of life, reduce complications.

- What should I do next? Now it is proposed to overcome cancer and to launch a total attack. It is hoped to get leadership support at all levels. I know that to achieve the purpose of cancer prevention, cancer control and treatment of cancer must be government leadership, government-led, experts, scholars efforts, the masses to participate in the mobilization of all, thousands of households to participate in order to do.

- Because cancer patients are getting more and more, the morbidity is on the rise, the mortality rate is high, it is recognized that in order to stop at the cancer source it should not only pay attention to treatment, but also pay attention to prevention; the research goal and focus should be on the study of prevention and treatment of cancer during the whole process of the occurrence and development of cancer.

Fourth, the "dawn of the C-type plan": the scientific and technological innovation, the outline to achieve, to avoid empty talk, to focus on hard work and to start

1, The combination of Chinese and Western medications

Comprehensive (Chinese and Western) anti - cancer strength

From Chinese medicine - higher than traditional Chinese medicine

From Western medicine - higher than Western medicine

Comprehensive Chinese and Western anti - cancer advantage strength - combined with innovation, innovation "Chinese medicine", innovation "Chinese - style anti - cancer"

(See another article)

13, the situation analysis (b)

Condense wisdom and move forward together; why is chinese herbal medication the advantage of our country in the study of cancer?

(1) Racing with the "new moon program (Cancer moon shot)", <u>why is not it led by our country, some of our famous university affiliated hospital oncology, cancer center or provincial tumor hospital? They have excellent equipment conditions and superb medical technology, but will it be led by the University of Traditional Chinese Medicine?</u>

Because the status of modern medications of the current China and the province of institutions of higher learning Affiliated Hospital of Oncology and Cancer Center is that:

- Life sciences, molecular biology, genetic engineering and proteomics groups all studied and were trained from the United States; we ourselves do not have innovative patents and inventions;
- Targeted therapeutic drugs and monoclonal antibodies are imported from the United States; we ourselves do not have innovative patents and inventions;

- cancer treatment equipment and precision instruments are imported from the United States and study and train from the United States ; we have almost no innovation patent and invention;

- new surgery or innovation of new surgical techniques studied and learned from the United States; we don't have our own patents and invention;

- Minimally invasive technology and minimally invasive equipment are imported from the United States and studied and learned from the United States; we do not have innovative patents and inventions.

In short, the modern medicine were from Europe and the United States, nearly a hundred years of modern American medicine developed and advanced it has developed to precision cancer medicine. **China's oncology lacks my own ontology innovation medicine, medication, technology, innovation academic, theory, innovation patent and invention.**

It must be self-reliant, independent innovation, the original innovation, to achieve breakthrough scientific and technological achievements, have our own medicine, medication and the scientific and technological achievements.

Innovation is not only technology, product innovation, but also basic theoretical innovation; the theoretical innovation is the biggest achievement. Scientific development is based on the basic theory of innovation, this is the largest invention and creation.

(2) Why is it led by the University of Traditional Chinese Medicine?

Because:

(1) We should develop the advantages of our country in the field of which our country have the advantage. In the field of cancer research, traditional Chinese medication is the advantage of our country, we should play this advantage in cancer research to explore the development of anti- Chinese herbal medication.

It should be carried out in-depth study, and have the active ingredient analysis, purification; perform for traditional Chinese medicine immunopharmacology research; do molecular level, gene level research, so that Chinese herbal medicine becomes the modernization and merges with the international standards.

(2) The combination of Chinese and Western medication is Chinese medicine characteristics and advantages: it comes from Chinese medicine, higher than traditional Chinese medicine, which comes from Western medicine, higher than Western medicine, is a combination of traditional Chinese medicine + Western medicine. 1 + 1 = 2, 2> 1, so that the cancer treatment after the combination of Chinese and Western is more perfect, reasonable, improve the efficacy. Because the traditional cancer therapy (surgery, radiotherapy, chemotherapy) are to reduce the immune function of the body, and immune regulation an ti-cancer traditional Chinese medicine is to increase the body immune function, and become a comprehensive treatment, postoperative immunization, radiotherapy + traditional Chinese medicine immunization (immunotherapy), Chemotherapy + traditional Chinese medicine immunization (immunotherapy), the effect is bound to improve.

1. Why in cancer research Chinese herbal medication is the advantage of our country?

Because the treatment must be aiming for the cause, pathogenesis, pathophysiology.

It should find the treatment methods and medications from the following multidisciplinary and cancer relationship:

A, Cancer and immune have a positive relationship so that it should be looking for immunomodulatory drugs;

B, some cancer have a positive relationship with the virus so that it should find antiviral drugs;

C, some cancer has a positive relationship with endocrine hormones so that it should be looking for drugs to control endocrine hormones;

D, some cancer has a relationship with fungi so that it should find anti-fungal drugs;

E, some cancer has a relationship with chronic inflammation so that it should be looking for anti-chronic inflammation drug.

These immune regulation, adjustment of endocrine hormones, anti-virus ... ... and other drugs are very rare and small in modern western medication; however China Fuzheng and firming solid, tonic Chinese herbal medications have the rich resources, and have good treatment results for immune regulation, hormone adjustment, anti-virus, and also have a long history and clinical experience and work; in recent years there are some researchers and graduate students who carried out the experimental analysis and research of some of the molecular level of Chinese herbal medication; the contents are rich. It should be said that in the study of cancer the rich resources of Chinese herbal medications are an advantage.

2   why in the field of cancer research Chinese herbal medications are the advantage of our country? We have the following experimental basis and the data and information accumulation from our clinical validation

Because our laboratory selected 48 taste from the 200 Chinese herbal medications which are indeed the traditional Chinese medications with the good anti-tumor rate.

The existing anti-cancer drugs kill both cancer cells and also the normal cells, and the adverse reactions are severe. Through the cancer-bearing mice in vivo tumor inhibition experiments, it was found the new drugs of only inhibition of the cancer cells without affecting the normal cells . We spent a total of three years to screen the commonly used traditional anti-cancer prescription and reported anti-cancer prescription used in 200 kinds of Chinese herbal medications for the tumor treatment in vivo tumor inhibition test. The 48 kinds with the good anti - tumor effects were screened out.

<u>The new drug research of searching and screening anti-cancer and anti-metastasis from Chinese herbal medications:</u>

The purpose is to screen out the intelligent anti-cancer drugs with no drug-resistant, non-toxic side effects, high selectivity, long-term oral anti-cancer and anti-metastasis and anti-recurrence.

To this end, we conducted the new drugs experimental study which was a full three years in the laboratory to screen anti-cancer and anti-metastasis:

A. The experimental study of the Chinese herbal medication inhibition rate was done in vitro with cancer cells culture method.

B. The experimental study of the cancer-bearing animal model was made and the Chinese herbal medication inhibition rate was done in vivo in the cancer-bearing animal model.

The experimental results:

In our laboratory 48 kinds of certain or even excellent inhibition of cancer cell proliferation were screened out from 200 kinds of Chinese herbal medications in the animal experiments and the tumor inhibition rate are 75-90% or more. But there are some of the traditional Chinese medications which are commonly used for the cancer treatment, after the experiments of the tumor inhibition rate in the animal in vitro and in vivo, they do not have anti-cancer effect; 152 kinds of no obvious anti-cancer effect were gotten rid of in these groups by the animal experiments.

48 Chinese medications with good tumor inhibition rate in the animal experiment was carried out to identify, and then optimized and combined, repeated the tumor inhibition test in vivo in the cancer-bearing animals, and finally developed the immune regulation anti-cancer traditional Chinese medications XU ZE China preparation (XZ -C$_{1-10}$).

XZ-C$_1$ can significantly inhibit the cancer cells, but does not affect the normal cells; XZ-C$_4$ can promote thymic hyperplasia and increase immune function; XZ-C$_8$ can protect the marrow to protect bone marrow hematopoietic function.

3 why is Chinese herbal medication the advantage of our country in cancer research,?

Because immune regulation traditional Chinese medications which can promote thymic hyperplasia, prevent thymus atrophy, improve immune were found from chinese herbal medications in our laboratory.

We conducted a full four-year experimental study in the laboratory. It was found from our laboratory experimental results that: the thymus has progressive atrophy, its volume reduces, the cell proliferation is blocked, the mature cells decreases. The thymus is extremely atrophic and the texture becomes harder in the late stage of the tumor,.

From the above experimental study it was found that: thymic atrophy and immune dysfunction may be one of the pathogenesis and pathogenesis of the tumor, it must try to prevent thymus atrophy, promote thymocyte proliferation, increased immune function. It should be explored at the molecular level from the body's immune function, especially cellular immune, T lymphocyte function and thymus immune regulation function and it should seek immunoregulation methods and effective drug research.

Where should the new ways of immunoregulatory treatment be found?

In order to prevent thymic atrophy, promote thymocyte hyperplasia, increased immune function, we searched from both the traditional Chinese medication and Western medication. Western medication which can improve the immune function and promote thymus hyperplasia is rarely so we changed from the Chinese herbal medication to find.

Why was the medications of promoting thymus hyperplasia, preventing thymus atrophy and enhancing immune functions searched from the Chinese medications?

Because the traditional Chinese medication tonic drugs generally contain the role of immune regulation. Chinese medication has tonic medications and polysaccharide Chinese medications.

A, tonic medications have the role of regulating the immune function. When the animal is in a low level of immune activity (such as the animals with removal of thymus, the aging animals, or chemotherapy drugs cyclophosphamide inhibition and the tumor animals), the tonic drugs can more significantly improve the body immune function.

B, anti-cancer immunization research of Chinese medication polysaccharide progresses quickly and a large number of immunopharmacological studies have been carried out at the molecular level and polysaccharides can improve the body immune surveillance system, include natural killer cells

(NK), macrophages (MΦ), killer T cells (CTL), T cells, LAK cells, tumor infiltrating lymphocytes (TIL), interleukins (IL) and other cytokines to achieve the purpose of killing tumor cells.

Both Chinese medication and Western medication have their own strengths, each has advantages and disadvantages, and it should take long and complement each other. Comparing Chinese medication immunopharmacology with western medication, each has its own characteristics and advantages, but also has its own shortcomings, and the advantages of traditional Chinese medication immunology are: a large number of Fuzheng Chinese medication(righting) has a role in regulating the immune function of the body. Traditional Chinese medication sources are rich, are effective good medications in the long-term clinical treatment, after extraction it can get the effective ingredients and significant pharmacological effects (including immunomodulatory effects), the study process is save labor and save time and high efficiency.

3, Why does our Hubei University of Traditional Chinese Medicine Experimental Institute propose the racing?

(1) In the past 28 years we have made cancer research achievements and scientific and technological innovation series:

It can participate in the games, participate in learning, motivate us to move forward

The goal of the competition is:

① **to extend the survival time of cancer patients (live long), good quality of life, fewer complications.**

② **reduce the incidence of cancer, improve the cure rate, and reduce mortality.**

(2) Since 28 years we have made cancer research achievements and scientific and technological innovation series:

A, The new discoveries of the experimental study and the new theories and new concepts which was put forward

A), "thymus atrophy and immune dysfunction are one of the pathogenesis and the cause of cancer"

---- put forward the new concept of cancer treatment principles

B), "the theoretical basis and experimental basis of protection of thymus and increase immune function of XZ-C immunomodulation therapy"

---- put forward the theoretical basis and experimental basis of immunoregulation therapy for cancer

B, It was put forward new concept and new initiatives of cancer treatment

A), "cancer treatment should change the concept and establish a comprehensive treatment concept"

- put forward the new concept of cancer treatment principles

B), "a new model of cancer multidisciplinary comprehensive treatment"

- Proposing the initiative: a new concept of cancer treatment combination model

C, cancer metastasis research and theoretical innovation

A), "in the human body there are three main forms of existence of cancer cells"

Advice on the theory of cancer metastasis therapy

B), "the whole process of cancer development," two points and one line"

Advice on the theory of cancer metastasis therapy

C), "three steps of anti-cancer treatment"

----Advice the theory innovation of cancer metastasis therapy

----- The "eight steps" of the transfer of cancer cells are summarized as "three stages" and trying to break each

D), "Open up the third field of anti-cancer metastasis therapy"

- put forward the theoretical innovation of cancer metastasis therapy, found and put forward the third field of human anti-cancer metastasis therapy

- Circulation system has a large number of immune surveillance cells and the "main battlefield" of annihilating cancer cells in the matastasis way is in the blood circulation

D, the exclusive scientific research and developed products: XZ-C immunosuppressive anti-cancer traditional Chinese medication product series

A), "the research overview of XZ-C immunomodulatory anti-cancer traditional Chinese medication"

--------In vitro culture of cancer cells, the screening experimental study of Chinese herbal medicine on the inhibition rate was conducted

------Set up the cancer-bearing animal model and conduct the experimental study of the Effect of Chinese Herbal Medication on Cancer inhibition rates in vivo in the cancer-bearing animals

B), "the experimental study and clinical efficacy observation of XZ-C immunoregulation anti-cancer traditional Chinese medication treatment of malignant tumors"

----Animal Experiment study and Clinical Application

---- XZ-C immune regulation of traditional Chinese medication is the results and the achievement of the traditional Chinese medicine modernization

C), "the cancer cases and some typical cases of XZ-C immunoregulation anti-cancer traditional Chinese medication treatment"

E, it was put forward cancer treatment reform and innovation

A), "cancer treatment reform and innovation research"

------Adhere to the road of scientific research and innovation of anti - cancer metastasis with Chinese characteristics

------ Cancer treatment reform and innovation research 1---8

B), "Walk out of a new way to overcome cancer"

- has been initially formed the theoretical system of XZ-C immune regulation, is experiencing clinical application and observation and verification

- has been an exclusive research and development products, XZ-C immunoregulation anti-cancer traditional Chinese medicine series, has a large number of clinical validation cases

- it has been initially walked out of a new way to overcome cancer in the past 20 years.

Now it is the fourth stage of our research work and is being carried out and proceeded; the research work is step by step and gradually deepening and the goal or the target of the study setting up is to reduce the incidence of cancer, improve the cure rate, prolong survival.

The current tumor hospital or oncology mode goes all out to focus on treatment and aims for the patients with the middle or advanced disease stages and the treatment effect is poor, and it exhausted human and financial resources, and failed to achieve lower morbidity, and the more treatment the more patients. The status quo is: the road which walked through in a century is focusing on treatment and ignoring prevention, or only treatment. Over the years we have just been working on cancer treatment . But in cancer prevention the work was done very little, almost did not do; therefore, the incidence of cancer continues to rise.

In short, cancer prevention is not attached importance and prevention is not paid attention to . Cliché prevention of the main, not to be concerned about and not taken seriously and not implemented .

How to do? How to reduce the incidence of cancer? How to improve cancer cure rate? How to reduce cancer mortality? How to extend my life? How to improve the quality of life?

It should launch to conquer cancer and launch the total attack and both of the cancer prevention and treatment are at the same attention.

The goal of conquering cancer should be: to reduce morbidity, improve the cure rate, reduce mortality, prolong survival, improve quality of life, reduce complications.

<u>The current global hospitals, hospitals in China are going all out to engage in treatment, heavy treatment with light defense, or only treatment .</u>

XZ-C that this hospital model or cancer treatment model, can not overcome the cancer, can not reduce the incidence. Global hospitals and our hospital must be on the overall strategy of changing from focusing on cancer treatment to focusing on prevention and treatment.

Therefore, we propose to launch the general idea and design of conquering cancer, XZ-C (Xu Ze-China) proposed to launch the general attack, that is, to start the comprehensive work if the three stages of the prevention cancer and cancer control and treatment cancer in full swing simultaneously.

Put forward the application of the "the necessity and feasibility report of the general attack on cancer"

Proposed the application report of "the XZ-C research program to conquer cancer and to launch a total attack"

In short, as mentioned above, China's modern medication in cancer treatment is more dependent on imported medication, and the self-invention and creation, patents, intellectual property rights is rarer and smaller.

<u>So how do you race? With what is it going to the game?</u>

As mentioned above, <u>in the field of cancer treatment, Chinese herbal medication is the advantage of our country</u>, 28 years in our experimental surgery Institute of experimental research and cancer specialist outpatient and 20 years a large number of cases of clinical validation, it was confirmed that in the treatment of cancer, Chinese herbal medicine is China advantage, can be to the international so that patients get benefit. Many cancer patients have significantly prolonged their survival time.

Therefore, the advantages of our country are:

1, Chinese medication, anti-cancer Chinese medication, immune regulation traditional Chinese medication, anti-cancer thrombosis of traditional Chinese medication with activating blood and removing stasis

2, Chinese and Western medicine combined with combining innovation 1 + 1 = 2, 2> 1

The advantage of the United States is: modern medicine, advanced treatment technology, targeted drugs

It should play the advantages of our country, should increase efforts to develop and explore the advantages of Chinese herbal medication

So I think: it should contest and should race

About Chinese medicine and Western medication, each has its own strengths, each has shortage, the two should be complementary advantages and combining the advantages ; one is running inner ring,and one is running outer ring; one mainly attack and kill cancer cells, and one mainly boost immune function and immune regulation, move forward together toward, and go to the science hall of overcoming cancer.

Racing with "new moon program" is not to challenge or fight, but to encourage themselves to achieve the "dawn of the C-type plan", move forward together toward the scientific hall of conquering cancer.

14, the situation analysis (c)

How to overcome cancer? Can you rely on traditional therapies (surgery, radiotherapy, chemotherapy) to overcome cancer?

In order to conquer cancer, where is the road? where to go? How to go?

The existing road, to analyze it; the prospects of how? How is the future?

1. the analysis of the situation of the occurrence and the development of cance for a century?

I am a medical practitioner who has been working for 60 years and has seen the situation in Wuhan for 65 years. It is deeply felt that the incidence of cancer is on the rise.

In 1951, Zhongnan Tongji Medical College was moved from Shanghai to Wuhan. At that time for the teaching, in order to find a lung cancer patients to show the students internship, even if a week earlier to call the hospitals, but also it was difficult to find. At that time all hospitals had no cancer section, only tuberculosis. Today (65 years later) cancer was common disease, frequently disease, all hospitals have oncology, and some large hospitals have cancer center, the more treatment the more patients.

It should be analyzed, why?

It should be analyzed, how to do? Where is the way out?

So I deeply appreciate that cancer should not only pay attention to treatment, but also to pay attention to prevention in order to stop at the source. The out-way of cancer treatment was in the "three early" (early detection, early diagnosis, carly treatment),and the out of the way of the anti-cancer was in the prevention.

It should be analyzed, how does Wuhan do? How can we reduce morbidity? how can the cure rate be improved?

How can it become "three early"? it should establish a full prevention+ control+treatment hospital and change the hospital model and change the treatment model.

How can we prevent? it should build science city to overcome cancer.

We will be in Wuhan, and in Wuhanthe the first "the scientce city of conquering" and the world's first "the science city of conquering cancer" was established.

2. the analysis of how the prospects of the current three traditional treatment is? How is the future?

Can three treatment methods be relied on to conquer cancer and even overcome cancer?

Cancer traditional therapy (surgery, chemotherapy, radiotherapy) have been for nearly a century, and the experience of success and failure of the lessons should be reviewed, reflected, summed up .

The traditional concept thinks about that cancer is the continuous division of cancer cells, proliferation, and the treatment target must be to kill cancer cells.

After half a century, how is the treatment result? The more treatment

and the more patients. Therefore, the above three treatment methods must be further studied and improved, andthe problems and drawbacks of the surgery, radiotherapy, chemotherapy should be analyzed and commented on.

A. One assessment of chemotherapy:

The problems and disadvantages of systemic intravenous chemotherapy

The current status of tumor chemotherapy was mainly systemic intravenous chemotherapy, and this systemic intravenous chemotherapy route of administration is:

Chemotherapy Cell toxic drugs → Elbow Vein →Upper Venous Vein → Right Heart → Left Heart →Aorta

↓

Spray to the whole body

↓

Cancer lesions get about 0.4% of the doses of the medications

the normal tumor-free organs and tissues (brain, heart, liver, lung, kidney, bone marrow … …) of the body recieved about 99.6% of the dose

However, this solid tumor intravenous chemotherapy route, although the world, China has been used for decades, we should think about it and analyze whether it is reasonable? Is it science? Does it damage the patient? Does it cause toxic side effects?

It should be analyzed and commented:

Comment 1: Comment on the route of administration of systemic intravenous chemotherapy

This route of administration was not fixed-point targeted administration, but through the heart pump to the chemotherapy cell poison with the blood spray to the body so that cytotoxic has the whole systemic distribution and so that the normal organs (brain, Lung, kidney, bone marrow) of the body obtain chemotherapy cytotoxic and are damaged, leading to toxic side effects. It is very unreasonable, very unscientific, the result is:

① very few foci cancer can get the medications, only about 0.4%, minimal effect (due to cancer foci accounted for a very small proportion of the body surface area)

② **99.6% of the cytotoxic drugs kill the normal body of normal cells causing toxicity of the brain, heart, liver, lung, kidney, bone marrow, gastrointestinal system, hematopoietic system, immune system, endocrine system .**

③ the current hospital chemotherapy drugs did not have the drug sensitivity test. If the drug is resistant, then the whole chemotherapy is to kill the normal tissue cells! especially to the inhibition of bone marrow hematopoietic cells and immune cells! On the foci it is no effect! (it is in vain of that is done once a chemotherapy!)

④ so does every chemotherapy kill cancer cells? It does not know how much to kill? It does not know and it can only be said to have once chemical work.

Therefore, this route of administration is unreasonable and unscientific and easily lead to iatrogenic side effects.

How to do? It should change the route of administration, to target organ tissue chemotherapy within the pathways, the drug directly to the "target organ", so the dose is very small, the effect is certain, no side effects, is conducive to the patient.

Comment 2: the dose calculation of the assessment of solid body tumor intravenous chemotherapy

This is the experience and methods of leukemia treatment extended to the solid tumor treatment and the guiding ideology is the whole body surface area of administration. It is unwise and unreasonable.

Why?

Because leukemia cells are distributed in the systemic blood circulation system, the treatment of the "target" also exists in the systemic blood circulation system, so the use of systemic intravenous chemotherapy is reasonable, wise, but also in line with targeted therapy.

However, solid tumors are confined to an organ whose target "target" should be an organ suffering from cancer and should be targeted at the target organ's intravascular route. It should not use the leukemia treatment experience of the body surface area calculated medication, it is unwise, unreasonable.

But now solid tumors are all having systemic intravenous chemotherapy, according to the body surface area to calculate dose, in order to achieve the purpose of cancer shrinkage, the inevitable need is to increase the amount of chemotherapy cells poisoning, it will lead to more toxic side effects and complications, damage the patient.

How to do?

It should change the route of administration and change into target organ intravascular chemotherapy; this dose is very small, the effect is certain, no side effects, and is conducive to patients.

Comments 3: the analysis and evaluation of the evaluation criteria of curative effect of systemic intravenous chemotherapy

① why the evaluation of the standard as a mitigation?

At present, the clinical use of chemotherapy drugs can shrink the tumor, but the effect is usually temporary, and can not significantly extend the patient's life. Therefore, the efficacy evaluation criteria are called "mitigation". Generally with days, weeks or months to calculate, such as complete remission which is completely disappeared tumor only sustains more than 4 weeks, that is, 4 weeks later it may recur and progress.

Mitigation is only temporary effect and can not be cured.

② **Why can it be only alleviated?**

a, the effective time to kill cancer cells of the patients with chemotherapy to kill is only 3-5 days of the intravenous infusion which have the role of killing cancer cells, and then no cancer cells to play the role, **it is only a short time**

to kill about (3-5 Day), can not once and for all, after 3-5 days the cancer cells continue to split and go on proliferation, so it can only alleviate a short time, can not be cured.

b, chemotherapy cell poison can only kill the differentiated mature cancer cells, can not kill yet undifferentiated unmatured stem cells; this time the chemotherapy kills the differentiate mature cancer cells and after some time, those who have not yet matured stem cells gradually mature,and continue to division, proliferation, and divide into two, two for the four clones, in this way it is the geometric progression so that the foci is "wild fire burned, spring breeze and health", goes on the recurrence, metastasis and progresses.

Therefore, chemotherapy can not be cured, can only alleviate. It can only palliative, can not cure, it can not rely on chemotherapy to overcome cancer.

Comment 4: Comment on why the adjuvant chemotherapy after the abdominal solid tumor surgery failed to prevent recurrence, metastasis?

Why does the adjuvant chemotherapy fail to prevent recurrence and metastasis after the surgery of abdominal solid tumor? It is because the whole body intravenous chemotherapy cytotoxic medications are injected from the superior vena cava instead of the portal vein, is difficult to reach the portal vein; the vena cava system and portal vein system are generally not connected, this route of administration is unreasonable and unscientific.

Where are the cancer cells in the abdominal solid tumor (gastric cancer, colorectal cancer, liver cancer, biliary cancer, pancreatic cancer, abdominal and other malignant tumors? It is mainly in the portal vein system, but in the current global and all of the hospital in China the abdominal solid tumor postoperative adjuvant chemotherapy is given by the elbow vein →superior vena cava → right heart → lungs → left heart→ aorta → spray to the body organs. But it can not directly go into the portal vein system because the vena cava system and the portal vein system are generally not connected.

Therefore, in the abdominal malignant tumors (stomach, intestine, liver, gallbladder, pancreas, abdominal and other cancers), after the abdominal surgery the vein route of administration of the adjuvant chemotherapy injected by the elbow vein →venous is unreasonable, is unscientific, does not meet the anatomy and physiological pathology, and does not meet the reality of cancer cell metastasis pathways, because this route of administration can not directly into the presence of cancer cells in the portal vein system.

For half a century, the thousands of cancer patients in all of the world and in China are suffering from the great pain of chemotherapy cells poisoning killing the normal cells of great pain. Clinicians should seriously think, analyze, reflect and evaluate.

How to do?

It should change the route of administration into the pathway of which chemotherapy medication is given inside the target organ vessels so that drugs can directly go into the portal vein, for the solid tumor medication should not be administered by the elbow vein, but should be changed to target organ intravascular administration, the drug targets reaching the target organ foci, which will greatly reduce the dose, improve the efficacy, will certainly reduce or eliminate the toxic side effects of chemotherapy, so that tens of thousands of cancer patients can avoid suffering from the pain and risk of the adverse reactions of chemotherapy and it is for the benefit of patients. To reduce or eliminate the toxic side effects of chemotherapy is bound to greatly reduce the medical costs and will be for the country, for patients to save more medical expenses and help solving the problem of that it is difficult to get medical treatment and the medical cost is expensive, this reform will be tens of thousands of cancer patient benefit.

Comment 5: There are some important errors and drawbacks in current chemotherapy

a, chemotherapy has the inhibition of immune function, inhibition of bone marrow hematopoietic function so that the overall immune function decreased.

Cancer thymus is inhibited, and chemotherapy inhibit bone marrow, as "worse", or "snow on plus frost" so that the entire central immune organs is damaged, and promote further decline in immune surveillance, may lead to cancer metastasis while chemotherapy is used; the more chemotherapy the more metastasis .

b, chemotherapy target is to kill cancer cells, is a one-sided treatment, ignoring the body's own anti-tumor ability, ignoring the host anti-cancer system anti-cancer cell system (NK cells, K cells, macrophages, LAK cells), anti-cancer cells Factor gene (IFN, IL2, TNF, LT and other factors), anti-cancer gene system (Rb gene, P53 gene), ignoring the body's anti-cancer mechanism and its influencing factors, ignoring the body's own anti-cancer internal factors with not activated and mobilized, but only blindly kill cancer cells, this one-sided treatment view is very unreasonable, it does not meet the biological characteristics of cancer cells and biological behavior.

B. Two reviews of radiotherapy:

Comments 1: radiation therapy is killing cancer cells at the same time, but also killing a large number of normal tissue cells so that patients are suffering from the torture of the radiation therapy complications, the quality of life decreased, the radiotherapy and toxic effects and damage are generally persistent and irreversible, and therefore it must pay attention to the prevention of the complications of tumor radiotherapy.

Comment 2: The main problem with cancer treatment is how to prevent metastasis, if this problem is not solved, the problem of cancer metastasis and cancer treatment can not be advanced.

Radiotherapy is for topical treatment and cancer metastasis is for systemic problems which is a major contradiction; how to play its role in anti-metastatic therapy must be carefully considered and studied in depth.

C. Three reviews of surgical treatment:

Comments 1: Surgery is the effective treatment of malignant tumors, even if the cancer treatment has developed the multidisciplinary treatment today, surgery is still one of the most important and the most common means the treatment of malignant tumors and is an important part of a multi-disciplinary comprehensive treatment.

Comment 2: Surgical treatment is the main treatment of solid tumors, but the "radical surgery" design ineeds to be further studied and improved to reduce postoperative recurrence and metastasis. It should pay attention to intraoperative "tumor suppression technology" to reduce or prevent intraoperative cancer cell shedding, planting, transfer. It should pay attention to surgical operation light, stable, accurate, to reduce intraoperative promotion of cancer cell metastasis and reduce cancer cells spread from the tumor vein. To prevent postoperative recurrence and metastasis must start from surgery. It must pay attention to the non-tumor technology and to prevent the transplant and implant metastasis in the incision and drainage sites.

Comments 3: after a century of historical evaluation the solid tumor surgery is still the most important and the most reliable and it is the main treatment method which can rely on and is the main science and technology and the main treatment method for conquering cancer in the future.

In short:

As mentioned above, the radiotherapy and chemotherapy exist the above problems and disadvantages, it is difficult to rely on overcoming cancer, and it must be another way and must find a new way to overcome cancer.

To recognize radiotherapy and chemotherapy problems and disadvantages, it is difficult to rely on conquering cancer. We must open another way and it is put forward: to overcome the cancer and launch a total attack, to build a science city to overcome cancer.

3. To analyze the prospect of the next step and the evelution of the prospective assessment of cancer treatment

-- Molecular targeted drugs attract attention
-- immune control drug prospects gratifying
--Immunotherapy opens a new era of tumor therapy

--Bioavailability and Combination of Chinese and Western Medication are two effective ways of anticancer metastasis
- Application of vaccine treatment is human hope
- the way out of cancer treatment is in the "three early"
- the way out of anti-cancer is in the prevention

1), the molecular targeted drug therapy is eye-catching

The Philadelphia chromosome opens the door to targeted therapy. In 1960, Philadelphia researchers found that there was a chromosomal abnormality in patients with chronic myeloid leukemia (CML). A few years later, the researchers found that this was the result of chromosome 9 and 22 chromosome long arm translocation. Since this chromosomal abnormality was first discovered in Phiadelphia, it was named Philadelphia (Ph) chromosome. The chromosome has also become the target of CML targeted therapy for 40 years. In 2001 the first confirmed to be against Philadelphia chromosome molecular defects - imatinib.

It is followed by human epidermal growth factor receptor 2 (HER2) as the target targeting drug trastuzumab, the treatment of HER2-positive breast cancer.

Tbevacizumab is targeted VEGF as the target and cetuximab is EGFR as the target fo the treatment of colorectal cancer.

Metabiib and erlotinib is for EGFR as a target for non-small cell lung cancer treatment.

Molecular targeted drugs are cell stabilizers, and most patients do not achieve complete remission (CR) or partial remission (PR), but are stable and improves the quality of life. In addition to gefitinib, erlotinib, imatinib, most of them need to be used in combination with chemotherapy drugs.

Molecular targeted drugs represent a new class of anti-cancer drugs, and imatinib (Gleevec) is a typical **example of the control of cancer by inhibiting the abnormal molecules that cause cancer, without damaging other normal nuclei.** There has been an increasing number of molecular targeting drugs used in cancer treatment such as Rituximab for the treatment of B-cell lymphoma; trastuzumab for the treatment of breast and Gifitinib and Erlotinib for the treatment of lung cancer. Targeted therapy brings anti-tumor hope.

2), immune regulation drug prospects gratifying

No matter how complex the mechanism behind cancer, immunosuppression is the key to cancer progression. Removal of immunosuppressive factors and recovery of immune system cells on the identification of cancer cells, can effectively resist cancer.

More and more research evidence shows that by regulating the body's immune system, it is possible to achieve the purpose of cancer control. Through the activation of the body's anti-tumor immune system to treat the tumor it is currently the majority of researchers excited areas, an important breakthrough in the next cancer field is likely to come from this.

Our laboratory is to explore the cause, pathogenesis, pathophysiology of cancer, and conducted a series of animal experimental research within 4 years in the laboratory, obtained from the experimental results of the new discovery, the new revelation: thymus atrophy, immune dysfunction is cancer Etiology and pathogenesis of one of the mechanism, so Xu Ze (Xu Ze) in 2013 at the International Conference on Cancer presented: cancer etiology, one of the pathogenesis, may be thymus atrophy, immune dysfunction, immune surveillance capacity decline and immune escape.

Therefore, the principle of treatment must be to prevent thymus atrophy, promote thymic hyperplasia, protect bone marrow hematopoietic function, improve immune surveillance, for the immune regulation of cancer provides experimental basis and theoretical basis.

Through the above four years to explore the recurrence, transfer mechanism of the basic experimental study, and after 3 years from the natural medications and herbal medication in the laboratory through the tumor-bearing animal experiments, from the 200 flavor of Chinese medicine it was screening out 48 of chinese medications which have a better tumor inhibition rate, and then through the animal cancer screening, they were composed of XZ-C1-10 anti-cancer immune regulation of traditional Chinese medications.

After 20 years of the clinical application in more than 12,000 cases of the middle and advanced cancer patients in cancer specialist outpatient clinic it was to confirm the observation and to confirm that "to protect thymus and to increase immune function" immunoregulatory treatment principle is reasonable, the effect is satisfactory. The application of immune regulation of traditional Chinese medication has achieved good results and improved the quality of life, significantly extended the survival period.

3). ASCO announced significant progress in clinical oncology in 2015

Immunotherapy opens a new era of tumor therapy

On February 4, 2016 at the Washington Capitol Hill in Washington, DC, the American Society of Clinical Oncology (ASCO) published the "2016 Annual Report about ASCO Clinical Oncology Progress with detailing the depth of the report on global clinical oncology research **in 2015: the summary was carried out ; at the same time, it was looking forward to the future direction of research and development. ASCO named the progress in 2015, that was, "tumor immunotherapy".**

Prof. JuLie M. Vose, Chairman of ASCO, said that the most important progress in 2015 was the discovery of immunotherapy, which she wrote in the foreword: "We are no longer determined by tumor type and staging as in the past Treatment, in the era of precision medicine, we according to each patient and tumor gene data selection or exclusion treatment.

There is no other significant progress that can be translated into clinical practice like immunology, so ASCO decided that the biggest progress in 2015 was immunotherapy."

Professor Don Dizon, chairman of the committee, also believes that the annual research results are increasing, but from the perspective of the benefit of patients, **the most important progress of the year should be immunotherapy.**

15, the situation analysis (d)

Preventing cancer and Anti-cancer, moving forward together and conquering cancer

(1) the goal of conquering cancer: reduce the incidence of cancer and improve the cure rate and prolong survival term

To achieve:

1/3 can be prevented

1/3 can be cured

1/3 can be treated, relieve pain, is a chronic disease and is the survival with tumor and prolong survival.

(2) the road of conquering cancer

the route:

① Conquer cancer and launch a total attack

What is the total attack?

That is the prevention of the cancer + the cancer control + cancer treatment and at the same time it launches the total attack and goes hand in hand.

② **to build the science and technology city to overcome cancer:**

 a. **the Innovative Molecular Oncology School of Medicine - and modern high-tech experimental talents**

 b. **the innovative hospital with the molecular tumor full prevention and treatment of the combination of Chinese medication and Western medication**

 c. **Innovative Molecular Tumor Research Institute**

 d. **Innovative Molecular Tumor Nanometer Pharmaceutical Factory**

 e. **Innovative Anti - Cancer Research Institute**

 f. **Animal Cancer Experimental Center**

(The following are provincial key disciplines)

(3) how to prevent Specific measures, feasible solutions (not empty talk) pragmatic, implementation

(4) how to control? Specific measures, feasible solutions (not empty talk) pragmatic, implementation

(5) how to rule? Specific measures, feasible solutions (not empty talk) pragmatic, implementation

(6) how to do? To avoid empty talk and focus on the hard work and start to go

(7) how to start?

① **first to do prevention, control, treatment of the hospital → the establishment of various disciplines(Department) → the establishment of the school group (study group)**

② **first to set up the medical and the teaching and the research (subjects and group) through-train; there are focused, there are basic, there are clinical, there are three basics, three stricts; there are theory and technology and experience.**

Cultivate the comprehensive talents: there are knowledge and experience and technology and theory; can change the current situation; there are separation and combination.

③ first to set up the graduate school and the personnel training methods and the ways;

A, first run graduate tutor courses and training courses; train personnel and seeds; train and guide talent and it is put forward learn and discuss the contents about how to overcome the cancer and to start the total attack

B, the talent seed plan: Recruitment of talent, experts, seeds which the experts and Professors are for the seed.

To Cultivate talent, that is, to sow:

To recruit students (master and Ph.D) to cultivate as the seeds; while working, they are learning, it needs 100, for all for the new seeds so that the generation and the generation are trained and it requires results and the achievements; the achievements are not just the paper, but that is fruitful and talents after three years or five years.

(8) how to carry out anti-cancer and cancer control work in Wuhan:

(1) more than two hospitals on the establishment of cancer

Each of the top three hospitals is responsible for three community anti-cancer work

Each top three hospital anti-cancer or prevention section, need to develop responsibilities, scope

Not just playing vaccination, should go deep into the community to carry out anti-cancer work

(2) the city's second, the top three hospitals to develop anti-cancer, anti-cancer responsibilities, division of labor is responsible for the regular inspection and supervision

① province each province top three hospitals responsible for two areas of prevention, control, governance

Each province's top three hospitals are responsible for two areas of medical care, difficult medical consultation, treatment, treatment, training, graded diagnosis and treatment, to solve the technical problems of quality, level

② the quality of the top three hospitals, the level of talent, technology must reach the quality of the top three hospitals must be worthy of the name, but also to solve the subordinate hospital personnel training, technical level

③ the establishment of consultation system, brainstorming, improve the level of medical care, to solve difficult problems, inter-city consultation, inter-hospital consultation.

④ Tongji, Concord, the people, the South, subordinate hospitals must solve the subordinate hospital referral, consultation, to solve difficult problems.

⑤ Tongji health system training province of anti-cancer, general practitioners, senior, intermediate health and epidemic prevention prevention scientific talents

⑥ each community set up anti-cancer, anti-cancer, anti-cancer, supervision, mission group, have responsibilities, tasks, division of labor

⑦ provincial and municipal health planning committee set up anti-cancer, cancer control office, organization mission, guidance, supervision

(9) how to carry out the prevention of the cancer and cancer control work in the community

To choose the several communities as the areas for cancer prevention, control cancer and the treatment cancer.

To establish the prevention of control and cancar control system of "China model"

(1) the research and development through the standardization of "three early" information and early warning system

In the community the person who has the following history is usually checked:

1. history of blood in the stool, hemorrhoids history that it should be colonoscopy
2. history of hematuria that it should have cystoscopy
3. there are lumps, nodules that it should be palpable or surgery
4. with the hepatitis B and cirrhosis. It should be checked every six months or once a year check

(2) the standardized community anti-cancer training

(3) the community registration, timely assessment

(4) focusing on the "three early" and the precancerous lesions and focusing on prevention, early diagnosis, early treatment.

Volume II

Conquer cancer and launch a total attack

The total design and the blueprint and the preparatory work of "The multidisciplinary and the scientific research base of cancer research group of overcoming cancer and launching a total attack ------- the Science City"

The table of Contents

一. "XZ-C proposed the research program of conquering cancer and launching the total attack

- The overall strategic reform and development of cancer treatment

二. It was proposed to establish the test area of conquering cancer work group (station) in the province / city

- Professor Xu Ze proposed the overall design planning and the blueprint to conquer cancer to launch a total attack

三. "the research base of the establishment of a comprehensive attack of conquering cancer – the Science City"

- The total design and the blueprint "The research base of capturing the cancer and launching a total offensive –the Science City"
- The total design and the preparation work of "the Science City"

四. The total design and the blueprint and the preparatory work of "the research base to capture the cancer and to launch a total offensive the Science City"

- XZ-C proposed **How to overcome cancer I see one**

五. XZ-C proposed how to overcome the cancer I see two:

- how to overcome cancer? To overcome cancer, we must create "Innovative Molecular Cancer Institute"
- to overcome the cancer and to build "the science city to overcome the cancer and to launch a total attack"

六. XZ-C proposed how to overcome cancer I see the three:

•How to overcome cancer? To overcome the cancer, we must create "the innovative molecular tumor hospital" (the global demonstration hospital of the prevention and treatment of cancer during the whole process of the occurrence and the development of cancer)

七. XZ-C proposed how to overcome the cancer I see four:

- How to overcome cancer? To overcome cancer, it must create "the animal experimental center of the experimental medicine cancer"

八. vXZ-C proposed how to overcome cancer I see six:

- How to overcome cancer? To overcome the cancer, we must create "the innovative molecular tumor nano-pharmaceutical factory" and "the research group and laboratory to analyze the anti-cancer and anti-cancer transfer active ingredients and the molecular weight and the structural formula and the immunopharmacology and the analysis of the molecular level"

九. XZ-C proposed how to overcome cancer I see five:

- How to overcome cancer? To overcome the cancer, we must create "the innovative environmental anti-cancer research institute"

一, XZ-C proposed the research program of conquering cancer and launching the total attack

The overall strategic reform and development of cancer treatment

Prof. Xu ZE, Honorary President of Wuhan Anti-Cancer Research Association, presented the following four research programs of the feasibility of reports and the total design to tackle the total attack on cancer in July 2015.

(1) For the first time in the international community it is put forward:

"The necessity and the feasibility of the report to capture the total attack of cancer"

- The overall strategy of cancer strategy is changed from focusing on treatment into focusing on prevention and treatment at the equal attention.

(2) for the first time in the international community it was put forward:

"To build the prevention and treatment hospitals during the whole process of cancer development and occurrence"

(Global demonstration of the hospital with prevention and treatment of cancer)

"the imagination and feasibility report of building the hospital with the prevention and treatment of cancer during the whole anti-cancer process"

- Describe the necessity and feasibility of establishing a complete prevention and treatment hospital

(3) For the first time in the international community it was put forward:

"To build the basic design and feasibility report of a total attack to capture cancer and science city"

- is equivalent to design the whole framework about design with Chinese charasteric of conquering cancer.

(4) For the first time in the international community it is put forward:

"In building a moderately society at the same time, the proposed" ride research "- for the medical science research of cancer prevention and cancer control and the necessity and feasibility report of cancer prevention and treatment"

- Adhere to the Chinese characteristics of anti-cancer and cancer prevention path

These four international research projects are the first time to be put forward in the international, are the international initiative, the international leader, open up a new field of anti-cancer research.

Change from paying attention to the heavy treatment and light defense into paying equal attention to both anti-cancer prevention and treatment, in an attempt to achieve lower incidence of cancer and improve cancer cure rate.

It is possible to overcome cancer and conquer cancer to open this new research field because for the centuries people are based on cancer treatment about cancer treatment, and the treatment method is based on killing cancer cells. But the chemotherapy is a first-class kinetics, it is impossible to kill cancer cells completely, the effective time to kill cancer cells in patients with chemotherapy to kill cancer cells was only 3-5 days during intravenous infusion, which has the role of killing cancer cells, and then there is no role of killing cancer cells, it is only a short time to kill about (3-5 days), can not once and for all, after 3-5 days the cancer cells continue to split, proliferation, so it can only alleviate a short time, cannot cure, can only kill a certain number of cancer Cells, there will still be cancer cells continuing to produce, therefore, its efficacy is defined as "remission", and the remission time is only 4 weeks or more, and it will still recur and metastasis . So chemotherapy cannot cure cancer and cannot be relied on to overcome cancer. Despite the use of more than half a century, cancer is still the first cause of death of urban and rural residents.

This research program is first proposed by Chinese people first proposed in the international community, and can benefit mankind, revitalize China, shock

the world. To propose to attack the cancer to launch a total attack needs to have courage, and needs for wisdom and strength and needs for scientific basis.

The first scientific research program is proposed a feasibility report and apply for the preparation by Professor Xu Ze in the international community for the first time. It will be conducted by the Wuhan anti-cancer research under the leadership of the provincial and municipal leaders.

The implementation of the "XZ-C attack on cancer to start the basic idea and design":

(Xu ZE) Professor proposed to overcome the cancer and to launch the general offensive ideas, strategies, planning sketches, and proposed the total design, guidance of the Science City of overcoming the cancer to launch a total attack, commanded "to build a science city which have the medical, teaching, research and development of conquering cancer and launch the total attack". First of all, to build "the hospital of the prevention and treatment of cancer during the whole process of cancer occurrence and development --- - global demonstration of the cancer prevention and treatment hospital."

The purpose is:

① reduce the incidence of cancer

② improve cancer cure rate

③ extend the survival period

④ improve the quality of life

⑤ reduce complications

二, it was proposed to establish the test area of conquering cancer work group (station) in the province or city

- Professor Xu Ze proposed the overall design planning blueprint to conquer cancer to launch a total attack

To set up the following groups:

1), the academic Committee to overcome the Cancer

2), the building work group of the Science City (the science city of conquering cancer and launching a total attack with the medical, teaching, research and development science school)

1, to set up the Academic Committee of overcoming cancer

The conditions of the academic members:

Genuine talent, academic achievement on the basic research or clinical work of cancer,, academic results, monograph, editor, patent, thesis, practical clinical experience, experimental research results, its research and academic is to capture cancer as the research direction. Leading talent of Leadership and organization of conquering cancer. It must both ability and political integrity.

academic committee

Consultant:

(Leading scientists who have academic achievements in cancer research)

Chairman:

Vice Chairman: 17 well-known experts, professors, academic leaders or leading scientists

Members: 36 are academic leaders, experts and professors

2, the building working group of the Science City (the science city with the medical, teaching, research and development to attack the cancer and to launch a total attack)

The building division of labor of the "Science City" with capturing the cancer as the research direction and the main task:

1. financing group: (financing, investment)
2. the building group: (site, house, decoration, equipment)
3. the academic group: (content: multidisciplinary subject set, multi-disciplinary research group set, compulsory courses and elective courses set, according to medical, teaching, research, hair were implemented, the laboratory set up and established)
4. the preparation of the Secretariat Office: Team leader:

3, the working group with research results, transformation and development of the province of attacking the cancer and launching a total offensive

Leading group

Leader:

Deputy head:

Co-leader:

Department of Education:

Science and Technology Department:

Health Commission:

Environmental Protection Agency:

Transformation, development office:

Secretariat:

XZ-C proposed to attack the cancer and launch a total attack, that is, prevention cancer, cancer control, cancer treatment three fleets go hand in hand; prevention and treatment at the equal attention both involved:

① education department: to cultivate the general offensive multidisciplinary senior personnel, the establishment of innovative tumor medical college and tumor multidisciplinary senior personnel training courses, teaching and research group (teaching and research) should have a better laboratory or laboratory.

② science and technology departments: to carry out the "three early" research, research early diagnosis of new reagents, new technologies, new methods, open up new areas of anti-cancer research, new technologies, new methods, new industries, eyes forward, Three early ".

③ Health and Social Health Department: cancer treatment, anti-cancer, cancer is the management of the work of the health sector, should be anti-governance and both.

④ environmental protection departments: should open up new areas of environmental protection and anti-cancer research, new technologies, new industries, because 80% of cancer and the environment is closely related. Should be from the clothing, food, live, anti-cancer, from the environment, small environmental anti-cancer, first monitoring, qualitative, quantitative, set the standard, the establishment of multi-project laboratory, macro, micro, ultra-microscopic research, Methods and measures.

4, the test area of the province or city to attack cancer work group (station)

the setting up working group of the "Science City"

the chief architect, president, chairman of the General Academic Committee is for Professor Xu Ze.

The preparatory group of the "Science City" to build scientific research program:

① innovative full-scale anti-cure hospital - are all disciplines and professors, each preparatory group has 12 professors, experts

② innovative tumor medical school - are all disciplines and professors, each preparatory group has 12 professors, experts

③ Innovative Cancer Research Institute - are professors and professors, each preparatory group has 12 professors, experts

④ experimental medical cancer animal experimental center - are all disciplines and professors, each preparatory group has 12 professors, experts

⑤ innovative nano-pharmaceutical companies - all disciplines and professors, each preparatory group has 12 professors, experts

5, Wuhan Anti Cancer Research Association and Shuguang Hing Conversion Medical Center

The working group of XZ-C research results transformation, development

(1) transformation of medicine, research and development working group:

Honorary leader:

Leader:

Deputy head:

Co-leader:

Director of the Centre:

Center Secretary-General:

Deputy Secretary-General:

(2) Purpose:

(3) Method:

三, the research base of the establishment of a comprehensive attack of conquering cancer - Science City

---The total design and blueprint of "The research base of capturing the cancer and launching a total offensive - Science City"

---The total design and preparation work of "Science City"

(A) how to overcome cancer? XZ-C (Xu Ze - China)

"Attack the cancer and launch a total attack"

1, why is it put forward to overcome cancer? Look at the present situation:

(1) the incidence of cancer is the status quo: the more the more patients

Today, the incidence of cancer in China is the annual incidence of new cases of cancer 3.12 million cases, the average daily new cancer patients 8550 cases, 6 per minute in the country diagnosed with cancer.

(2) the status of cancer mortality is high and has been the first cause of death in urban and rural areas in China

Today, China's cancer mortality rate is 2.7 million deaths per year due to cancer deaths, an average of 7,500 people died of cancer every day, every 7 dead people that one died of cancer.

Cancer in China is so high incidence, the more the rule of the patient, the high mortality rate, should be a major issue of national economy and people's livelihood, should be a major issue of people's health, should be the people's major suffering and disaster.

Human beings should not sit still, physicians should not do nothing, leadership should not do nothing, I think we should put forward "to overcome cancer." "Declaring war on cancer" is the time, should gather wisdom, overcome cancer.

2, why did Professor Xu Ze propose to overcome cancer and to launch a total attack? Look at the current status of cancer treatment:

(1) the current status of cancer treatment:

Although the application of the traditional three treatment for nearly a hundred years, tens of thousands of cancer patients to bear the release, chemotherapy, but the results? So far the cancer is still the first cause of death, although the patients are carried out a formal, systematic radiotherapy or chemotherapy, or radiotherapy + chemotherapy, it still failed to prevent cancer metastasis and recurrence, little effect.

(2) the status quo of the mode of the current tumor hospital or the oncology

(1) go all out to focus on treatment, for the middle and late cancer, depleted human and financial resources, and failed to achieve lower mortality, prolong survival, reduce morbidity, cancer is still the first cause of death in urban and rural areas.

(2) only treatment, or paying more attention to heavy treatment and less attention to defense, the more the more patients.

(3) ignored the "three early", ignoring the prevention.

(4) many large hospitals, university hospitals have not established a laboratory, can not carry out the basic research of cancer or clinical basic research, because if no basic research breakthrough, the clinical efficacy is difficult to improve, "Oncology" is still today's medicine The most backward of the subjects. why? Because "oncology" of the etiology, pathogenesis, pathophysiology are not yet clear. People on its pathogenesis, cancer cell metastasis mechanism is still lack of understanding, and therefore the current cancer treatment program is still quite blind, it must establish a laboratory for basic research and clinical basic research.

The status quo is: a, through a century road, the hospital model is: heavy treatment and light defense, or only treatment, the result is: the more treatment and the more patients.

B, through a century road, the treatment model is: to aim at the late invasion and metastasis of the advanced patients and it exhausted human and financial resources ; the result is that the mortality rate is high.

How to do? It should change the current treatment mode and the hospital mode, and it is put forward to overcome cancer and to launch the total attack.

3, what is the total attack of conquering cancer?

XZ-C proposed to the general idea and design of capturing cancer.

The total attack is to conduct the work in full swing, simultaneously for the three stages such as cancer prevention, control and treatment during the whole process of cancer development and occurrence.

That is:

Prevention of cancer - before the formation of cancer

Cancer control - malignant transformation of precancerous lesions

Cancer treatment - has formed a foci or metastases

The Objective: To reduce the incidence of cancer, reduce cancer mortality, improve the cure rate, prolong survival, improve the quality of life, reduce complications.

四. The total design and the blueprint and the preparatory work of "the research base to capture the cancer and to launch a total offensive – the Science City"

XZ-C (XU ZE - China) proposed:

How to overcome cancer I see one:

1. how to overcome cancer? To overcome cancer, it must create "the innovative molecular cancer medical school"

- to overcome the cancer and to build "to overcome the cancer launched a total attack of the science city" one

(1) why is it to create "innovative molecular cancer medical school"?

Because: (1) the current status of cancer scholars are mainly the radiotherapy and chemotherapy talent and in order to attack the cancer and launch a total attack, it needs the multi-disciplinary talents.

① **to overcome cancer, the talent is the key.** It is to train the relevant personnel who can participate in the capture of cancer, launch the total attack. The talent must be genuine talent and have the technology and theory and must both ability and political integrity and medicine is benevolence, the moral is the first.

Personnel must have knowledge of undergraduate knowledge, life science knowledge, knowledge of Chinese medicine, molecular biology, genetic engineering, environmental science, environmental science, medical multidisciplinary knowledge, immunology, virology, endocrinology, immunopharmacology and so on.

② **to overcome cancer, talent is the key, how to train talent is the key.** Research of cancer talent requires a number of disciplinary knowledge and technology, to genetic engineering, molecular biology immunology, virological experimental personnel, knowledge must also have technology, hands-on ability, technology needs knowledge, so that under the guidance of the theory, The development of high-end technology, the need to tackle the first-class talent, we must concentrate on, calm down, concentrate on this work. Where does talent come from? It is based on their own training and that they create their own machine to hatch the talent.

③ **to overcome the cancer, start the total attack and move forward together with the prevention of the cancer + control cancer + the treatment of the cancer and the three are together, so the teaching plan must develop cancer prevention science talent, the cancer disease control personnel and the teaching content and knowledge and the course related anti-cancer and preventive medicine.**

At present, anti-cancer, cancer control talent is scarce, urgent need to accelerate training to meet the urgent need to launch a general attack.

In view of more than 90% of the cancer caused by environmental factors or closely related to the current we are ongoing energy-saving emission reduction, sewage pollution control, this policy and work and anti-cancer, cancer control work has a great relevance, Related talent.

④ the current educational content can not keep up with the development of the times. **To overcome the cancer it must develop the modern high-tech disciplines and it must have a good laboratory, but in the current it lacks of the laboratory talent. For attacking the cancer and launching a total attack and anti-cancer and controlling cancer, it is lacking of the laboratory experimental modern high-tech talent and the intermediate specialist talent who can go deep into the community to prevent cancer, cancer control capacity.**

It should strengthen the establishment of laboratory personnel for the tertiary institutions. Modern life science and technology progress rapidly and the genetic engineering and the molecular biology and the cell inheritance rapid develop.

Because Professor Xu Ze (XZ) proposed to attack the cancer and launch a general attack, which is unprecedented in human work, must develop the high-tech talent and technology with the basic medicine, clinical medicine, life sciences, Chinese and Western medicine, preventive medicine, experimental medicine, molecular level skills and it must personally practice, create experience, develop medicine. Therefore, at the same time it is to establish the graduate school, to cultivate thesenior scientific and technological personnel for attacking the cancer .

(2) how to set up "innovative molecular level cancer medical school"?

(1) to overcome cancer, talent is the key, how to train talent is the key? People who study cancer must require multidisciplinary talent and technology. The current world countries are concentrated on a large number of scientific research elite research, therefore, the education sector to accelerate the development of anti-cancer research multidisciplinary senior personnel services.

We build "innovative molecular cancer medical school" which is to attack the cancer and launch a total offensive training research personnel training services. Professor Xu Ze proposed to attack the cancer launched a general attack, is unprecedented in human work, must create their own experience, must practice in person, this is a new cement road, every step will leave the eternal scientific footprints, so I suggest a Department of Education Department of the Office of the Department of Cancer Medical College of the leadership, to create experience.

(2) the current global and China's oncology is the main treatment of talent, and attack the cancer launched a total attack, compared to cancer + cancer + cancer (anti-+ control) to carry out simultaneously, troika, go hand in hand, you need Prevention of talent, prevention

of scientific talents, public health department of talent, prevention of medical college talent, urgent need to prevent and control talent.

(3) **the current cancer treatment of the object is mainly invasive, middle or late transfer or recurrence of the patient, the main treatment for the traditional three treatment, surgery, radiotherapy and chemotherapy, and attack the cancer to attack the total attack was anti + + control, Focus on the left shift, the main attack of the object is mainly "three early", early in situ cancer, precancerous lesions, "three early" diagnosis and treatment technology. Early can only qualitative, and some can not locate, it only needs a small surgery, generally it does not need the big surgery and the early cancer prognosis is good and can be complete cured and "three early" in situ cancer, precancerous lesions, severe atypical hyperplasia do not have to put Chemotherapy.**

(4) **how to overcome cancer? Training talent is the key.**

How to train talent? How to cultivate modern high-tech talent, to attack the cancer launched a total attack, the goal catch up with the international advanced level, to obtain the original innovation, the leading international level of scientific and technological achievements, the key is the educational institutions, the teaching and research group should have a good laboratory to cultivate cancer HiTech Personnel.

Because the innovative molecular cancer medical school teaching content includes: modern medical science knowledge and technology, life science knowledge and technology, modern biomedical knowledge and technology, traditional Chinese medicine knowledge, experimental medicine knowledge and technology ... ... **these modern science is the developing science. Science - is the endless frontier, the rapid development of modern high-tech, with each passing day, the quality of**

university teachers and teaching quality must also keep up with modern high-tech development, advancing with the times.

University teachers should have a dual task on the shoulders, one is to improve teaching, the second is the development of science.

University teachers should have a good laboratory for scientific research, based on the known science, to explore the unknown science, for the future science, emerging disciplines, marginal disciplines, interdisciplinary, scientific frontier, for innovation and development.

To conquer cancer must have the talents with multiple skills with the following skills: immune and caner; virus and cancer; endocrine hormones and cancer; fungi and cancer; molecular biology and cancer; genes and cancer; environment and the relationship between cancer and cancer; Cancer; traditional Chinese medicine and cancer; chronic inflammation and cancer.

It is necessary to cultivate high-level professionals with the prevention of control and cancer control and treatment of cancer . Education is the backing of cancer. The education must cultivate talents for the purpose of attacking cancer, and the people must have this professional theoretical knowledge and professional skills., Talent must both ability and political integrity, medicine is benevolence, legislation for the first.

(3) how to run an innovative molecular cancer medical school in order to train the personnel for attacking the cancer and launching a total offensive? It should build a good laboratory.

It is necessary to have a good laboratory, to carry out scientific research, to be based on known science, to explore unknown science, and to face emerging science in the future.

China's universities and Europe and the United States compared to the gap between the size of the school and the number of teachers and students, the main gap is the lack of high-tech laboratories, the US technology boom, high-tech development, Attention to science and technology experiments, attention to the laboratory. Each year, a large number of international students, visiting scholars to study in the United States, are basically in the laboratory work and study. China University and the United States and Britain and other countries of the University of the main gap lies in the United States and Britain and other universities modern high-tech laboratory everywhere, excellent equipment, teaching and research group of basic teaching work in the laboratory, research, research, training graduate students, students to teach students to innovation, To develop new areas of research, a talent, a master.

Massachusetts Institute of Technology, the scale is small, the number of teachers and students only a few thousand people, but the school had 38 Nobel Prize winners, won a total of 39 Nobel Prize in Science, one of them won two Connaught Award. Ranking the highest in the world famous universities. Because the school has many modern high-tech high-level laboratories, laboratory talent, there are many academic masters, pioneered a number of cutting-edge research areas, strict style of study, rigorous and rigorous.

This shows that the laboratory is the incubation of scientific research results, the laboratory is the training of personnel incubator.

University professors should not only talk about the knowledge of the textbooks, but also should talk about today's new progress, the development of new trends, new achievements and unknown knowledge, a mentor should have a good laboratory, it is possible to guide graduate students to conduct scientific research, Papers, development science.

To have the Development of science, scientific and technological innovation, the laboratory is the key condition.

It should vigorously build laboratories and train more the high-tech talent and have more innovative results.

(1) training talent is two ways

    ① founder of Cancer Medical School
    ② founder of Cancer Graduate School

(2) Method:

    ① to overcome the cancer to mobilize the total attack academic committee members and Wuhan anti-cancer research professor and interested in conception of cancer professor, 100 professors, mentor with 100 graduate students and Master and Ph. D students.

    ② Graduate School is teaching, experiment, practice (morning clinical, surgery, outpatient, afternoon into the laboratory
    To Guide academic thinking, scientific research ethics, experimental methods, scientific research

    ③ academic committee professor according to the clinical problems must solve the clinical basis of the problem ... ... and so out of 100 topics, postgraduate academic committee to discuss the subject to decide to get the Master and Ph.D students.

50 master questions - must be a result, to solve practical problems, clinical can be practical, the patient benefit

50 doctoral thesis - heavy experiment, heavy practice, heavy technology, heavy theory, re-scientific thinking, heavy theoretical basis, must be a result, innovative thinking, or a patent, clinical application value, achievements, results, patents, papers, Must be innovative, we must pay attention to scientific research ethics.

Medical is benevolence, legislation for the first

Master and Ph.D students must have both ability and political integrity.

(3) Graduate School and the Provincial Natural Science Foundation, Science and Technology Department, Association for collaboration

(4) within three years it must product 100 research papers or achievements, or patents, or Chinese herbal anti-cancer new drugs, focusing on "three early" new reagents, new technologies, new methods, new drugs.

The new drugs, new methods, new technologies, new concepts, new theories, Chinese and Western medications for anti - cancer metastasis and anti-cancer recurrence and the prevention of cancer

(2) how to set up "innovative molecular cancer medical school"? How to implement and create? It should apply for provincial education department leadership and support.

Five. XZ-C puts forward how to overcome the cancer I see two:

How to overcome cancer? To overcome cancer, we must create "the Innovative Molecular Cancer Institute"

- to overcome the cancer, to build "to overcome the cancer and launch a total attack of science city" one

(1) Why should we start the "the Innovative Molecular Cancer Institute"?

Because:

1, "oncology" is still the current medical science in the most backward of a discipline. why? Because the "oncology" etiology, pathogenesis, pathophysiology are not yet clear, there are a lot of basic theoretical problems yet not to understand clearly on the biological characteristics of cancer cells; the molecular mechanism of cancer cell metastasis is still lack of understanding; it is involving in the virus, immune, fungal, endocrine hormones, the environment and other carcinogenic factors; it must have the multidisciplinary research.

The study of oncology is the most complex subject in medical research. It involves multidisciplinary knowledge and theory. It is necessary to set up a specialist group closely related to cancer to conduct an in-depth study in order to help overcome the total attack of cancer.

2, Therefore, the creation of "Innovative Molecular Cancer Institute" is to overcome the cancer and launch a total attack for the exploration of cancer etiology, pathogenesis, cancer cell metastasis mechanism, immune mechanism, in-depth study and for the organization of further study of science closely related to cancer . it is based on the knowledge and theory of the discipline, known medicine, to explore the subject of unknown knowledge, future medicine, edge disciplines, interdisciplinary, to understand the causes and mechanisms of cancer, so as to provide effective intervention for cancer prevention snd treatment measures in order to help overcoming cancer.

(2) Why should we build a cancer research institute?

Because: in order to overcome the cancer, we must build "innovative molecular tumor research institute" closely with clinical practice, cancer research.

To overcome cancer, where the road? I believe that the road in the scientific research, the road on the prevention and treatment of cancer scientific research, the road to explore the cause of cancer, pathogenesis, pathophysiology of experimental basic research, the road in the study of cancer, the development of The whole process of scientific research, the road in the traditional therapy reform and development, the road in the multi-disciplinary research, the road in the study of cancer metastasis, recurrence of prevention and control, the road in the "three early" study.

Through the scientific research of cancer prevention and treatment, mankind will overcome cancer, and ultimately will overcome cancer.

① how to overcome the cancer I see one: the road to scientific research is to explore the cause of cancer, pathogenesis, pathophysiology of experimental basic research

I believe that the development of cancer science research is the urgent need in the current status of oncology, we must recognize the status of cancer disciplines what problems are and how to do.

Although cancer treatment has been more than a century, has now entered the second decade of the 21st century, but "oncology" is still the most backward of the current medical disciplines, why? Because "oncology" Pathogenesis and pathophysiology are not yet clear. The scientific research of Oncology is a virgin land and needs to have a lot of basic scientific research and clinical basic research.

Although the application of the traditional three treatment (surgery, radiotherapy, chemotherapy) has been used for nearly a hundred years and tens of thousands of cancer patients had radiotherapy and chemotherapy, but how are the results? so far the mortality rate of cancer is still the number one in the cause of death of urban and rural residents in China. How should the road be walked? It should be in-depth reflection, in-depth analysis, in-depth study.

Why so? the reasons are for the following main points:

① the cause of cancer is not clear, the pathogenesis is not clear, pathophysiology is not clear, there are a lot of basic theoretical problems yet to understand clearly.

② the lack of understanding of the biological characteristics and biological behavior of cancer cells.

③ the molecular mechanism of cancer cell metastasis is still lack of sufficient understanding.

② how to overcome the cancer I see two: the road to scientific research is to carry out multidisciplinary research, the formation of the relevant specialist group, special in-depth basis and clinical research

Anti-cancer research needs to involve multidisciplinary, not only clinical medicine, there are many marginal disciplines, interdisciplinary, basic disciplines involved. Cancer metastasis and recurrence research involves medical, surgical, radiation, endocrine, drug, immune, molecular biology, virus, biological information, genetic engineering, life sciences, molecular chemistry, enzyme chemistry, environmental protection, Chinese medicine, laboratory and so on. The city has the above disciplines of talent, there is a certain basis, we can organize all the scientific and technological strength and the team work, take the scientific research cooperation joint research road, together to improve the level of anti-cancer metastasis and relapse for the benefit of millions of cancer patients.

③ it should set up the following special group which are closely related with the cancer to do the basis and clinical research in-depth.

In view of the fact that the study of oncology involves multidisciplinary knowledge and theory, it is necessary to set up the relevant specialist group, to further study, based on the known knowledge of the discipline, known medicine, to explore the unknown knowledge of the discipline and the edge disciplines and the interdisciplinary; in order to help overcome the cancer, it should set up the following specialized groups; in the future it may be the formation of new disciplines or interdisciplinary, new industries.

(1) **Immunology and Cancer Research Group: Laboratory;**

(2) **Virus and Cancer Research Group: Laboratory;**

(3) **endocrine hormone and cancer research group: laboratory;**

(4) **mycotoxin and cancer research group: laboratory;**

(5) **Environmental and Cancer Research Group: Laboratory;**

(6) ....

(7) ....

(8).......................................;

To overcome cancer, we must build "the Innovative Molecular Cancer Institute."

First, it is to establish the multidisciplinary group related to cancer research; the purpose is to study the "three early" new reagents, new technologies, new methods to improve the "three early" diagnosis and treatment. The current CT, MRI ... ... and other diagnostic methods are very advanced, the hardware is very good, but once cancer is diagnosed, it is in the middle and late; it should try to study the method of early diagnosis, early treatment method, the early diagnosis method, early treatment method for precancerous lesions and precancerous state.

In the current it is mostly the morphological or affect the diagnosis which are required to grow to a certain volume which can be diagnosed, if from the serum, immune ... ... to find a study, it may be able to find a diagnosis such as Kang Hua's anti-syphilis for the diagnosis of the syphilis and Feida response for the diagnosis of Typhoid and other early diagnosis methods.

(3) how to create "innovative molecular tumor research"? How to implement and create?

To build an innovative molecular tumor research institute

Sixth floor 11 12

Fifth floor 9 10

Fourth floor 7 8

Third floor 5 6

Second floor 3 4

First floor 1 2

First rent a 6-storey building, in close connection with the actual needs of the clinical, first to carry out a number of multi-disciplinary and cancer-related research, first try, then gradually enhance scientific research projects, additional research group.

Rent three years a year to pay a year rent.

First floor

(1) immunology and cancer research group and laboratory

(2) virus and cancer research group and laboratory

Second floor

(3) endocrine hormone and cancer research group and laboratory

(4) Environmental and Cancer Research Group and Laboratory

Third floor

(5) Chinese medicine and cancer research group and laboratory

(6) "three early" and cancer research group and laboratory

Fourth floor

(7) fungi and cancer research group and laboratory

(8) Molecular Biology and Cancer Research Group and Laboratory

Fifth floor

(9) Genetic Engineering and Cancer Research Group and Laboratory

(10) precancerous lesions and cancer research group and laboratory

Sixth floor laboratory, office

The Above to carry out a number of scientific research group project, and "to build cancer, the development of the whole process, hospital" department connected.

To build an "innovative molecular tumor research institute" is to overcome the cancer to attack the total clinical prevention, prevention and treatment of clinical problems, according to the clinical problems of research.

Why to build innovative molecular tumor research institute, to carry out cancer scientific research? It is the urgent need of the current status of oncology and we must recognize what the problems are the status of cancer disciplines? how to do?

Although cancer treatment has been more than a century and it has now entered the second decade of the 21st century, but "oncology" is still the most backward of the current medical disciplines, why? Because the etiology and pathogenesis and the pathophysiology of oncology are not clear. The scientific research of oncology is in a virgin land and need to have a lot of basic scientific research and clinical basic research.

Although the application of the traditional three treatment (surgery, radiotherapy, chemotherapy) has been used for nearly a hundred years and tens of thousands of cancer patients underwent chemotherapy, but what are the results? so far the mortality rate of cancer is still the number one of cause of death in the urban and rural residents in China. How should the road go? It should be in-depth reflection and in-depth analysis and in-depth study.

Therefore, it is necessary to build an innovative molecular tumor research institute, carry out the basic research of cancer and anti-cancer metastasis and recurrence and it must be carried out in the study of cancer animal model to study the mechanism of the cancer metastasis and because if there is no basic research breakthrough, the clinical efficacy is difficult to improve.

Xu ZE (Professor) pointed out: the research topics and the research routes all should follow the following scientific research line:

- All studies are from clinical → experimental → clinical → re-trial → re-clinical. Return to clinical to solve the problem, so that patients benefit.
- The theory and practice are closely integrated, the topics are from the clinical, to find the clinical focus of the problem and clinical breakthrough, after experimental and clinical validation, and then applied to clinical, to solve clinical problems.
- the evidence-based medicine, seeking truth from facts, strong scientific, with the facts to speak and to argument; there are measurable experimental research and clinical validation of information and it should attention to the accumulation of raw data.
- The efficacy evaluation criteria: the long live, the long survival time, the good quality of life, the clinical observation of 3-5 years, or even 8-10 years, to the initial evaluation of long-term efficacy.

Innovative Molecular Cancer Institute

The study of oncology is the most complex and difficult problem in medical research. It involves multidisciplinary knowledge and theory. It should be organized with the following special groups, which are closely related to cancer, and specialize in basic and clinical research; it should be based on the known knowledge of the discipline, known medicine, to explore the unknown knowledge of the discipline and the future of medicine and the edge disciplines and the interdisciplinary in order to help overcoming cancer. In the future it may form the new disciplines and the new industries.

Based on 28 years of scientific research experience, Professor Xu Ze think of that the following disciplines are related cancer occurrence and development and pathophysiology and pathogenesis and metastasis and recurrence and treatment so that it is proposed to first set up the following disciplines research groups.

The following specialized groups should be organized:

(1) Immunology and Cancer Research Group (Section):

Recent clinical research tasks should be (to carry out the following work)

① the detection of immune status of cancer patients, assessment.
② cancer patients with immunoregulatory treatment efficacy monitoring.
③ quantitative monitoring of immune function in patients with chemotherapy and chemotherapy.

(2) Virus and Cancer Research Group (Section):

① fund the establishment of the virus and cancer cell culture center laboratory and identify professionals and academic leaders.
② financing the establishment of cancer cell culture room.
③ financing the establishment of animal animal model laboratory.
④ to be with the United States Yale University Dr. Lee to carry out HPV detection.

(3) hormones (endocrine) and cancer research group and laboratory

① clinical testing of hormones
② hormone imbalance and the occurrence of cancer clinical laboratory observations

③ the application of hormones and carcinogenic problems

④ precancerous lesions and hormone observation

(4) Environmental and Cancer Research Associations (Section) and Laboratory

① common malignant tumor risk factors for investigation, control, into the intervention study

② monitoring of pollution-induced cancer data, research and development of cancer prevention, cancer control measures

(A) food, food; (b) water pollution, beverages

(C) House decoration; (d) Quantitative data monitoring of carcinogens for air pollution, plants and automobile exhaust

③ **monitoring of environmental pollution carcinogenic data, research anti-cancer measures, research and development intervention means**

④ **pollution abatement, environment-friendly, set up "8 +1" anti-cancer, anti-cancer alliance**

⑤ **to founded the prevention of cancer, anti-cancer newsletter - "mass medicine" to prevent cancer from the big living environment and a small environment anti-cancer.**

The above special schools belong to the hospital disciplines and are located in the hospital. After about a year it will try to establish the special subject of the Institute and for the total establishment of the Institute.

The above research institutions: departments → research group → Institute → Institute of the purpose, tasks, planning, implementation, coordination of projects, topics, objectives; scientific research, scientific and technological innovation. It is to have "To overcome the cancer" as the direction of scientific research to improve the overall level of medical care so that patients benefit.

Above the special research group Discipline research total design, discipline general manager: xxxx

We have to build "innovative molecular tumor research institute" which is to overcome the cancer and launch a series of multidisciplinary research. Professor Xu Ze proposed to attack the cancer and launch a total attack, is unprecedented in human work, must create their own experience, must practice in person. Therefore, I suggest that a provincial science and technology department of the Office of the cadres of the Cancer Institute of the leadership (secretary) support and create experience.

Six, XZ-C proposed how to overcome cancer I see the three:

How to overcome cancer? To overcome the cancer, we must create "the innovative molecular tumor hospital" (global demonstration of the hospital with the prevention and treatment of the whole process of the cancer occurrence and development)

- one of << to conquer cancer and to build "the science city of overcoming cancer and launching a total attack of" >>

(1) Why is it to create "the hospital of the innovative molecular tumor with the prevention and treatment during the whole process of cancer occurrence and development"?

Because:

1, in the current global there are the problems in china cancer hospital and oncology department and the hospital model.

A), go all out, the focus of treatment is the cancer patients in the middle and advanced stages and metastatic and recurrence ; the efficacy is poor; it exhausts the human and financial resources and fails to achieve lower mortality and to improve the cure rate and to reduce morbidity; the death rate is still the first cause of death of urban and rural residents.

B), only treatment without prevention, or attention of treatment and no prevention; the more treatment and the more patients.

2, Cancer hospital or hospital oncology department and the hospital model in the current global and in China are the treatment of hospitals; the objects of the treatment of patients are in the middle and late stages and metastatic; the effect is very poor.

The hospital models: are the treatment hospitals and attention of treatment and light defense, or only treatment and no prevention.

The treatment model: both for advanced patients with advanced cancer metastasis.

It should (must) reform:

To reform of the hospital model: it should be changed to prevention and control and treatment at the same equal.

To reform of treatment model: it should be changed to focus on early, precancerous lesions ... ... and so on, the way out of cancer treatment is in the "three early", must study the diagnosis of the new technologies, new methods, new reagents of "three early" ; the early cancer can be cured.

③ Therefore, to create "the hospital of the innovative molecular tumor with the prevention and treatment during the whole process of occurrence and development;" in order to overcome cancer, it should reform the hospital model and change the treatment model, XZ-C proposed to overcome cancer and launch a total attack.

What is called as conquering cancer and launching the total attack?

The total attack is to carry out in a comprehensive work of three stages of cancer prevention and cancer control and cancer treatment during the whole process of cancer occurrence and development, and synchronized, troika, go hand in hand, keep pace, reform the current hospital mode, change the current treatment model.

Namely: the reform of the current treatment-focused model. To change the current hospital model of focus on treatment in the middle and late stage; to reform treatment model of focus on treating the middle and late stages; reform only treatment and not prevent into prevention and control and treatment at the same equal leve.

How to implement this new unification model?

It should be established the hospital of the prevention and control and treatment during the whole process of occurrence and development of cancer .

(2) how to create "innovative molecular level cancer hospital"? How to implement and create?

Preparations work in two steps:

First of all, rent a house to do the hospital, in order to carry out early work, first try

Followed by the election area to build a new hospital, about 2-3 years later, it can be fully carried out the work

(1) to build the hospital of the full prevention and treatment with innovative molecular tumor

1 2 11 12

3 4 13 14

5 6 15 16

7 8 17 18

9 10 19 20

First rent two builds with 6-storey floors to have enough parking spaces

1st floor outpatient high risk group physical examination

2 floor clinics rent three years a year to pay a year rent

3rd floor outpatient clinic

4th floor three early

5 floor three early, precancerous lesions

6 floor office, laboratory, school group

Gradually selecting the sites to build a new hospital and there must have enough parking spaces

500-1000 beds, facing the world

Please 1-2 retired Chief Executive Officer, the office director to preside over the preparatory work.

Contents:

- the branch with the prevention of cancer and the control Ca Branch, three early outpatient, three early wards, precancerous lesions ... ... and so on
- the establishment of multidisciplinary related groups and laboratories
- Each equipment and the instruction of physical exam and screening (all of the equipments merge with the United States)
- The study project of the prevention of the cancer, three early, precancerous lesions protocol is provided by Professor Xu Ze, Xu jie, Chen etc.
- Ask the provincial health committee or a leading cadre of the University of Traditional Chinese Medicine to participate in this comprehensive prevention and control hospital leadership (secretary) and create experience.

Study: three early diagnosis: new reagents, new methods, new technology

Three early treatment: new technology, methods, arrangement prescription

Treatment methods of precancerous lesions and observation methods

The Surgery requirements Quality: the prevention of cancer recurrence and metastasis an cultivation need to start from the surgery, it should attach importance to "Non-tumor technology."

Non-tumor technology research: it is the requirements of international high level; in China there are more patients and it should be more experience in surgery, excellence, each case are preoperative discussion, postoperative discussion, analysis, regular follow-up.

To create:

1, three early study group:

2, Precancerous lesion study group:

3, Cancer metastasis study group:

4, Anti-cancer research group:

5, Cancer Research Group:

6, Intravascular "target" organ treatment group:

The establishment of Global Demonstration Hospital - Prevention, Control and Treatment at the same attention

1, condense wisdom

> **1), condense wisdom, condensetechnology, condense high technology and scientific research and integration (mature experience, technology) and**

condense patents and condense monographs and condense the project topics and condese forward-looking and the exploratory prevention and control and treatment research(Research topics, goals, programs, indicators, outcomes, closely integrated with clinical practice)

(2) the cooperation projects and cooperation issues

Put forward a number of topics proposed from the clinical → after experimental study → back to clinical, to solve practical problems→ improve the quality and level of medical care to benefit the patient.

Raised a number of questions, the subject (three early, precancerous lesions, invasion, transfer). To put forward the extisting question is why? Study why? To solve why? How to do? Thus it will be helping to solve the practical problems of clinical care, improve the quality of medical care.

(3) to Create:

1), Medical Research Group - Medical and Research

A, each case of surgery are discussed the specific requirements, measures, drugs, technology, methods to prevent postoperative recurrence and metastasis and to prevent the complications, excellence;

B, adhere to the rounds of the system, consultation system, preoperative discussion system, postoperative follow-up system

② teaching and research group - teaching research group - teaching and research - training graduate students, students, young doctors

③ the prevention research group-----the prevention and control research group--- the prevention of cancer, cancer control and research should develop the prevention of cancer and cancer control research new areas, new technologies, new industries; should be from the clothing, food, shelter and walking to research the prevention of cancer and to prevent cancer from the big environment and the small environment ; first monitoring, qualitative, quantitative, set the standard, the establishment of multi-project laboratory, the specific methods and measures to prevent cancer.

- emphasis on improving the quality of medical care, good service attitude, layers of responsibility, adhere to the rounds of the system, preoperative discussion system, postoperative discussion system, discussion and consultation system.
- Responsible system, chief physician responsibility system, physician responsibility system at all levels
- Emphasize wholehearted service for the patient, the urgency of the patient, the pain of the patient, the patient as a loved one, care for patients, care for patients, respect for patients
- Bonus is not linked to medication. Reward and medical quality, service attitude linked, medication, prescription, open check not rebate, not linked with the bonus
- Improve the physician's integrity, respected and reverent
- The doctor should be responsible for the words and deeds, and should be respected by the patient and his family
- Every prescription must have a reasonable theoretical basis for each doctor's advice
- nurses should do care, visit the ward, guide patients with medical care, do not engage in the form, to engage in the actual benefit of patients
- To restore the level of medical care in the 1950s, 1960s and 1970s
- Hospital guidelines should be: to improve the quality of medical care, improve service attitude, to help patients recover
- To restore the physician's rounds at all levels, to fulfill the duties of physicians at all levels.

The chief physician should solve the problem that the deputy chief physician can not solve.

Deputy chief physician to solve the problem that the attending physician can not solve.

The attending physician should solve the problem that the resident can not solve.

- The department should have the medical routine of the undergraduate course, so that the technology has rules to follow.
- Section director should set the routine, grasp the regular (Section director is the technical director, not only the executive director, should grasp the medical, teaching, research).
- Doctors have a learning system to continuously improve their academic level, technical level and level of diagnosis and treatment
- Have academic reporting system, medical record discussion system, in short, should pay attention to medical quality, service attitude, academic improvement.

"To build the hospital with the innovative molecular tumor full prevention and treatment"

To build the hospital of the prevention and treatment of cancer during the whole process of the development and occurrence ------ the global demonstration hospital with cancer prevention and treatment

- Selecting the Location of the new hospital

1, The bases: according to the prevention and treatment of cancer, the strategic thinking of the prevention and treatment of cancer during the whole process of the cancer occurrence and development it is to build a new type of tumor prevention and treatment hospital.

2, the method: change the contents of the cancer treatment reform, innovation and development in the third monograph "cancer treatment of new concepts and new methods" into clinical practice; into the implementation in the majority of cancer patients who can benefit. It is the establishment of transformation of medicine and the research and development work group and the establishment of the transformation of medical center and medical is benevolence and the legislation is for the first.

3, the planning:

(1) size

① the number of beds prepared

The first stage (1-3 years) 100-300 beds

The second stage (3 years -) 500 beds

The third stage of 1000 beds, facing the world

② the coverage of an area of 15000m2 30000m2 45000m2

(300 beds) (500 beds) (1000 beds)

Have enough parking spaces

(2) the personnel and departments: staffing: medical, nursing, medical technology, prevention, control personnel

① Outpatient first outpatient second outpatient third clinic

(Specialist characteristics) (specialist focus) (specialist characteristics) (remote outpatient service)

② ward (40 beds per ward)

③ departments are senior professors and academic academic leaders responsible for the technology should be the domestic first-class

Department of internal medicine, surgery, gynecology, three early, anti-cancer, cancer control, precancerous lesions, radiation diagnosis,

Ultrasound, electrocardiogram, chamber chamber, operating room, pathology room ...

Immunology and Cancer Research Group and Laboratory

Virus and cancer research group and laboratory

Endocrine hormone and cancer research group and laboratory

Fungi and Cancer Research Group and Laboratory

Environmental and Cancer Research Group and Experiment

Three early study group and laboratory

Precancerous lesion research group and laboratory

④ hospital departments set up, set the following multi-disciplinary testing:

A, immunology and cancer discipline

B, molecular biology, cytokines and cancer disciplines

C, virus and cancer discipline

D, endocrine hormones and cancer disciplines

E, fungi and cancer disciplines

F, tumor marker detection, angiogenesis factor detection

G, trace element detection

H, coagulation factor and blood viscosity, blood rheology, thrombosis, anti-tumor bolt test

I, endoscopic examination

J, Ca Cell culture and chemotherapy sensitivity test

K, pathology + immunohistochemistry

L, gene detection

M, carcinogens monitoring

We build an innovative molecular tumor full anti-hospital, is the overall strategy of cancer treatment reform to focus on the treatment of prevention and treatment.

After Professor Xu Ze experienced 28 years of the camcer basic and clinical research, it was deeply understood: to achieve the purpose of prevention and control of cancer must start the total attack, that is, the prevention cancer + control cancer + cancer treatment three stages of work imultaneously; three Driving goes hand in hand in order to achieve lower morbidity, improve the cure rate, reduce mortality, prolong survival. If it is only treatment, or heavy treatment and the light defense, it will never be able to overcome cancer. Because it can not reduce the incidence, the more treatment and the more patients.

We have to build "the hospital with the innovative molecular tumor prevention and treatment" is to overcome the cancer to start the overall clinical practice and the prevention of cancer + control cancer + treatment cancer at the same levle, to cxplore a large number of three early diagnosis and treatment, technology, medicine, basic theory of the experiment and new research, to find out new drugs, new technologies, new theories, to find out the new technologies, new drugs, new methods, new methods, new techniques, new theories of the treatment of precancerous lesions. With the current advanced imaging and morphological diagnostic techniques CT, MRI, B sound, etc, once the cancer is diagnosed, it is already in the late, it is difficult for three early diagnosis and treatment. Professor Xu Ze proposed to attack the cancer and launch a total attack which is unprecedented in human work, must create their own experience, must practice in person. This is a new cement road and every step will leave the eternal scientific footprints. Therefore, I suggest that a provincial health and health committee of the Office of cadres as a hospital leadership during the whole tumor prevention and treatment to create experience.

To apply for the preparation of a XuZe plan as shown in the new model of the hospital of the prevention and treatment of cancer during the whole process of the occurrence and development which is unlike now to the invasion of the main model of the hospital. This new type of prevention and treatment of hospital is in close connection with clinical practice and aims for the current problems and shortcomings of the traditional therapy to put forward a series of initiatives and the reform and development and to change in the current global setting up the hospital model with the attention treatment and ignorance of the prevention of the caner.

Anti-cancer out of the way is in the prevention of cancer; the treatment out of the way is in the three early, so it may reduce the incidence of cancer, improve cancer cure rate, prolong survival.

Why is it "to build a global demonstration hospital of the prevention and treatment during the whole process of the occurrence and the development of cancer "?

Because in the current in the global and China the cancer hospital or hospital of the Department of oncology are all the hospital treatment model.

① treatment of objectives: the patients are invasive period, the late patients.

② diagnostic methods: are CT, MRI, B super ... ... and other advanced technology imaging and morphological footprints; it should have a certain volume, physical, shape in order to show the size of the occupancy; if there is no size of the volume of the entity, the imaging X film can not be shown. Therefore, in the current it is considered that less than 5cm of liver cancer is as "small liver cancer." Therefore, CT, MRI, B sound, although very advanced technology, but once cancer is diagnosed, that is, it is in the late and can not be found early. We must try to study the new technologies of the "three early" diagnosis and treatment.

③ the hospital mode: are the treatment of hospitals with the heavy treatment and light defense, or only treatment .

④ the hospital mode reform: should be changed to the prevention and control and treatment at the same level and attention.

⑤ the way out of cancer treatment is the "three early": must study the new technologies and the new methods of three early diagnosis and treatment.

Table:

	XZ-C put forward to the hospital model the current global tumor hospital (treatment with the prevention Hospital) and treatment During the whole process of cancer occurrence and development	the current global tumor hospital (treatment Hospital)
hospital mode	prevention+control+ treatment	only the attention of treatment without prevention or ignore defense
The goal or Target	the whole process of occurrence and development	mostly invasive stage or middle and late stage
The objective	three early, precancerous lesions	CT, MRI,B sound(location and occupany
skills of diagnosis	foci cancer needs to be studies	
Treatment	biology treatment and immune Treatment and different induction and surgery treatment and Chinese medication, the combination Of the Chinese and western medications, Laser	surgery radiotherapy and chemotherapy
The expected Results	can be cured	can not be cured, just ease, in the relief of 4-6 weeks above, then development and metastasis and invasion again
The expected goal	decreasing the cancer incidence rate Increasing the cancer cure rate Can conquer cancer	can not decrease the cancer incidence rate; the more treatment and the more Patients; can not conquer cancer

As mentioned above, the overall strategic of the reform of cancer treatment should shift the emphasis on treatment to both prevention and treatment.

Why is it proposed to build the hospital of the prevention and treatment of cancer during the whole process of the occurrence and development?

The following is a brief description of the whole process of the the occurrence and development of cancer; it is to clarify the necessity and feasibility of the prevention and treatment during whole process

Cancer's production and growth will go through stage of susceptibility, precancerous lesion and invasive stage. All the present tumor hospitals or tumor departments mainly focus on the cancer treatment in middle or advanced stage. The Therapeutic effects are poor. If patients in middle or advanced stage can accept surgical operation, then they will be treated surgically. But if not, they will only receive palliative treatment. Therefore, cancer treatment lies in "early detection, early diagnosis and early treatment". Generally, patients in the early stage will get a better therapeutic effect. The increase of therapeutic effect will certainly reduce the fatality rate of cancer. Consequently, we must put much emphasis on the study of early-stage diagnostic and therapeutic methods, and on the treatment of precancerous lesion for lessening medium-term or terminal patients in the invasive stage.

Occupying lesion can be seen through CT or MRI, middle or advanced stage

stage of susceptibility	precancerous lesion	early stage	no metastasis	have metastasized	
				local position	amphi position
①	②	③	④	⑤	⑥

① Cancer prevention

② Outpatient service of "three kinds of earliness"

③ Surgical operation

④ Place surgical operation first, radiotherapy, chemotherapy and biological TCM second

⑤ Possible to undergo surgical operation

⑥ To give treatment as carcinomatous metastasis

If patients have been treated well in the stage of precancerous lesion or early stage, then the number of patients in middle or advanced stage of invasion and metastasis will fall off. Thus, the cancer incidence rate will also decline. Therefore, we hold that the present tumor hospitals in various places mainly focus on the cancer treatment in middle or advanced stage. Even though the therapeutic result is effective, it can only bring the reduction of cancer mortality rate. But if ignoring the stage of susceptibility, precancerous lesion or early stage, it will be impossible to reduce the cancer incidence rate. Therefore, we must put much emphasis on the whole process of cancer production and growth. After all this is the real global change of strategic importance.

The writer has engaged in surgical oncology for over fifty years. More and more patients suffer from cancer, and the cancer incidence rate also rises. The writer deeply feels that people should emphasize not only therapy but also prevention. Only in this way could the cancer be killed in the source. Cancer treatment lies in "three kinds of earliness" (early detection, early diagnosis and early treatment); anti-cancer method lies in prevention.

As stated above, the strategic center of gravity of tumor treatment and prevention moves forward. There are two aspects in its meaning. One is to prevent cancer by changing life style and improving environmental pollution; the other is to cure precancerous lesion for inhibiting cancer's development to the invasion stage, middle stage or advanced stage.

In 1990, our institute's specialist out-patient department of tumor surgery once opened the outpatient service of "three kinds of earliness" to carry out various endoscopies and biopsies, through which have found many atypical hyperplasia of stomach, intestinal metaplasia, atrophic gastritis and hyperplasia of mammary glands, etc. These "precancerous lesions" are difficult to treat.

Then how to handle these precancerous lesions or precancerous conditions so as to prevent their cancerations urgently needs clinical researches to look for better treatment methods.

Put emphasis on fundamental and clinical researches of precancerous lesions with diagnosis and treatment techniques.

"Three kinds of earliness" is the key to cancer treatment. While how to handle precancerous lesion is the key stage for cancer prevention and treatment.

The present cancer diagnosis mainly depends on image examinations of type-B ultrasonic, CT and MRI. But as soon as the cancer comes to light, it has reached the middle or advanced stage. Many patients have lost the chance of radical excision. Although the complex treatment has been done, the therapeutic effects are still poor. If the cancer is in the early stage or belongs to the carcinoma in situ, then the curative effect of operation will be better and the cancer can be cured. Therefore, the cancer treatment should strive for "three kinds of earliness", which refers to early detection, early diagnosis and early treatment.

Because cancer's pathogenic factors are not very clear, the primary prevention is still quite difficult.

Studies in recent years indicate that malignant tumor rarely has a direct carcinomatous change in normal tissues. Before the occurrence of tumor in clinical diagnosis, cancer often goes through quite a long evolution stage, which is the stage of precancerous lesion. Early identification and control of these precancerous lesions will bring positive significances for the secondary prevention of cancer.

What is precancerous lesion? The precancerous lesion is a histopathology concept, which refers to a kind of tissues with the dysplasia of cells. Precancerous lesion has the potential to become cancerous. If there is no cure in a long period, precancerous lesion will evolve into cancer. In other words, precancerous lesion just has the possibility of changing into cancer. But not all the precancerous lesions will eventually become cancer. Through proper treatments, precancerous lesions may return to their normal states or have a spontaneous regression.

Canceration is a developing process with several stages. There is a stage of precancerous lesion between normal cells and cancer. It is a slow process from precancerous lesion evolving into cancer, which needs many years or even more than ten years. The length of canceration course is closely related to the strength of carcinogenic factors, individual susceptibility and immunologic function. Therefore, the study of precancerous lesion is of great importance to cancer's prevention and control.

More than one third of cancers can be prevented.

The tumor formation is a long process with several factors and stages. Precancerous lesion is of reversibility, so cancer is preventable.

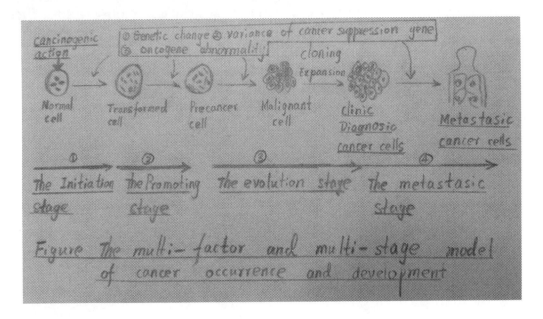

Figure 1 Multi-factor multi-stage model of tumorigenesis

Early primary cancer growth

In the initial stage of primary cancer, the growth of tumor cells is provided by the infiltration of microenvironment through the adjacent tissues and organs. This stage of the tumor diameter is generally not more than 1 ~ 2mm. The number of tumor cells does not exceed 10^7, pathologically known as carcinoma in situ. Clinically it is reported more that there are the cervical carcinoma in situ, esophageal carcinoma in situ, stomach in situ cancer. Carcinoma In situ have the good prognosis after surgery or endoscopic resection.

The development and occurrence of the tumor experience the susceptibility stage, precancerous lesions and invasive stage, and our current treatment is mainly concentrated in the invasive stage, that is, advanced stage of cancer. This situation, from the perspective of conquering the tumor, is still at the primary level. The ultimate goal of human control of the tumor should not be in the late stage, the future will move from the late stage of the tumor to the early, precancerous lesions or even susceptible stage. This is also consistent with the strategy of "China's long-term scientific and technological development plan (2006-2020)" proposed "disease prevention and treatment center of gravity forward" strategy.

5-year survival rate of cancer of the status quo is still hovering at a low level in the present in the global

It can be said that today's clinicians in the clinical treatment of cancer options and methods available more and more. But we have to face a reality, a large number of clinical epidemiological analysis shows that the diagnosis and treatment of the ability and means of maturation and development, and the overall effect of tumor improvement seems not fully synchronized. According to the American Cancer Society (The American Cancer Society) data (Figure), nearly a decade, a variety of malignancy diagnosis and treatment level than in the past has been greatly improved, but its 5-year survival rate is still hovering in a Lower level. Such as the 2004 global colon cancer 5-year survival rate of 62%, although the colon cancer diagnostic techniques and surgical treatment has made considerable progress, but only increased to 65%, did not make a breakthrough. Liver cancer etiology, epidemiological studies and a variety of treatment techniques have been greatly improved, but the current 5-year survival rate of only 18%, 10 years ago, only increased by 11 percentage points, how to improve the prognosis of patients is still troubled Hepatobiliary surgeon's problem. The mortality rate of gastric cancer has been high, although the level of surgical technology continues to improve, but the 5-year survival rate of gastric cancer from only 10 years ago, 23% to 29%. In addition, the 5-year survival rate of pancreatic cancer than 10 years ago little change in the 5% up and down; esophageal cancer 5-year survival rate has been maintained at 14%; breast cancer 5-year survival rate from 10 years ago, 87% Down to the current 79%, cervical cancer from 71% to 69%, lung cancer 5-year survival rate from 15% to the current 14%.

The Comparison of 5 - year Survival Rate in Global Malignant Tumor is the following:

At present, most clinicians are more concerned about the specific treatment of cancer and treatment technology research and research, surgery can be bigger and bigger, the treatment program can also be more and more complex, but the lack of cancer etiology of the fundamental means of treatment is a Objective reality.

The diagnosis of cancer is mainly by CT, B ultrasound imaging can only be diagnosed, but once found in the late, many patients have lost the chance of radical resection, although the comprehensive treatment, the effect is still very poor, if Can improve early diagnosis, early cancer or carcinoma in situ, the surgical treatment is effective, can be cured.

Therefore, the treatment of cancer in the early three early, early detection, early diagnosis, early treatment, the prognosis is good.

The stage of applying and preparing the science city (the medicine and the teaching and the research and the development) of conquering cancer

(1) Why is it I to become the total designer, the President, the Chairman of the General Academic Committee of the "Science Center for Cancer Science"? Because all of these total basic assumptions and basic design are put forward by me. Each department (medical school, research institute, hospital, experimental

center) is my basic ideas and design and planning and blueprint. I put the purpose, the goal, the task, the method, the step, the scientific research route, the scientific thought, and the preliminary development of the mission of the Science City; I will design the president, the common dean, executive dean, executive president and vice president and the task, responsibility and the division of labor clearly and the implementation of their duties; to do their duty, to build. The goal is to achieve results and produce the achievement, unified arrangements and the unified deployment.

How is this scientific research ship of "the Science City of overcoming the Cancer" operated?how is it to operate these small ship such as Target, course, task, destination? how to plan a boat? It must be clear the goal to achieve the purpose of conception of cancer and it must be coordinated and be the collaboration; the goals are consistent to overcome the cancer and to launch a total attack.

(2) Wuhan anti-cancer research teams of overcoming cancer are the research team which is the old, middle and green combination

① old: more than 65 years old, 70 years of age, 80 or more for the older generation has more than 40 years of rich clinical experience, teaching, research are experienced; ②: 55-65 years old, more than 30 years of mature clinical experience; ③Green: 35-55 years old, with momentum, energy, enthusiasm, is the main, is the focus, you can further development, development, innovation.

(3) New China's medical creation and development are developed by our own.

After the liberation of 1949, the new Chinese medicine is poor and white. At that time surgery is only to do hernia, hemorrhoids, anal leakage … … and other surgery. In 1951, Peking Union Hospital, Professor Guan Hanping performed subtotal gastrectomy, the city's surgeon visit. After the liberation of 20 years there was no connection with and the United States, Britain, France and other diplomatic relations and it could not study and visit from other countries and no English magazines, books; it all relied on our own self-reliance development and relied on the clinic work after the success in the animal experiments. The Chinese are smart and hard. **In the 1970s, China achieved many major medical results. In the 60 - 70 years China put a lot of medical satellites and created a medical miracle. Shanghai Ruijin Hospital saved the Qiu Kokang 85% of the area of three burns; Shanghai six hospital had the arm recovery success; the artificial insulin synthesis had the success; Tianjin General Hospital has the half cycle; in Beijing, Xi'an, Nanjing, Henan Anyang cardiopulmonary bypass had been applied in clinics after the animal experiments; In Shanghai Ruijin, Wuhan Tongji liver transplantation was applied for the clinics after the animal experiments ... ... are shocked the world. Chinese people can create miracles in medicine. Go their own way, others have already and we have to learn and have to have; others do not have and we should create our own characteristics or advantages and it should be combined with innovation, and international medicine modernization and strive to take our own characteristics of independent innovation path, promote the 21st century and the new development of modern oncology.**

(4) why do I study cancer? I am a clinical surgeon. As a general and chest work, why do I study cancer and propose to launch a total attack and to build "the science city of overcoming cancer ", it is because:

① in 1985 I conducted the petition on 3000 cases of thoracic and abdominal cancer patients which I operated by my own, the results are found that most patients were the recurrence or metastasis within 2-3 years. Therefore, we must study the prevention of postoperative recurrence and metastasis methods to improve postoperative long-term efficacy.

② I suddenly had acute myocardial infarction in 1991. After the treatment was improved and it was the recovery, I should not be on the operating table and was to calm down and hid in the small building to concentrate on scientific research.

③ through experimental studies it was found that thymus atrophy and immune dysfunction are one of the etiology and pathogenesis of cancer and it needed to expand and in-depth study.

④ through experimental research and clinical validation, after 28 years of more than 12,000 cases of clinical validation observation, we found the new road of the modernization of Chinese medication in the molecular level of the combination of the Chinese and Western medication with this innovative "Chinese-style anti-cancer" and the new road of Chinese medication immunoregulation to prevent thymic atrophy, promote thymic hyperplasia, protect bone marrow hematopoietic function, improve immune surveillance at the molecular level of combination of Chinese and western medication to overcome cancer so that it persisted and continued to study. Therefore, it is proposed to overcome the cancer to launch a total attack, to build the "Science City" of conquering cancer to overcome cancer in an attempt to achieve: reduce the incidence of cancer; improve cancer cure rate; extend the survival of cancer patients; to reach "three early" (early detection, early diagnosis, early Treatment), early can be cured. To achieve the prevention and control and treatment at the same attention . Both Prevention and treatment can overcome the cancer, reduce the incidence of cancer.

All basic research must work for clinical and improve patient efficacy so that patients benefit. The evaluation criteria for the efficacy of cancer patients should be:

① live a long time, extended survival

② good quality of life

③ no complications - to reduce complications, and even no complications

Of course, to overcome the cancer is just one of the road, there may have a vaccine, gene targeting ... ... and other roads to be explored and researched.

Through the research of the prevention and treatment and cancer prevention and control and treatment at the same attention, human beings will overcome cancer, and ultimately will overcome cancer.

It is to avoid empty talk and to pay attention to the heavy hard work and to start to go. No matter how far away the cancer path is, it always should go. Wanli Long March always go, thousands of miles began with a single step.

1, Why should we build a prevention and control and treatment demonstration hospital?

The purpose is:

① change the hospital mode

To Change from paying attention to heavy treatment and ignoring the defense into prevention +control+ treatment at the same attention

② change the treatment mode

- from only treating the middle and late and metastasis and severe ---- poor efficacy, more complications.
- to focus on "three early" precancerous lesions, in situ cancer ----the effect is well and it can be cured

③ change the drug burden

- Late stage, aggressive, metastatic, severe, radiotherapy, chemotherapy, targeted drugs - ---- the cost is high and it used the expensive medications
- Early stage, precancerous lesions, carcinoma in situ, polyps------ it needs the minor surgery + immune regulation or differentiation induction, traditional Chinese medicine, less money, no need to have radiotherapy and chemotherapy, reduce the burden on patients and the state.

The aims:

① **The way out of cancer treatment is the "three early"**

Anti-cancer out of the way is in the prevention

② the target of the prevention of cancer and anti-cancer and the evaluation criteria are:

To Reduce morbidity, reduce mortality, prolong survival, improve quality of life, reduce complications

③ **What is the results of the treatment of cancer patients? It usually considered to be:**

Patients with long survival time, good quality of life, fewer complications.

2, why should it build the new hospital and the existing top three hospital can not be used?

Because:

① **The new hospital mode is the hospital model which the mode has been changed.**

The prevention and + control+ treatment at the same lever

To Focus on three early, precancerous lesions, carcinoma in situ, polyps … … and so on

The hospitals can not think of making money as the goal and it should mainly be for the service and public welfare.

The Hospital income is greatly reduced.

② due to focus on three early, precancerous lesions, carcinoma in situ, polyps ... ... and so on, It only needs to have the small surgery, endoscopy ... ... immunotherapy, differentiation induction therapy, Chinese and Western treatment ... ... and so on

Then, the radiotherapy and chemotherapy are not used or greatly reduced.

Because it is early, PET / CT ... ... and so n do not have been used or greatly reduced; CT, MRI greatly will be reduced.

Hospital income is greatly reduced, patients and countries are greatly reduced economic load

③ For reducing the hospital income, it can be added by improving the diagnosis and treatment fees and the testing technical fees and the surgery costs, etc.

So it is to try a new demonstration hospital to achieve early diagnosis, early treatment and the combination of prevention and control ad treatment to improve efficacy, prolong survival, improve quality of life, reduce complications, reduce medical costs, reduce patients and Health insurance costs, reduce the severity of patients (because of early detection, early treatment, good effect); due to the good efficacy the doctor-patient relationship is good too.

Seven. XZ-C proposed how to overcome the cancer I see four:

How to overcome cancer? To overcome cancer, it must create "the experimental medicine cancer animal experimental center"

- to overcome the cancer, to build "the science city of overcoming the cancer and launch a total attack" one

(1) Why creates a "Experimental Medicine Cancer Animal Experimental Center"?

① in order to overcome cancer → conquest cancer → capture cancer, we must first understand the basic understanding of cancer: the cause of cancer, pathogenesis, pathophysiology, immunopathology, cancer cell biological behavior? Transfer mechanism? Why is it implanted and does it grow? The Recurrence mechanism? A series of oncology and tumor-related issues have not yet clear, oncology for scientific research is a virgin land and it needs to be a lot of basic scientific research and clinical basic research. To carry out the basic research of cancer science is the urgent need of the current oncology discipline.

Therefore, we must establish "the experimental medicine cancer animal experimental center".

② to carry out the basic research of oncology, a good laboratory is the key. The scientific design, scientific vision, must be finished through laboratory experiments in order to draw conclusions and the results.

We believe that the establishment of the scientific basis(Science City) for the development of launching the total attack must first vigorously build the laboratory, so that many basic problems have experimental research, open up the basis of tumor research, should encourage the development of new areas of research and produce the talent and the results to help capturing cancer.

③ to overcome the cancer and to launch a total attack and to build experimental medical cancer animal experimental center, the good equipment laboratory is the key.

For the study of the new drugs of the prevention of cancer and anti-metastasis it must do the nude mice animal model experimental study. The Experimental surgery is extremely important in the development of medicine and it is a key to open the medical closed area, many diseases prevention and treatment method is applied to the clinical after in many animal experiments it achieved the results of stability and promote the development of medical career .

How can technology have the innovation? How can we overcome cancer? A good laboratory should be built.

Therefore, the development of science, scientific and technological innovation and the production of the result and the patent, the laboratory is a key condition.

How to carry out basic research on cancer? How to develop new research areas of cancer?

How can the original innovation of cancer research be done? A good laboratory should be established.

(2) how to set up "the experimental medicine cancer animal experimental center"?

The Experimental animal experimental center should not be located in the city center and downtown and it can be located in the suburbs and the University City.

Location: to be in the University City Huangjia Lake

Animal buildings should be closed to the veranda, surrounded by isolation and it should be met to national laboratory requirements management.

The "Science City" total design blueprint

Of overcoming the cancer and launch a total attack

The preparation work of "Science City" one

How to overcome cancer? To overcome the cancer, it must be founded "experimental medicine cancer animal experimental center"

To overcome the cancer, to build "Science City" one

How to create "experimental medicine cancer animal experimental center"? The detail plan will be published in the future.

Xu Ze (XU ZE) Professor proposed:

- To study the study of cancer etiology, pathogenesis, recurrence, metastasis mechanism must be carried out experimental laboratory experiments.
- In order to study and carry out effective measures to control invasion, recurrence and metastasis, it is necessary to carry out experimental experimental animal experiments.
- In order to find new anti-cancer, anti-metastasis and anti-recurrence of new drugs from natural medicine, it is necessary to carry out experimental experimental study of experimental medicine, manufacture of animal model of cancer, and to carry out the experimental study on the inhibition rate of Chinese herbal medicine in vivo.
- How do you conduct basic research? How to open up new research areas? How can the original innovation results? Should be built well laboratory.
- How can technology be innovated? How can we overcome cancer? It is key to establish a good laboratory.
- "Science City" of the Institute of Innovative Oncology; Innovation Cancer Institute; innovative tumor prevention and treatment of the hospital, should be based on their own training personnel, the key is to build a good equipment laboratory. I am deeply aware of the importance of the laboratory.

Based on their own training personnel, the key is to build a good equipment laboratory. I am deeply aware of the importance of the laboratory, I was the first batch of college students after the liberation of college students, I did not study, did not study, but I made a number of international level results, the key is that I have a good laboratory, I participated in the era of extracorporeal circulation animal laboratory, 80 years I established a cirrhosis of the liver laboratory, the early 90s I established the Institute of Experimental Surgery, to capture the main direction of cancer, my animal laboratory, equipment conditions are better Mice, rats, rabbits, rabbits, dogs, monkeys and other animal experiments, a better animal aseptic operating room, can be a dog's chest, abdomen, a variety of major surgery, and animal observation after the ward, Design, design, through the experimental operation, to achieve results or conclusions.

Therefore, the laboratory is a key condition, if there is no laboratory through the experiment, can only design, imagine, can not become a factual result.

Eight, XZ-C how to overcome the cancer I see six:

How to overcome cancer? To overcome the cancer, we must create "innovative molecular tumor nano-pharmaceutical factory" and "to build the research group and laboratory of researching anti-cancer, anti-cancer transfer active ingredients, molecular weight, structural formula, immunopharmacology, molecular level analysis"

(1) Why should founder the innovative molecular tumor nano-pharmaceutical companies and anti-cancer, anti-cancer transfer active ingredients, Chinese medication immunopharmacology research group?

Because to conquer cancer must study and develop the new and effective drugs of anti-cancer and anti-cancer metastasis. XZ-C thinks of that to capture cancer must have two wheels, one is life science, biomedical (modern medicine) and it A wheel ; one is the clinical basis, immune Regulation, anti-cancer bolt (Chinese herbal medicine) and it is B wheel.

Its purpose is: in-depth development of Chinese herbal medications of anti-cancer, anti-cancer transfer which is indeed effective drugs to coarse storage fine and the natural medicine herbs are as the resources and conduct the modern research to become precision medicine.

To further study the anti - cancer Chinese regulation and control immune medication at the molecular levels .

To further explore the anti - cancer anti - cancer Chinese herbal medications on early in situ carcinoma and precancerous lesions.

(2) how to set up innovative tumor nano-pharmaceutical companies and Chinese herbal active ingredients analysis group and laboratory?

The experimental surgery is extremely important in the development of medicine, it is a key to open the medical closed area, many disease prevention and control methods are applied to the clinical after in the several animal experimental research, it achieved a stable effect and it is to promote the development of medical career.

Therefore, In order to have the development of science, science and technology innovation, the laboratory is the key condition. To be Self-reliance and to train our own innovative talents! the laboratory is a key condition.

To build the analytical research group and laboratory of anti-cancer and anti-transfer active ingredients of traditional Chinese medication

The aims:

(1) to further develop the molecular level experimental and clinical research and clinical application of XZ-C immunoregulation anti-cancer traditional Chinese medication cytokines.

(2) to further explore the anti-cancer anti-cancer Chinese herbal medication on early in situ carcinoma and precancerous lesions prevention and treatment and clinical application

The purpose:

In-depth study of Chinese herbal medication anti-cancer, anti-cancer transfer is indeed effective drugs, to coarse deposit, to become the precision medications.

It is as the natural medication herbs for the resources and conduct the modernization research so that it becomes the precision medications.

The methods and the steps:

(1) animal experiments: a, in vitro experimental screening

b, in vivo experimental screening

(2) the molecular level experimental study:

The Induction of anticancer lesions differentiation

The anti – cancer and anti - cancer metastasis Chinese herbal medication screening

(3) the gene level experimental study of anti – cancer and anti - cancer transfer Chinese herbal medication screening

The topic selection and the material selection: it first selects from the clinical application of effective Chinese herbal medication for further study and first it is to isolate the active ingredients.

The laboratory:

(1) Equipment: Equipment for drug composition analysis

(2) the personnel: the scientific and technological personnel to preside over the analysis of drug ingredients .

(3) The topic selection and the material selection

(4) The expected results

XZ-C proposed that for 30 years we carried out the following series of research work during the process of developing XZ-C immunoregulation anti-cancer Chinese herbal medications:

(1) in the exploration of the experimental study of the mechanism of cancer incidence and invasion and recurrence and metastasis mechanism:

From our laboratory experimental results it was found that: in the cancer-bearing mice the thymus was atrophic atrophy and volume reduction; the cell proliferation was blocked,; the mature cells decreased. To the late stage of the tumor, the thymus was extremely atrophic and the texture becomes harder.

From the above experimental study it was found that thymus atrophy and immune dysfunction may be one of the pathogenesis and pathogenesis of the tumor, it must try to prevent thymic atrophy, promote thymocyte proliferation, increased immune function . It should seek immune regulation methods and effective drug research from the body's immune function, especially cellular immunity, T lymphocyte function and thymus immune regulation function and explore at the molecular level.

It should further study to find the new ways of cancer treatment and the new methods from the thymus function and tissue structure, immune dysfunction and how to promote immune function so that the immune function can be the reconstructed and how to "protecting the thymus and increasing the immune function".

(2) the new drugs experimental study from the natural medications to find and to screen the anti-cancer and anti-metastasis

In our laboratory it was conducted the following the screening tests of the new anti-cancer and anti-metastatic drugs from traditional Chinese medications:

(1), the use of cancer cells in vitro culture method to conduct the screening experimental study of the Chinese herbal medication inhibition rate:

In vitro screening test: the use of cancer cells in vitro culture to observe the direct damage to cancer cells.

The screening test in the tube: in the culture of cancer cells in the test tube, were placed crude crude drug (500ug / ml), to observe whether the inhibition of cancer cells, we will be traditional Chinese medicine that anti-cancer effect of 200 kinds of Chinese herbal medicine, In vitro screening test. And under normal conditions with normal fibroblasts, test the toxicity of the drug to this cell, and then compared.

(2) Building cancer-bearing animal model for the screening of the tumor inhibition rate of Chinese herbs in the cancer-bearing animal experiments

The inhibition test in vivo screening test: each batch experiments with mice 240, divided into 8 groups, each group 30, the first group was the control group 7, group 8 with 5-Fu or CTX control group, the whole group of small mice was inoculated with EA C or S 180 or H22 cancer cells. After inoculation 24h, each rat was oral fed the crude product of crude drug powder, long-term feeding the screened herbs, observed survival, toxicity and observed the the survival rate and calculated the inhibition rates.

So, we conducted experimental study for four consecutive years, and has conducted a 3-year incidence of tumor-bearing mice and transfer mechanism, the experimental study of the mechanism of relapse, and experimental studies to explore how cancer causing death of the host each year with more than 1,000 tumor-bearing animals model, made a total of nearly four years, 6000 tumor-bearing animal models, mice each were carried out after the death of the liver, spleen, lung, thymus, kidney pathological anatomy, a total of 20,000 times slice to explore to find out whether There may be slight carcinogenic pathogens, with microcirculation microscope 100 tumor-bearing mice were tumor microvessels bell establish and microcirculation.

Results: In our laboratory animal experiments screened 200 kinds of Chinese herbs and screened48 kinds of certain and excellent herbs with inhibition of cancer cell proliferation, inhibition rate of more than 75 to 90%. But there are some of commonly used Chinese medicine which consider to have the anticancer roles, after animal in vitro and in vivo inhibition rate anti-cancer screening, showed really no effect, or little effect which 152 kinds of medications having no anti-cancer effect had removed from the phase-out of animal experiments.

It was screening out of the real 48 kinds of traditional Chinese medications with having good tumor suppression rates, and then it optimized the combination and repeated tumor inhibition rate experiments in vivo, and finally developed immunomodulatory anticancer Chinese medication XU ZE China1-10 with Chinese own characteristics China (ZC $_{1-10}$).

Z-C$_1$ could inhibit cancer cells, but does not affect normal cells; Z-C$_4$ specially can increase thymus function, can promote proliferation, increased immunity; Z-C$_1$ can protect bone marrow function and to product more blood.

The Clinical validation: Based on the success of animal experiments, clinical validation was conducted. Namely the establishment of oncology clinics and Western medicine combined with anti-cancer, anti-metastasis, recurrence Research Group, retained patient medical records, to establish a regular follow-up observation system to observe the long-term effect · face from experimental research to clinical evidence, the discovery of new clinical validation process issue, went back to the laboratory for basical research, then the results of a new experiment for clinical validation. Thus, a clinical experiment again and again clinical experiment, all experimental studies must be clinically proven in a large number of patients observed 3--5 years, or even clinical observation of 8 to 10 years, according to evidence-based medicine, and can have long-term follow-up assessment information, verified indeed have a good long-term efficacy, the efficacy of the standard is: a good quality of life, longer survival. XZ-C sectional immune regulation anti-cancer medication had been verification after these were applied for 30 years in the more than 2000 of the advanced cancer patients and achieved remarkable results. XZ-C sectional immune regulation anti-cancer medicine can improve the quality of life of patients with advanced cancer, enhance immune function, increase the body's anticancer abilities, increased appetite and significantly prolong survival.

Now is the fourth stage of our research work, is carrying out and carry out research work, step by step, the research goal or "target" located in the anti-control, governance and focus on the study of "three early" and "precancerous lesions Study on the Prevention and Treatment of Early Cancer and Precancerous Lesions of Chinese Herbal Medicine for Cancer Prevention and Control and Its Clinical Application.

The exclusive research and development products: XZ-C immunoregulation anti-cancer traditional Chinese medicine products (Introduction)

(see attached)

12, the preparation for the publication work: the prevention of the cancer and anti-cancer:

Wuhan Anti-Cancer Research Association will publish the following publications and monographs

1, to popular the prevention cancer research and the science map.

2, to publish the science books prevention cancer and anti-cancer "mass medicine" quarterly

3, to publish the magazine publication "cancer recurrence, transfer of basic and clinical" bimonthly

4, to publish "Proceedings - cancer treatment innovation" monograph

5, to publish "tumor-free technology" - how to do cancer radical surgery, anti-recurrence, anti-transfer monograph

6, to publish the "three early", "precancerous lesions" publications

7, to publish "from the clothing, food, live, anti-cancer knowledge" publications, quarterly

Note: Xu Ze: Honorary President of Wuhan Anti-Cancer Research Association, Senior Professor of Surgery, Hubei Provincial Hospital of Traditional Chinese Medicine, China • Hubei • Wuhan

Department of Surgery, Affiliated Hospital of Hubei University of Traditional Chinese Medicine

Department of Experimental Surgery, Hubei University of Traditional Chinese Medicine

Mobile: 13871018507 E-mail: xuze88cn@163.com

Nine, XZ-C put forward how to overcome the cancer I see five:

How to overcome cancer? In order to overcome cancer, we must create "the innovative environmental anti-cancer research institute"

- One of the science cities to overcome cancer

(1) Why create an innovative environmental protection institute?

Because: in the current the incidence of cancer is on the rise, which 90% is related to the environment.

The occurrence of cancer is closely related to people's clothing, food, live, walking and living habits.

The current environmental pollution is serious, and the degradation of ecosystems may be related to the increase in cancer incidence.

We have reviewed and reflected 60 years of cancer research work and clinical research and clinical and deeply appreciate the cancer not only to pay attention to treatment, but also to pay attention to prevention; in order to stop at the source, it must do the prevention and treatment at the same time ; the way of out of the anti-cancer is the prevention and the prevention is as the main.

So how to prevent? What is it to prevent? The various environmental carcinogens must be measured, qualitative, targeted, quantified, and sought to remove them.

Therefore, we must establish anti-cancer research institute, should do the prevention research from the clothing, food, shelter, walking and from the big environment and the small environment to the micro, ultra-microscopic anti-cancer research.

How to carry out the prevention cancer research? First of all, it should master and understand the situation of containing carcinogens in the clothing, food, shelter and walking? whether does it contain carcinogens? The qualitative and the quantitative monitoring, and then set the standard, set the bottom line, to discuss and to put forward anti-control measures.

(2) How to set up "the innovative environmental protection cancer research institute"?

The prevention cancer research is a major event and in the current the global does not have anti-cancer research institute. We will apply that in the Science City of overcoming cancer it is to create "the world's first anti-cancer research institute" to do the macro, micro, ultra-microscopic environmental protection carcinogens monitoring and the analysis to implement the anti-cancer system engineering.

How to overcome cancer? To overcome the cancer, we must launch a total attack. The total attack is to carry out the entire work at the three stages: the prevention and control and treatment of cancer during the whole process of the occurrence and development of cancer simultaneously and the prevention and control and treatment of cancer are the same attention and level and it must pay attention to the prevention of cancer. The prevention is the most important. How to prevent? What is it to prevent? How to prevent? As discussed in more detail below. How to overcome cancer? To overcome cancer, it must create "innovative anti-cancer research institute."

With the improvement of people's living standards, a variety of high-tech products bring us a better life ; at the same time it may also bring a lot of negative effects. A variety of chemical, physical, biological environment, a large number of carcinogens, a variety of carcinogenic substances enter into our human body or a variety of carcinogenic factors affect our body, leading to an increasing incidence of cancer.

Look at the current situation: the incidence of cancer in the status quo is more and more patients, the current incidence of cancer in China is 312 million of the new cases of cancer in the annual incidence and the average daily new cancer patients are 8550 cases and in the country every minute there are 6 Diagnosed as cancer.

Now XZ-C proposed the scientific research programs of attacking cancer and launching a total attack; the prevention cancer and anti-control and treatment at the same level and attention and troika and go hand in hand.

So how to prevent? How to control? What is it to prevent? What is it to control? How much is it to prevent? How much is to control? The target or goals of the prevention of cancer or control of cancer must be clear; a variety of environmental carcinogens must be measured and be qualitative and be quantitative and be positioning.

Because cancer is thought to be mainly caused by factors such as the environment, diet, hobby and so on; people will attach great importance to the carcinogenic factors in the environment and strive to clear them.

In order to carry out the prevention of cancer and cancer control work, Professor Xu Ze proposed:

(1) it should prevent cancer from the clothing, food, live, walking and from the big environment and the small environment.

(2) it should set up the following anti-cancer research group, please graduate students to carry out and complete the scientific research work.

Professor Xu Ze, as the chief designer, put forward the following research projects and the topics in order to overcome cancer and it must carry out the following research work:

(1) to understand what needs to be the prevention? What needs to be controlled? How to prevent? How to control? It must be qualitative and be quantitative and be positioning and be monitoring and be clear and be specific data, we must master the first-hand information in order to do the scientific and accurate anti-cancer work, we must attach importance to the accumulation of raw data, as accurate scientific data and experimental anti-cancer in accordance with.

(2) how to achieve this plan and to do his scientific research work? It can be put into the training of graduate students and it can be conducted by the doctoral students, master's degree candidates; it can be both to cultivate the field study of graduate students, but also received anti-cancer, carcinogens qualitative, quantitative analysis and analysis of components, and further propose anti- method.

The Method: by the school graduate students to set up the subject and have the purpose and there are tasks arranged arrangements.

(My graduate students is this case, the tutor general subject is like a table banquet, each graduate student is a small sub-title, as frying a dish, Ph.D is frying a large market and the master students is frying a small dish), so give full play to graduate students, but also cultivate the scientific thinking and the scientific and practical ability of graduate students and products out of the paper and products a talent and product a result.

We must pay attention to scientific and technological papers and it is not written by the pens; however it is come from the scientific and technological work. It is necessary to pay attention to the original information, attention to scientific and technological innovation, attention to advanced, innovative and practical. We must pay attention to scientific research and honesty.

How to prevent cancer from the clothing, food, live and walking? First of all, it should grasp and understand the clothing, food, live, and other crops containing carcinogens; whether it contains carcinogens and the qualitative and the quantitative and the monitoring and then set the standard, set the bottom line, to discuss, put forward the prevention and control measures.

It is proposed to build the following research groups:

(1) The research group: [clothing] clothing, cosmetics and other carcinogens monitoring and prevention and control of cancer:

purpose:

method:

technology:

Equipment conditions:

personnel:

The expected results and achievements: whether there are the carcinogenic substances, qualitative, quantitative, set the bottom line, set the standard micro, ultra-microscopic monitoring;

The analysis and the conclusions: the prevention and control measures are proposed, or it is further to do experiments and to do animal models.

Graduate student (master, Ph.D)

tutor:

(2) [food] food carcinogens monitoring, prevention, control research group → the research Institute

Pickles: pickles, dried salted fish, sausages, mustard, bacon, fermented bean curd, pickles, canned fish ... ... carcinogens content monitoring, qualitative, quantitative micro-research

Fried: ... ... and other carcinogenic content monitoring, the qualitative and the quantitative micro-research

Speculation: ... ... and other carcinogenic content monitoring, qualitative, quantitative micro-research

Smoked: ... ... and other carcinogenic content monitoring, qualitative, quantitative micro-research

Cooking: ... ... and other carcinogenic content monitoring, qualitative, quantitative micro-research

Steaming: ... ... and other carcinogenic content monitoring, qualitative, quantitative micro-research

Smoke stove: ... ... and other carcinogenic content monitoring, qualitative, quantitative micro-research

Leftovers: ... ... and other carcinogenic content monitoring, qualitative, quantitative micro-research

Overnight leftovers: ... ... and other carcinogenic content monitoring, qualitative, quantitative micro-research

Grain: ... ... and other carcinogenic content monitoring, qualitative, quantitative micro-research

Oil: ... ... and other carcinogenic content monitoring, qualitative, quantitative micro-research

Vegetables: ... ... and other carcinogenic content monitoring, qualitative, quantitative micro-research

Mcat: ... ... and other carcinogenic content monitoring, qualitative, quantitative micro-research

Fish: ... ... and other carcinogenic content monitoring, qualitative, quantitative micro-research

The supermarkets sell a variety of food (packaged)

(3) [live]: housing, decoration (painting, paint ...) materials, furniture ... ... carcinogens monitoring and the prevention and control research group

Materials, air, microscopic, ultrastructural carcinogens

Whether the excessive (for several large advertising companies ...)

Trace element determination and monitoring

(4) [line]: automobile exhaust, automotive equipment carcinogens monitoring and the prevention and control research group

Cars, trains and other equipment, air

train:

aircraft:

Battery car

(5) Water, pollution (sewage of various factories, air) carcinogens monitoring and the prevention and control research group

(6) Fertilizer, pesticide, soil grain, genetically modified food, whether carcinogens monitoring and the prevention and control research group

(7) whether the computer and the mobile phone have the role of causing cancer or damage monitoring and the prevention and the control research group

(8) the research group of the monitoring of whether air, air conditioning, hood, ray, radiation, nuclear radiation measurement have the carcinogen and the cancer prevention and control

(9) Chinese food, Western food are together with micro-qualitative, quantitative monitoring whether there are the carcinogenic and the qualitative and the quantitative and the standard

- Objective of the study: To determine whether carcinogens and their contents are available, qualitative, quantitative and standard
- Method: Arrange the doctorate, postgraduate program, project

The primary screening and research is to find the problem → ask questions → research problems → solve the problem

Participants: chefs, nutritionists, mentors, graduate students, cafeteria, hotels, restaurants, snack, hot noodles, powder

The researchers come to the scene to study the subject design, experiment, practice to carry out scientific research work

Tutor - graduate - nutrition expert trinity monitoring, research, analysis

- The general arrangement of the subject, the purpose, the request can be a college, responsible for the one hand.
- 100 graduate students, ie 100 papers, preliminary carcinogen composition, quantitative, qualitative monitoring, analysis with funding.

- For the support of the Department of Education, the Office of Science and Technology, the Office of Environmental Protection, the Health and Health Committee
- For college support, guidance, leadership, it will be able to obtain a large number of epidemiology, nutrition disciplines, preventive medicine, public health, environmental science principles of scientific research, to prevent cancer, cancer control first-hand information.

"Three Early" Research

The research of the three early:

Specimens: blood, urine, saliva, feces, sputum

Inflammation Tumor

Boundary monitoring

Before treatment After treatment

Early diagnosis technology, early diagnosis of reagent research, looking for early diagnosis methods, reagents:

1, to monitor changes in trace elements:

Normal: 500 cases

Precancerous lesions: 500 cases

A variety of cancer patients: 500 cases

Various patients: 500 cases

A variety of tumor specimens were cut: 500 cases

2, immune monitoring

Normal: 500 cases

Precancerous lesions: 500 cases

A variety of cancer patients: 500 cases

Various patients: 500 cases

A variety of cancer specimens: 500 cases

A variety of cancer preoperative: 500 cases

Postoperative: 500 cases

Before chemotherapy: 500 cases

After chemotherapy: 500 cases

1 time

2 times

3 times

4 times

Before radiotherapy: 500 cases

After radiotherapy: 500 cases

3, the endocrine hormone monitoring

Monitoring of ovarian function and milk Ca: 500 cases

Ovarian function and cervical Ca, ovarian cancer monitoring the search for baseline and bottom line boundaries and monitoring: 500 cases

4, hemorheology monitoring and metastasis correlation analysis: 500 cases

Correlation analysis of blood coagulation monitoring and metastasis: 500 cases

Analysis of microcirculation monitoring and microvascular thrombus embolism: 500 cases

5, the gene detection and clinical manifestations (symptoms, signs) combined with the relevant analysis

Genetic analysis and pathophysiology, metabolic function, compensatory function combined analysis

Is genetic testing or fruit? Combined with analysis

6, the tumor markers and clinical analysis, grading combined study

7, CEA ↑ AFP ↑ PSA ↑

It is on behalf of Ca Cells? It can kill cancer? Can it work and be effective? How to handle?

8, the early diagnosis: it is only qualitative, not positioning, how to deal with? What medication are used to deal with?

Volume III

In order to conquer cancer, it must start the total attack and the cancer prevention and the cancer control and the cancer treatment at the same weight and level

How to overcome cancer? How to prevent cancer? I see

Table of Contents

First, how to prevent cancer I see one:

(1) the situation analysis 1, ---the incidence of cancer is rising

(2) the situation analysis 2, --- the cancer incidence is related to the environment

(3) the situation analysis 3, ---it should improve the carcinogenic factors of the external (external environment) and the internal (internal environment) to prevent

(4) the situation analysis o 4,--- the formation of the environmental and the cancer research group

(5) the situation analysis 5, ---the relationship between the environment and cancer

(6) the situation analysis 6,---which are the carcinogenic factors in the environment? How should I prevent?

Second, how to prevent cancer I see two:

(A) The problems were found and asked from the follow-up results

(B) XZ-C proposed to overcome cancer and to launch a total attack

(C) XZ-C proposed to create a scientific city as a scientific and research base to overcome the cancer

(D) XZ-C proposed to create anti-cancer research institute and anti-cancer system engineering

(E) The anti-cancer research work cannot walk slowly and should run forward and save the dying and help the hurting

(F) how to improve the research work of the cancer cure rate

Third, how to prevent cancer I see three:

(A) why does it need to launch a total attack in order to conquer cancer?

(B) the catastrophe of cancer covers the whole world

(C) XZ-C proposed to the advice and suggestions of the establishment of the anti-cancer research institute and the anti-cancer system engineering

Fourth, how to overcome cancer?how to prevent cancer?I see four

How to prevent cancer from "two types of society"?

(A) the construction of "two-oriented society", which has the great relevance to the cancer prevention and anti-cancer

(B) the environmental pollution can increase the incidence of cancer

(C) why should we build a "two-oriented society" environment-friendly society?

(D) I think the current energy-saving and the emission reduction and the pollution prevention and the pollution treatment; to create a "two-oriented

society" is I level prevention to prevent cancer and to anti-cancer. Its purpose and effect can achieve Class I prevention.

(E) So far there is no practical solution to carry out the cancer prevention and the cancer control; it can be not only from the technical and the tactical to proceed but it should focus on from the strategic; the implementation is the people-oriented and fundamentally it emphasizes the harmony between people and the environment. The scientific research must be carried out to explore the innovation.

First, How to prevent cancer? I see one
How to prevent cancer? What does it prevent? How to prevent?

Professor Xu Ze proposed how to overcome cancer? how to prevent cancer? I see:

A. How to overcome cancer? how to prevent cancer? I see one:

(A) the situation analysis: (1) - how to prevent cancer? cancer incidence is rising.

1, from 85 years old of my social experience this year I see: I am deeply aware that the current incidence of major cancer diseases that threaten people's health is on the rise.

(1) I was in Wuhan in 1951 to enter the Tongji Medical College in Central South study, graduated from Tongji Medical College in 1956, assigned to the Hubei College of Traditional Chinese Medicine hospital surgery, has served as director of surgery, Professor in Hubei Institute of Traditional Chinese Medicine Experimental Institute.

In 1951 Zhongnan Tongji Medical College from Shanghai to Wuhan, when in order to teach and to find a case of lung cancer to show the students, it was difficult to find one a week earlier to make the hospital phone call.

At that time (the 1950s - sixties) in all hospitals in Wuhan there are no tumor department, nor tumor doctors, only a hospital in Wuhan there is a physician to see blood disease; in Tongji Hospital there is a gynecologist to see gynecology Tumor.

But now (65 years later) cancer is a common disease, frequently disease, and is seen in each hospital more common, cancer patients are queuing up, each of the top three hospitals has cancer department and is busy with cancer treatment. I made 60 years of tumor surgery,the more patients the more treat, we physicians should seriously think and review and reflect, why is it? Why is the more patient and the more treatment? What are the causes or factors that lead to an increase in morbidity? What should I do?

I have been engaged in medical clinical work for 60 years and to carry out "to overcome the cancer "as the direction of the experimental research and clinical validation work has been 30 years, so I deeply appreciate not only to pay attention to cancer treatment, but also should pay attention to cancer prevention; in order to stop at the source and to promote the incidence of cancer decline, the out of the way of cancer treatment is in the "three early" (early detection, early diagnosis, early treatment), and the out of the way of anti-cancer is in the prevention.

B. How to overcome cancer? how to prevent cancer?I see two:

(B) the situation analysis: (2) - cancer incidence is related to the environment.

So, how should it prevent? What is it prevented? How to prevent? Where is the target of the anti-cancer or "target"? How to control? What is it controlled? How to control?Where is the target or "target" of cancer control?

It must have a specific anti-cancer object, a clear goal, there are operational, and it must be consistent with the motivation and the effect.

Currently the more number of patients the more treatment, the incidence is on the rise, which 90% is related to the environment, which is why? Professor Xu proposed anti-cancer goal or the "target" should study and explore carcinogenic factors (the external environment and the internal environment) of the environment.

① Why will the rising incidence of cancer be related to the environment?

Because cancer is the abnormal proliferation of cells and is caused by the external factors (the external environment) or the internal factors (the internal environment). Cells in the normal development process is always in the dynamic balance among proliferation, survival, death control. However, sometimes under the influence of the external (external environment) or internal factors (within the environment) a cell proliferation activity disorders are breaking the normal mechanism of limiting and rapidly proliferates to form tissue mass, and the formation of abnormal proliferation of cell groups are called tumor. Tumor has the benign or the malignant, only rapid proliferation without metastasis is known as benign tumors; not only abnormal rapid proliferation, but the cells can occur proliferation and metastasis is known as malignant tumors which malignant tumors are cancer.

② the cause of cancer is related to the carcinogenic factors of the external environment and the internal environment

After years of world research, people now have a consensus:

That is that cancer is a process of evolution of multiple factors, multiple stages, and polygenes that the external factors are one side and one body organism (substance) are one side.

The so-called external factors, refers to the genetic factors other than the body, including both outside the human body living environment, chemical factors, physical factors, biological (bacteria, viruses, etc.) factors, as well as human lifestyle and eating habits, including the body Internal environment, such as hormone status, disease infection, and mental factors.

And genetic refers to the genetic material DNA or gene, leading to the occurrence of cancer has two most basic factors: one is the intrinsic genetic factors; the other is the external environmental factors. Most of the cancer is the result of the combined effect of these two factors.

③ If we have a better understanding of the cause of cancer, then in the future will be able to put forward more valuable <u>advice: how to prevent which carcinogenic factors, how to monitor which carcinogenic factors, and even clear which carcinogenic factors, so that we stay away from cancer, prevention cancer</u>. For example, should not smoke, should not eat pickles and smoked products, should avoid strong sun, which is the future to reduce the incidence of cancer is an important way.

<u>From the above analysis (1)</u>

It prompts and suggests:

1, In Wuhan City in 50 years - 60 years in 20 century, there is few patients with cancer; there is neither tumor, nor tumor specialist.

But now (65 years later) cancer was common disease and frequently disease, the patient lines up registered, each of the top three hospitals have oncology and are busy with cancer treatment.

<u>It is proved that the incidence of cancer is on the rise.</u>

2, the analysis: what causes or what factors lead to cancer incidence increased?

why? What should I do? Whether from this point in-depth analysis, to find out the factors leading to rising incidence of cancer, so as to find out the anti-cancer, cancer control methods.

The analysis from the above situation (2)

It suggests and prompts:

1, cancer is abnormal cell proliferation malignant transformation, is caused under the influence of the outside (the external environment) or the internal factors (the internal environment).

The so-called external factors refers to the genetic factors other than the body, including: the living environment outside the body of the chemical factors, physical factors, biological (bacteria, viruses) and other factors, as well as human lifestyle, eating habits, including the body's internal environment, Such as endocrine hormones, mental factors.

2, the analysis of what causes or what factors lead to cancer incidence increased?

Today people living standards continue to improve, a variety of high-tech products to bring us a better life at the same time, but also brought a variety of chemical, physical, biological environment, a large number of carcinogens. A variety of carcinogenic substances into the human body or a variety of carcinogenic factors affect the human body. People seem to be shrouded in the ocean of environmental pollution carcinogens.

It seems that the rise in cancer incidence is due to find, anti-cancer target or "target" is also very clear, very specific, how should cancer prevention? How to control What is it? Is clear, concrete, and operational.

But some people talk about cancer discoloration, it seems that all the vegetation; and others are numb, in the life of their own way.

Cancer is not terrible, the terrible is that we do not have a simple basic knowledge of cancer prevention, because most of the cancer can be prevented.

How to overcome cancer how to prevent cancer I see the three:

(C) Analysis of the situation: (3) - should be from the external factors (external environment) and internal factors (internal environment) of the carcinogenic factors to prevent.

How to prevent? We should prevent from the external (external environment) and internal factors (internal environment) to improve the carcinogenic factors.

Professor Xu Ze proposed: the establishment of innovative anti-cancer research institute, and innovative anti-cancer system engineering, which is unprecedented work, must practice in person, for human health benefits.

How to implement the creation of this anti-cancer research institute.

Professor Xu Ze XZ-C proposed anti-cancer design, proposed anti-cancer system engineering:

(1) personal prevention: to improve anti-cancer knowledge (see another article)

(2) The government should carry out anti-cancer projects

What is anti-cancer project?

① that is, the various departments of the carcinogenic factors, to be monitored, qualitative, quantitative, set the bottom line standards, to be prevented, and even legislation, the division of labor is responsible.

B, which is responsible for the government, arranged to arrange anti-cancer system engineering rules.

C, the division of labor departments, anti-cancer research institute for technical monitoring.

D, macro, microscopic, ultramicro, sampling, providing effective reporting.

② from which departments, scope, testing? Xu Ze proposed from the clothing, food, live, line … … whether the detection of carcinogenic factors.

A, [clothing]: - light industry sector is responsible for receiving the investigation, testing: clothing, cosmetics, toys … … and so on to Ca detection, over the warning to be warning or stop.

B, [food]: the agricultural sector, the food sector is responsible for receiving investigation and research, water, soil, fertilizer, agricultural transgenic, food, fish, meat, chicken, duck, packaged food, food, oil, feed…Detection of carcinogenic factors

C, [live]: - housing construction department is responsible for receiving the investigation, testing: decoration materials, supplies, design and other carcinogenic factors to monitor, exceeding the standard to be warning, to stop.

D, [line]: - the industrial sector is responsible for receiving surveys, trains, cars, aircraft … … tail gas hazards, testing should not be exceeded should be legislation.

E, environment: environmental protection departments should be responsible for, support, reception, anti-cancer research monitoring, investigation, garbage disposal, air pollution, water pollution, factory chimney … … pollution, from the macro, micro-monitoring, qualitative, quantitative detection Carcinogens content, exceeding the standard to be a warning or stop.

F, the education sector: large, medium and small teachers should be teachers

Large, middle and primary school students

Textbook content plus: physical health

Health care, basic moral knowledge

Anti-cancer, anti-cancer and other knowledge

<u>G, Professor Xu Ze proposed to promote scientific research ethics, medicine is benevolence, Lide first</u>

<u>Scientific research ethics: products should have moral standards</u>

<u>Standard: should not harm human health as the standard for the bottom line</u>

<u>Basic ethics: all products and people harmless, do not harm people's health, especially for children</u>

(To be beautiful, the flowers of the living environment, living environment)

<u>H, health administrative departments defend life to protect health, and it should lead, guide, support to guide anti-cancer measures, anti-cancer engineering, anti-cancer testing, anti-cancer monitoring,</u> cancer is a whole human disaster, the global people are eager to one day to overcome cancer ; there is eagerly hope that experts and scholars can find anti-cancer measures to keep people away from cancer.

Cancer is a disaster of all mankind, must struggle with the world, the people of the world struggle, <u>human beings should not sit still, physicians should not do nothing, health administration should not do nothing, should lead and guide the series of anti-cancer research project, common forward</u> and work together, Complementary advantages, leadership and guidance to overcome cancer, launched a total attack.

Environmental pollution, air pollution, water pollution, cancer incidence increased, this is not a country, a region, but the global existence of the problem, which is a by-product of industrial development, should be analyzed, should be invited to the World Health Organization leadership Research, to prevent all environmental pollution of the carcinogenic projects, to defend the survival of mankind on the living environment, the survival of mankind in a harmonious and friendly environment, away from cancer.

Four, how to overcome cancer? how to prevent cancer? I see four:

<u>(4) The analysis of the situation: - the formation of the environmental and cancer research group</u>

<u>How to implement the anti-cancer research institute to create the work? It should be set up environmental and cancer research group:</u>

(1) the investigation and detection of common cancer risk factors, in-depth intervention study

(2) to monitor pollution carcinogenic data, research and development of cancer prevention, cancer control measures

For

A), food, food, packaging, additives

B), water pollution, beverages

C), housing decoration, materials

D), air pollution, factory chimneys, car tail steam

E), soil, fertilizer, transgenic

(3) to monitor environmental pollution carcinogenic data, to study anti-cancer measures

To research and develop the intervention methods.

(4) To founded anti-cancer, cancer control newsletter (publications) - "anti-cancer mass medicine"

From the big living environment and a small living environment to do anti-cancer, away from cancer

(5) the several work:

A), monitoring of the environmental pollution carcinogenic (data)

B), sampling the incidence of cancer high incidence

C), founder of anti-cancer anti-cancer newsletter reported

D), research and development of anti-cancer technology, tools, products

E), science (anti-cancer) publicity and education

F), "three early" universal study

G), how to early self-discovery

(6) the several aspects:

A), from the clothing, food, live, anti-cancer

B), from the living environment anti-cancer

C), from the living environment to prevent cancer

D), from life behavior, life hobby, lifestyle anti-cancer

(7) the 21st century anti-cancer three points:

A), smoking (smoking cessation) - "smoking has no harm to harm"

B), limit alcohol - limit the amount of alcohol

C), lose weight - not obese

Five, how to implement the building work of the prevention cancer system engineering of the prevention cancer research? we must first understand the relationship between environmental pollution and cancer research history

Xu Ze in his third book "new methods of cancer treatment and new methods" in Chapter 38:

<u>the situation analysis: (5) ---- the relationship between environment and cancer</u>

In the process of finding the cause and occurrence of cancer, human beings have carried out extensive exploration and accumulated rich knowledge. It was found that more than 90% of the cancer caused by environmental factors or closely related.

The environment in which human beings live includes the natural environment and the social environment. The natural environment, which surrounds people around the various natural factors, such as everyone should breathe the air, drink water and eat food, these common material environment is known as the big environment.

Everyone has to engage in certain work, take a certain way of life, such as occupation, lifestyle and hobbies constitute a living environment called a small environment.

No matter the big environment or small environment, both of them are external environments upon which mankind depends for survival and activities.

The physical condition of the human body itself is called the inner environment.

The external environmental substances through the body's intake, digestion, absorption, metabolism and excretion have a close relationship with the internal environment which has a huge impact on the human body.

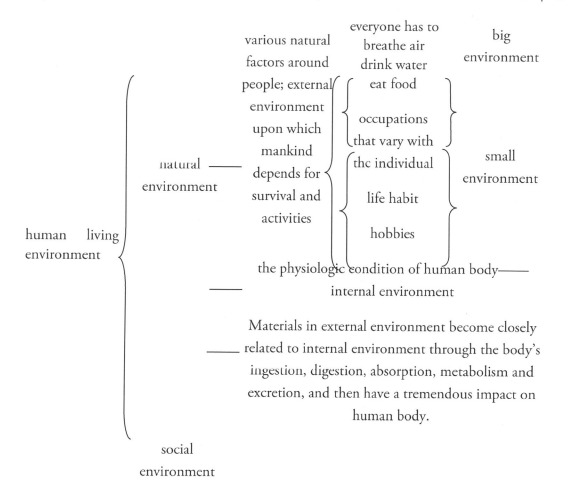

Human living environment

The Natural environment   ## the social environment

the various natural factors
around the people is
the external environment
for the survival and the human activities :

a. Drinking and food and Everyone has to breathe the air are Called **the big environment**

b. the occupation which Vary from person and living habit and the hobby are called **a small environment**

The state of the body itself - called **the inner environment**

<u>How to prove the relationship between environmental pollution and cancer? there are many examples on the history.</u>

In 1775, English doctor Pott proved that cleaners of chimney have higher risk of suffering from scrotal skin cancer, as they always contact coal tar, which was the first historical case that combined cancer with environmental factors.

After 100 years, Germany doctor Volkman also recognized that the high rate of suffering skin cancer for workers was possibly related to the contact with coal tar.

In 1907, some scholar found that exposure to sunlight is related to skin cancer and reported firstly the epidemiologic research on sunlight and skin cancer. Researchers found that crews were always exposed to solar radiation that led to chronic skin diseases, which was often seen. Later, researchers proved that <u>sunlight and ultraviolet rays were likely to result in skin cancer</u> with animal model.

In 1915, the first animal model of inducing tumors by chemical agents was established. Besmearing tar repeatedly could make rabbits suffer from skin cancer, which provided experimental reasons for the theory of chemical carcinogenesis based on that cleaners of chimney were easy to suffer from carcinoma of scrotum in 1775. Later<u>, people confirmed that and got the effective constituent by abstraction, named coal tar.</u>

In the 1920s, bladder carcinoma was popular with the workers <u>who produced alpha naphthylamine, ethyl naphthalene and benzidine dye. Almost all the workers who had done this suffered from bladder carcinoma later.</u>

In 1930, <u>the first chemical carcinogen benzopyrene was separated from coal tar.</u> The known substance of carcinogenic environment, coal tar was separated into different constituents, which were confirmed that they could result in cancer by experimental analysis with animal model.

In 1938, according to researches, it could be found that the process of chemical carcinogenesis was divided into two stages, the stage of activation and the stage of promotion. Non-specific stimulators could activate and promote the occurrence of cancer under small dose of carcinogen like besmearing tar or mastoid tumorous virus.

In 1940, researchers discovered that limitation of heat could reduce the occurrence of tumors for mice. It was proved that the intake of heat could encourage the occurrence of several kinds of tumors like breast carcinoma, liver cancer and skin cancer induced by benzoapyrene. Until today when obesity is popular worldwide, this project is attached with importance again by people.

In 1950, research on epidemiology discovered that smoking was related to lung cancer. By reviewing the lung cancer sufferers with the habit of smoking, it could be proved that smoking had close relation to lung cancer. Later, from the research on the obvious relation between smoking and the mortality of lung cancer among male doctors, it has been proved that smoking is a dangerous factor for many kinds of cancer and it can increase the mortality of cancer by 30%.

In 1958, it was been proved that food additive forbidden by reforming organization for food additive could induce the occurrence of cancer for human beings and animals.

In 1964, American surgeon Luther L Terry proposed that smoking was connected to lung cancer.

Vinyl chloride is the main raw material of the plastics industry, until 1974 scientists know that this chemical is a potential strong carcinogen, it can cause liver cancer.

In recent decades, according to epidemiologic research, it can be found that if workers in many occupations contact the carcinogens in manufacturing environment, the incidence rates of some parts will greatly increase. Elimination or avoiding these contacts can reduce the incidence rates gradually or even make them disappear, which plays an important role in the occurrence of tumors.

The long-term effects of various environmental factors other than the human body are the leading causes of the majority of cancer, and therefore should minimize the impact of these environments, living and behavioral factors on the human body, away from cancer.

Various environmental factors outside human bodies are the major reasons resulting in the occurrence of cancer. Therefore, it is necessary to reduce the effects of these environmental, living and behavior factors to human bodies so as to get away from cancer.

The following is talking about the severe cancerogenic effects of environmental pollution like air pollution, water pollution and soil pollution, etc. to human beings.

1, **The environmental pollution in the air pollution and cancer**: human life in every second per minute are inseparable from the air. Air pollution can lead to the occurrence of many diseases, especially respiratory diseases, including the most serious lung cancer.

At the beginning of 20th century, lung cancer mainly happened in such occupational environments like mines, exploitation and smelting. After world war one, the morality of lung cancer began to increase. In late 1930s, with the development of modern industry air pollution, occupational carcinogens and the consumption and production of tobacco and cigarette increased greatly. Meanwhile, the morality of male who suffered from lung cancer in western industrial developed countries rose rapidly. In the UK, the death rate of lung cancer was 10/100,000 in 1930, 53/100,000 in 1950, 99.7/100,000 in 1966 and 120.3/100,000 in 1975. From 1930 to 1975, it has an increase of twelve times in 45 years.

During 1934 to 1974, lung cancer rose from the fifth to the number one place in causes of death of American male. Its mortality rate rose from 3.0/100,000 to 54.5/100,000, up 17 times as compared with before. Female lung cancer went up from the eighth to the top three. Its mortality rate rose from 2.0/100,000 to 12.4/100,000, up 5.2 times as compared with before.

In the early 1980, lung cancer in 24 countries and regions involving UK, France, Netherlands, Germany and USA and others generally occupies the number one in the cause of death of malignant tumor patients. Since the mid-20th century, the tendency of high incidence of lung cancer in western industrial developed countries has been rising.

Dangerous gases in industrial developed countries, produced from power generation, steel-making, cars, planes, fuels, energy sources and volumes of smoke, are emitted into the atmosphere and pollute air. Human respiratory tract is irritated by breathing into polluted air, which causes the continuing rise of the incidence rate and mortality rate of lung cancer.

2, the environmental pollution in the water pollution and cancer:

Human activity in production and life depend on water at all times. Water quality pollution is mainly caused by industrial and agricultural production as well as urban pollution discharge. In China, township enterprises are having a fast development, which worsen industrial pollution. According to the survey, many major rivers are facing a serious pollution increasingly. Fertilizers, farm chemicals and pesticides in agricultural production lead to the serious pollution of water quality.

Some rural areas of China have a habit of using pond water. The research of Qidong County in Jiangsu Province has found that the high incidence of liver cancer in this area is related to drink pond water. Fusui County in Guangxi Province also has the similar report. All of these explain that water pollution is relevant to the incidence of liver cancer. Haining County in Zhejiang Province also finds that people drinking pond water are over seven times easier to suffer from colon cancer than people drinking well water.

In recent years, due to the advance of analysis technology of water quality, more than 100 different kinds of organic substances in water are found to have actions of carcinogenesis, cancer-promoting and mutagenesis. Animal experiments have proved that drink water mixed with the following chemical compounds can cause liver cancer, such as benzene hexachloride, carbon tetrachloride, chloroform, trichloroethylene, perchlorethylene, and trichloroethane, etc. Furthermore, there are some limnetic algae toxins, such as blue-green algae has an obvious action on the promotion of liver cancer.

Mulberry fish pond area of Shunde in Guangdong Foshan is low lying and easy to generate water-logging and water accumulation, so the water quality pollution is more serious. The incidence of liver cancer of local population is higher. While neighboring residents in Siping drink deep phreatic water. The water quality is good, so the incidence of liver cancer is lower. According to the research data of WHO and International Association for Cancer Research, drinking off-standard water can induce or promote the generation of cancer. The test indicates that drink water with a large amount of nickel is easy to induce oral cancer, throat cancer and carcinoma of large intestine; water with more cadmium is easy to induce esophageal carcinoma, laryngeal carcinoma and lung cancer; water with more plumbum is easy to induce stomach cancer, intestinal cancer, oophoroma and all kinds of lymph cancer; water with more iron and zinc is easy to induce esophageal carcinoma.

3, the environmental chemical pollution and cancer - chemical carcinogen:

Chemical carcinogen refers to chemical substances that can induce the generation of tumor.

In the mid-20th century, the problem of chemical carcinogenesis attracts widespread attention, mainly because modern tumor incidence rate and mortality rate continue to rise. The age of suffering from cancer has a younger tendency. Environmental chemical pollution is also found to have a close relation to the incidence rate of tumor. World Health Organization also indicates that 80%~90% of human cancers are relevant to environmental factors, which are mainly chemical factors.

The following chemical substances have been studied and proved to have carcinogenic action.

Chloroethylene: In 1974, people began to realize that this substance is the cause of professional cancer. Experimental study has found liver cancer, brain cancer, renal carcinoma, lung cancer and cancer of lymphatic system in experimental animals exposed to Chloroethylene. But the related personnel cannot timely realize the hazardness of these substances from experimental results. Therefore, they fail to take measures to protect workers in time. Until recently, workers start to stop using the spraying agent of Chloroethylene; and plastic factory also change manufacturing technique to prevent workers from exposure.

Here to point out that Chloroethylene is an important raw material for record, packaging material, Medical test tube, household appliances, bathroom equipment and other kinds of plastic products. Plastic products themselves have no risk, but the liver cancer risk of workers in Chloroethylene factory is 200 times higher than that of common people.

Benzene: It is a kind of harmful chemical material, which can destroy the hematopiesis of marrow. If exposed in the environment filled with benzene, people may suffer from aplastic anemia that can change into leucocythemia after a long period. The first case of "leucucythemia led by benzene" was discovered in 1928.

Researches from other countries have also proved that benzene is a sort of harmful material with occupational hazards. Italian scientists have reported before 200 years that the risk of suffering from leucocythemia for the workers in printing houses and shoemaking factories was 20 times higher than that of others.

Some activities and addictions in daily life are usually related to environmental cancerogen palycyclic aromatic closely. Palycyclic aromatic produced by smoking is the key factor of inducing lung cancer for human beings. Meanwhile, palycyclic aromatic with carcinogenicity produced in cooking foods of oil and fat including frying, grilling and smoking, etc. are threatening extremely the health for human beings, which should be attached with great importance.

In addition, benzoapyrene in asphalt and hot-mix asphalt is closely related to the high risk of cancer occurrence for roadmen and worker dealing with the water proofing of roof. Farm labors often contact several kinds of pesticides, herbicide and chemical fertilizers which contain some known carcinogens and some that can induce cancer in experimental animals and others that are proved to be mutagenic agents after short-term test. And the pesticides can enter food chain and accumulate in biological system.

4, the physical factors in environmental pollution and cancer - ionizing radiation:

With the development of technology, frequent nuclear tests, the applications of nuclear energy and radioactive nuclides are increasing, so as the radioactive substance poured in human environment. Therefore, people pay increasingly more attention to environmental pollution by ionizing radiation.

The ionizing radiation means the rays radiated by some radioactive substance in the process of transmutation. This kind of rays can give the absorbed substance adequate energy to divide ionize molecules and atoms. Some ionizing radiations are electromagnetic radiations like X-ray and γ-ray.

The sources of artificial radiation include nuclear tests which increase the radioactive environmental pollution, the exploitation, processing and retreat of nuclear fuel, for instance, in the exploitation of mineral radon gas and radioactive dust can pollute atmosphere. As the sources of energy in the world are less and less, more and more nations have been beginning to build nuclear power stations currently. This nuclear power industry can all discharge radioactive waste gas, water and residue which will pollute environment if mishandled.

Although radioactive nuclide can be applied extensively in industry, agriculture and medicine, the radioactive waste can still pollute environment.

The major effects of ionizing radiation to human bodies are body damages including chronic radiation diseases, malignant tumors, cataract, and decrease in the capacity to bear children, etc; radiation carcinogensis with longer delitescence like leucocythemia, skin carcinoma, lung cancer and osteocarcinoma; and hereditary damages which make descendants possessed with hereditary disease.

5, the carcinogen from the environmental pollution into the food:

With the development of science and technology, food processing process is increasingly industrialized, the external environment or manufacturing food processing process itself, may lead to a variety of foreign substances, including chemical, biological carcinogenic substances, Contaminated food.

In the processing of food raw materials, add artificial additives, the use of smoke, frying, baking and other practices, the result is in the food may occur carcinogenic.

Food products often have to go through the storage and transportation to reach the hands of consumers, so that carcinogens contaminated food and provide another source.

It is a very important issue to study the sources of pollution of human food products and how to eliminate such pollution.

How to prevent? What is the The important link of the prevention of the cancer?

As early as the 20th century, 80 years of domestic and foreign experts, scholars believe that more than 90% of the cancer is caused by environmental factors, protection and recovery of a good environment, is an important part of the prevention of cancer.

How to prevent cancer? How to prevent? It must first understand what the carcinogenic factors are and its carcinogenic process in order to put forward preventive measures.

(6) the analysis of the situation(6)----- which are carcinogenic factors in the environmental factors? How should I prevent?

1, chemical factors are the main cause of human cancer, 90% of human cancer are caused by the environmental factors, of which more than 75% are the chemical factors.

The earliest observation of chemical factors and human cancer can be traced back to the 1870s. Percivall Port has been found to have increased the rate of scrotal cancer in men who had had chimney sweepers during childhood. Although the nature of the carcinogen was not clear at that time, the discovery of Port suggested that occupational exposure was associated with the onset of the tumor. After that, many examples of the relationship between a variety of chemical carcinogens and human tumors, therefore it provides a series of experimental evidence for the scientists to understand the chemical cancinogenesis.

2, what is chemical carcinogens? It refers to a chemical substance that has the ability to induce cancer formation.

In the mid-20th century the chemical carcinogenesis caused widespread concern and it was found that environmental chemical pollution is closely related to the incidence of cancer. The World Health Organization also pointed out that 90% of human cancer is related to the environmental factors which is mainly chemical factors.

Treatment should first understand the cause of the disease, the prevention of cancer is also the first to understand in the environment which carcinogenic factors are and how to avoid?

Common chemical carcinogens are mainly related to the following 11 categories of chemical substances.

The types of chemical carcinogens are:

Species	Examples of
1, alkylating agent	mustard gas, chloromethyl ether, formaldehyde, ethylene oxide, diethyl sulfate, ethylene, benzene, butadiene, carcinogenic alkylating agent
2, polycyclic aromatic hydrocarbons	such as benzopyrene, dimethyl benzene anthracene, diphenyl anthracene, 3-methylcholanthracene and coal tar pitch
3, aromatic amine	benzidine, ethyl naphthylamine, nitrobenzene
4, metal and metal	arsenic, nickel, chromium, beryllium, cadmium, selenium
5, mold and phytotoxin	aflatoxin, microcystin and so on
6, nitrosamines and nitrosamides	
7, asbestos and silica	
8, hobby	cigarettes, tobacco, betel nut, excessive alcohol and beverages
9, the thermal cracking products of food	
10, the drug	includes certain hormones
11, cancer products	have some chemicals only promote cancer, should be classified here, such as croton oil and its purified phorbol ester. Some promote cancer also has a starting effect

3, there are the wide ranges of chemical carcinogens:

For the study of chemical carcinogens **systematically and in-**depth, it is necessary to classify and to sum up the three main categories, that is, according to the role of chemical carcinogens, according to the relationship of chemical carcinogens and human tumors, it is classified by chemical nature.

(1) according to the role of chemical carcinogens classification

According to the role of chemical carcinogens can be divided into the three categories: direct carcinogens, indirect carcinogens, the cancer promoter .

① direct carcinogens refers to these chemicals which after entering into the body without metabolism the things can directly work on the cell and can induce normal cell carcinogenesis of carcinogens. This type of chemical carcinogen which has the strong carcinogenic effects and the carcinogenic effect is fast, commonly used in in vitro cell malignant transformation study such as various carcinogenic alkylating agents, nitrosamide carcinogens and the like.

② **indirect carcinogens** refers to the chemical substances which after entering into the human body, by the microsomal mixed function of oxidase activation it changes into a chemical form of active form which is the carcinogenic carcinogens with chemical carcinogens. Such chemical carcinogens are widely present in the external environment. There are the common types such as carcinogenic polycyclic aromatic hydrocarbons, aromatic amines, nitrosamines and so on.

③ the promote cancer, also known as tumor promoters promote cancer alone in the body without carcinogenic effects, but can promote other carcinogens induced tumor formation. Common promotional items are croton oil (phorbol diester), saccharin and phenobarbital and so on.

(2) according to the relationship between chemical carcinogens and human tumors

According to the relationship between chemical carcinogens and human tumors can be divided into affirmative carcinogens, suspicious carcinogens and potential carcinogens. Surely carcinogens are chemical carcinogens that are identified by epidemiological studies and that clinicians and scientists acknowledge that they have carcinogenic effects on humans and animals, and that have carcinogenic effects in a dose-responsive relationship; suspicious carcinogens have in vitro transformability, and Contact time is associated with carcinogenesis, animal carcinogenicity is positive, but the results are not constant; in addition, these carcinogens lack epidemiological evidence; potential carcinogens generally in animal experiments can be some positive results, but in the crowd There is no data to prove whether the person is carcinogenic.

(3) by chemical classification

Chemical carcinogens can be divided into organic chemical carcinogens and inorganic chemical carcinogens by chemical properties, the former a wide range, such as the majority of compounds in the table, which mainly include carcinogenic metals and metals and crystalline silicon and asbestos, So both foreign and endogenous chemical carcinogens are organic chemical carcinogens.

4, organic carcinogens

Organic carcinogens can be divided into seven categories: polycyclic aromatic hydrocarbons, heterocyclic amines, N-nitroso compounds, dioxins and their analogues, pesticides, azo dyes, bio-alkylating agents, triazenes Compounds and the like.

(1) polycyclic aromatic hydrocarbons

PAH is a series of polycyclic aromatic hydrocarbons (PAHs) compounds produced by pyrolysis or incomplete combustion of coal, petroleum, coal tar, tobacco and some organic compounds, many of which have carcinogenic effects. It is the most widely distributed environmental carcinogen. In recent years, a large number of studies have shown that air, soil, water and plants are subject to polycyclic aromatic hydrocarbons pollution, and modern vehicles - cars, aircraft and other motor vehicles discharged from the exhaust also contains a considerable number of multi-ring Aromatics. So in the frequent traffic streets, polycyclic aromatic hydrocarbons pollution is quite serious. With the development of industry, the problem of carcinogenic polycyclic aromatic hydrocarbons is bound to become a growing concern. It is also the most closely related to human carcinogens. Some of the activities in human daily life and some hobby are often associated with the production of polycyclic aromatic hydrocarbons. Such as smoking is an important way to produce polycyclic aromatic hydrocarbons, in recent years has been proved to be an important factor in the induction of human lung cancer; another example in the fried food, fried, smoked and other cooking process also has carcinogenic polycyclic aromatic hydrocarbons, And is considered to be one of the major causes of increased gastric cancer rates in some areas. Therefore, polycyclic aromatic hydrocarbons (PAHs) are the most widely distributed carcinogens that are closely related to human beings and have a great impact on human health. We must pay enough attention. The 1973 International Cancer Research Center (IARC) panel of experts pointed out that some polycyclic aromatic hydrocarbons are harmful to humans.

5, the source of environmental pollution

Natural polycyclic aromatic hydrocarbons mainly exist in coal, oil, shale oil, tar, asphalt and so on. Polycyclic aromatic hydrocarbons can also be produced in the combustion of hydrocarbon-containing materials.

In the polycyclic aromatic hydrocarbons compounds, benzo [a] pyrene research is the most detailed and in-depth, has established a relatively accurate determination method, and polycyclic aromatic hydrocarbons in the carcinogenic effect of a strong substance, so the following mainly benzene Pyrene [a] pyrene as an example to illustrate the environmental pollution of this class of chemicals.

(1) the Pollution of the atmosphere

Outdoor air can be contaminated by fixed sources of pollution (such as thermal power plants, industries, enterprises) and mobile sources of pollution (such as aircraft, automobiles, etc.), especially in cars and trains, the discharge of pollutants is very low, very close to people's breathing zone, and often close to the residential area, so sometimes cause serious pollution. Most of the polycyclic aromatic hydrocarbons in the crystalline state attached to the dust, the need to absorb a lot of air, filter a certain amount of dust, and then measured. From the historical data, the atmosphere of benzene pyrene [a] pyrene concentration is the highest in London, UK, car exhaust emissions from the internal combustion engine will contain polycyclic aromatic carcinogens.

(2) Contamination of soils

There are many types of PAHs in the soil. Such as the eastern United States rural soil containing benzo [a] pyrene, phenanthrene, fluorenene anthracene, pyrene, Qu Shang anthracene anthracene and so on. Different chemical companies, the surrounding soil pollution is also different, in the vicinity of the oil plant soil was measured per kilogram of soil containing 200 mg of polycyclic aromatic hydrocarbons, in the vicinity of the coal tar plant can be up to per kilogram of 650 Mg. France has reported that benzo [a] pyrene carcinogens are isolated from limestone 50 meters from the deep strata.

(3) Water pollution

The water environment includes ground water (rivers, rivers, lakes, reservoirs and oceans) and groundwater. The most eye-catching water in the residential area. From the ground water has been detected dozens of polycyclic aromatic hydrocarbons, of which seven or eight kinds of carcinogenic effects, such as benzoanthracene, benzofluoresene, dibenzoanthracene, flexor pyrene, benzo [a] pyrene.

4) the pollution of food

Food also contains a variety of polycyclic aromatic hydrocarbons, such as anthracene, benzanthracene, dibenzoanthracene, benzo [a] pyrene and so on. As benzo [a] pyrene is an important component of smoke, so smoked foods can often detect a certain amount of benzo [a] pyrene.

The source of benzo [a] pyrene in food is mainly:

In vivo synthesis

The benzo [a] pyrene, such as benzo [a] pyrene, was detected in the marine plants of the unaffected seawater aquatic plants in the Greenland Bay and from the contaminated areas and the content is sometimes similar that of the contaminated area, Indicating the possibility of synthetic polycyclic aromatic hydrocarbons.

From the contaminated soil, the waters absorb the rich, such as potatoes in the contaminated soil, and the wheat containing benzo [a] pyrene is higher. The content of benzo [a] pyrene in aquatic plants and small plankton is directly related to the content of river water. The content of benzo [a] pyrene in plankton in river water is several times higher than that in upstream clean water. Marine organisms have the ability to enrich polycyclic aromatic hydrocarbons, marine fish containing benzo [a] pyrene up to 2 to 65 micrograms per kilogram.

Plant foliage is contaminated by atmospheric deposition.

Animal foods also contain polycyclic aromatic hydrocarbons.

Food processing, storage of contaminated food additives and packaging, bio-vegetable oil does not take mechanical crushing, but by adding organic solvents, such as ethane, the oil extracted, this time, the addition of organic solvents such as polycyclic aromatic hydrocarbons can be It is brought into vegetable oil. Another example is the use of paraffin coated on paper can also be included in the polycyclic aromatic hydrocarbons pollution of packaged food.

Smoked, barbecue, coke and other processing methods, or directly to the polycyclic aromatic hydrocarbons containing smoke to the food, or because of high temperature leaving the food carbohydrates or fats into polycyclic aromatic hydrocarbons.

How much is the amount of polycyclic aromatic hydrocarbons consumed daily from a food? It is estimated that the Germans from the value of oil every day intake of carcinogenic polycyclic aromatic hydrocarbons 0.3 micrograms, from cereals, potatoes, vegetables, fruits, intake of 10 micrograms, of which benzo [a] pyrene about 3% to 50%.

Therefore, the general population exposure (non-occupational exposure) polycyclic aromatic hydrocarbons may be as follows: the polluted atmosphere (the main release source for the car, factory and residential timber, coal, mineral oil); contaminated indoor air (the main release source Open stove and cigarette smoke); smoking; use of polycyclic aromatic hydrocarbons containing products; house dust; from contaminated soil and water absorbed by the skin; contaminated food and drinking water.

(5) carcinogenic mechanism of polycyclic aromatic hydrocarbons

As early as the 1940s, Schmide noted the relationship between carcinogenic activity and electrical properties of polycyclic aromatic hydrocarbons, and many others proposed different models to explain the structure and activity of PAHs, briefly described below.

Carcinogenic agents in the body of the carcinogenic mechanism is still very little to know.

6, N-nitroso compounds

N-nitroso compounds (NOC) are widely found in nature, human mainly through diet, drinking water and other ways to absorb into the body. N-nitroso compounds are a class of organic compounds with similar structures. Since gastric cancer, which is caused by gastric cancer, has been widely validated in animal experiments. Therefore, whether human gastric cancer is associated with epidemiology is concerned. By 1983, more than 300 kinds of nitroso compounds had been studied, of which 90% were carcinogenic.

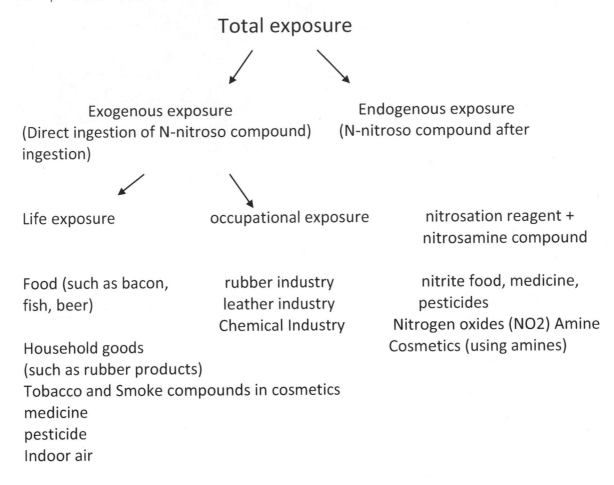

Figure . contact with N-nitroso compounds

(1) the source of N-nitroso compounds in the environment

Human contact with N-nitroso compounds in the environment, Wang Lansheng, etc. made a detailed induction (Figure 2-1), a total of two types: exogenous exposure and endogenous exposure. Exogenous exposure refers to the direct intake of N-nitroso compounds from the environment, but also can be divided into two types of life exposure and occupational exposure; endogenous exposure refers to the presence of nitrosamines and nitrosation reagents in food, medicine and cosmetics N-nitroso compounds.

(2) N-nitrosamine marinated meat in food:

Wang Lansheng and other agricultural products in 395 German meat and meat products in the N-nitrosamine were systematically analyzed, the results show that only nitrite or nitric acid Salt-treated samples will undergo nitrosamine contamination. Among them, salted pork and ham are the most polluted by nitrosamine.

Bacon, ham, beef sausage, Italian sausage, meat and so on, usually do not change its original N-nitrosodimethylamine concentration, but the concentration of N-nitroso pyrrolidine will increase.

The main source of intake of N-nitroso pyrrolidine from food is fried bacon, and the United States and Canada are similar, and the amount of volatile nitrosamines in the raw bacon is small. The amount of nitrosamines produced in the fry is affected by the cooking method, temperature and cooking time. For example, pyrrolidine nitrosamines produced by frying bacon with a pan are much less than those produced by cooking in a microwave oven. The bacon samples do not substantially produce pyrrolidine nitrosamines at 99 ° C and fry for 105 minutes. 204 ℃, fried 4 minutes to produce pyrrolidine nitrosamines.

Janzowshi et al. Studied 33 fried bacon, ham, sausage, sausage samples and found 9 of them containing non-volatile carcinogens N-nitroso-3-hydroxypyrrolidine. Lee also detected the carcinogen in the fried bacon.

Fish: fish and fish products have been found in the trace of volatile nitrosamines, Kawabate and so on an important Japanese food - into a dry fish for a detailed study, with gasifier cooking these fish, N-nitrosodimethylamine was increased and no N-nitrosopyrrolidine was detected. The amount of N-nitrosodimethylamine was increased in the squid with the gasifier, and the N-nitroso pyrrolidine was also added to the cooked whale. N-nitroso was detected in all tested fish samples Dimethylamine.

Chinese fish, with nitrate containing sodium chloride pickled, can be detected N-nitrosodimethylamine, salted fish in Guangzhou volatile nitrosamines N-nitrosodimethylamine and N - nitrosodiethylamine and N-nitroso morpholine content is very low, cooked after the content will increase. N-nitrosodi-N-propylamine and N-nitroso-di-N-butylamine were not detected in the raw fish samples but could be detected in the fish after cooking.

Western fish only contains a small amount of nitroso carcinogens, and mainly N-nitrosodimethylamine. In the UK, 80% of the 94 samples contained nitroso carcinogens. However, most of the content is very low. Similar results have been reported in the United States, Canada, Sweden and Germany.

Dairy products: some dairy products, such as dry cheese, milk powder, milk wine, there is a trace of volatile nitrosamines.

Fruits and vegetables: some vegetables and fruits contain amines, nitrates and nitrites, therefore, in the processing of vegetables and other processing, long-term storage, fruits and vegetables in the amine and nitrite and other reactions, Trace nitrosamines.

In some areas of China, the incidence of esophageal cancer is high, in the region of corn bread found in a characteristic N-nitroso compounds, namely N-nitroso-N-(3-methylbutyl) -N- Methylacetone nitrosamines.

Beer and other beverages: Wang Lansheng and other food nitrosamine pollution in the study, the most surprising discovery is that beer often contains N-nitrosodimethylamine.

Some European beers are also contaminated. The study found that beer through cellar maturation is the only source of N-nitrosodimethylamine. Raw beer will only have a small amount of N-nitrosodimethylamine can be ignored, nitrification reagents in the curing process (1500 ~ 1800 ℃) in the form of nitrogen oxides exist to improve the curing conditions can significantly reduce the malt beer in the nitramine concentration.

Other alcoholic beverages such as wines, cider, rice and spirits are usually free of volatile nitrosamines. Seven of the Scottish whiskey with six N-nitrosodimethylamine were tested; Waller et al. Studied 145 French apple brandy and found 50% N-nitrosodimethylamine.

(3) Tobacco and Smoke

Hoffmann, Brunemann, Hecht and his colleagues first studied the nitroso compounds in tobacco and smoke. The tobacco that has just been harvested does not contain nitrosamines. However, in its drying, aging, fermentation process will form nitrosamines. Smoking can form nitrosamines, the formation of the amount of nitrate and tobacco related to the content.

Tobacco Specificity Nitrosamines are the only known class of nasal carcinogens, and nitrosamines in snuff can be extracted from tobacco blocks and can also be detected in saliva with snuff and chewing tobacco blocks.

(4) Pesticides

Since Roos et al. Have confirmed that pesticides have been contaminated with nitrosamines for the first time, this has been extensively studied. In the United States, more than 300 compounds were studied. It has been shown that pesticides containing the following genes are potential amylamine carriers: dinitroaniline derivatives (especially 2,6-dinitroaniline), dimethylamine salts with phenoxy chains, diethanolamine salts in acidic pesticides And triethanolamine salts (such as maleic acid hydrazide), quaternary amine compounds and morpholine derivatives.

The nitrosamines in pesticides can exist in the form of impurities and can also exist in the form of contaminants, with the following forms of formation: side reactions in the production process; the use of contaminated chemicals in the synthesis; preservatives (especially nitrous acid Salt); nitrosation reagents in the environment; intermolecular rearrangement. In addition, many chlorine-containing pesticides can be nitrosated under experimental conditions to form N-nitroso compounds amine precursor.

The US Environmental Protection Agency has made a decision to reduce the exposure of humans to pesticides that can produce nitroso compounds. As a result, many pesticide manufacturers have reduced or even eliminated the pollution of nitrosamines in pesticides by preventing nitrosation and direct chemical damage.

(5) Cosmetics

Diethanolamine, triethanolamine and some salts (eg, dodecyl sulphate) are widely used in many industrial emulsions such as cosmetics (such as ointment, cream, shampoo, lipstick). The contamination of nitrosamines in cosmetics may be due to the use of contaminated paints or the results of contact with nitrosation reagents such as NO2 during production. <u>Analysis of cosmetics widely used in the United States, 27 of the 29 samples were detected N-nitrosodiethanolamine. N-nitrosodimethanolamine can be detected in the urine after exposure to N-nitrosodimethanolamine-contaminated cosmetics, indicating that the compound is easily absorbed through the skin.</u>

(6) carcinogenic mechanism

<u>The carcinogenic effects of nitrosamines are related to their chemical structure, route of administration, drug dose and animal species.</u>

On the carcinogenic mechanism of nitrosamines, the more common view is the nitrosamine compounds in the role of mixed functional oxidase can be generated diazoethane, and then by dealkylation to form free methyl. The latter causes the nucleic acid and protein of the cell to be alkylated, in particular the alkylation of RNA and DNA guanine. <u>Nucleic acid after alkylation changes the genetic characteristics of cells, through somatic mutations or cell differentiation disorders, leading to the occurrence of cancer.</u>

<u>For nitrosamide, it is generally believed that it can be directly carcinogenic.</u>

In some parts of China, South Africa and Iran, the incidence of esophageal cancer is quite high. <u>Our scientists have revealed the incidence of esophageal cancer and nitrite in the urine of nitroso amino acids, including nitroso-sarcosine-related relationship, and nitrosyl sarcosine is esophageal cancer carcinogens.</u> In China, high risk areas of esophageal cancer, the potential risk of endogenous nitrosation is also very high. In China and South Africa, mildew food in the nitrosamine pollution has been considered an incentive for esophageal cancer. In southern China, <u>nasopharyngeal carcinoma is more common, studies have shown that the incidence of nitrite and proline-related, more intake of salted fish is an important risk factor. In the salted fish can be detected in nitrosamines such as N-nitrosodimethylamine, etc., with the Guangdong salted fish fed rats can induce nasal cancer, these proved that nitrosamines are nasopharyngeal carcinogenic factors.</u>

Fish, meat and other foods in the nitrate and nitrite salt salted fish and meat is an ancient method, its effectiveness is reduced by the nitrate nitrate nitrite, nitrite can inhibit some of the spoilage bacteria Growth, so as to achieve the purpose of corrosion.

About 50 years ago, it was found that only a small amount of nitrite treatment of food, can achieve a lot of nitrate effect. The nitrite is then gradually substituted for nitrates as preservatives and colorants. **China's provisional meat products in the residual amount of sodium nitrite shall not exceed 30 mg / kg, canned meat can not exceed 50 mg / kg.**

There are a lot of nitrates and nitrates in the nature of the amines in the environment, and secondary amines (secondary amines) may also be present. Nitrite and secondary amine do not have carcinogenic effects, but in the acidic conditions can be biosynthesis of nitrosamines compounds.

Gastric cancer is one of the most common multiple malignant tumors. The etiology of gastric cancer may be related to the level of nitrate and nitrite in the environment, especially the content of nitrate in drinking water.

According to the etiology of esophageal cancer, the incidence of esophageal cancer is related to the environmental factors. In addition to aflatoxin, soil nitrogen and nitrosamines may be important environmental factors. In the areas of Hepatocarcinoma high incidence the non-staple food, especially pickles, contains the nitrosamine; in the areas of the high incidence of liver cancer the determination of nitrosamine in the pickles showed that the detection rate of nitrosamines is up to 60%. From the domestic and international epidemiological survey results, some of the human cancer may be related to N-nitroso compounds.

Chile's nitrate production ranks first in the world, agriculture, the use of a large number of nitrate fertilizer, so that the higher levels of nitrite in food, the body of the opportunity to increase the rate of nitramine, so that Chile's first gastric cancer mortality in the world may be related to this. Linzhou City, Henan Province, China is also one of the world's high incidence of esophageal cancer, with high incidence of sauerkraut soup concentrate or pickled cabbage extract, successfully induced rat esophageal cancer.

A lot of evidence shows that N-nitroso compounds are carcinogenic causes of various human cancers, including oral cancer, lung cancer, esophageal cancer, pancreatic cancer, liver cancer, nasopharyngeal carcinoma and bladder cancer.

7, the measures of preventing the harm of nitroso compounds

The nitrosation of nitroso compounds can be influenced by a variety of compounds and environmental conditions. Such as vitamin C, vitamin E, tannic acid and phenolic compounds can inhibit its synthesis. Sucrose has a blocking effect on the synthesis of nitroso compounds at pH 3. When the molecular concentration is twice as high as that of nitrite, the blocking effect is the best. In the system to make sausage, such as the addition of nitrilate at the same time to add vitamin C to prevent the formation of dimethyl nitrosamines. But vitamin C has no effect on the formation of nitrosamines. Chen Bingqing concluded that the prevention of nitroso compounds harm the main measures are the following:

(1) to ensure that food is fresh, which is essential to reduce the content of nitroso compounds in food To prevent food poisoning can prevent other microbial contamination, because some bacteria can be reduced nitrate nitrite, but also decomposition of protein, which is defaulted asthe amine compounds, and also become theenzymatic nitrosation. Therefore, in food processing, it should ensure that food is fresh; to prevent microbial contamination.

(2) through the diet to prevent and reduce the harm of nitroso compounds, vitamin C can block the process of nitrosation in the stomach. Vitamin C can inhibit the precursor formation of nitrosamines, both in vivo and in vitro are effective. Vitamin C can block the synthesis of nitrosamines in the stomach, reducing the level of exposure to nitrosamine in the stomach, the performance of gastric nitrosamine content decreased. Some natural fruit juice also contains ascorbic acid other than the inhibition of nitrosation of unknown ingredients. Soy products can also effectively inhibit the synthesis of N-nitrite, the inhibition of the order of the order is soy milk powder> bean paste> tofu, soy products can reduce the nitrite content and induced liver cancer have a significant preventive effect. Tea in the body played by the antioxidant effect, the way is not a single, not only can be directly removed from the same base can also be induced by the elimination of free radical enzyme epidemic, inhibit carcinogen activation and promote activation of carcinogens degradation, And other integrated process to block lipid peroxidation, inhibition of peroxidation damage, which play the role of anti-cancer. **Chinese scholars found that garlic and allicin can inhibit nitrate nitrate in the stomach, so that significantly reduced the amount of nitrite in the stomach. In addition, kiwi fruit, seabuckthorn fruit juice also has a blocking effect,** the former also inhibit the N-nitrosodimethylamine mutagenic effect.

(3) **strict control of the food processing process to minimize the use of nitrate and nitrite, in order to reduce the amount of nitrosylated precursor, in the processing process is feasible, try to use nitrite and nitrate alternatives.**

Dioxins and their analogues

Since January 1999, Belgium, the Netherlands, France and other countries have been due to dietary contamination of dioxin, which led to poultry, meat products and dairy products containing high concentrations of carcinogens - dioxin events. After the incident, attracted wide attention from all over the world.

Urban fixed waste incineration of fly ash contains dioxins. Contains polyvinyl chloride and other garbage incineration may be higher.

Car exhaust gas due to the incomplete combustion of gasoline, car exhaust can release dioxins.

In industrialized countries, dioxin is mainly derived from municipal solid waste incineration, chlorine-containing chemicals, pulp bleaching and vehicle exhaust emissions. And China has a different source of pollution with the industrialized countries, due to the need to prevent the use of schistosomiasis to prevent the use of a large number of PCP-Na snails, resulting in China's Yangtze River Basin rivers and lakes serious pollution. In addition, small paper mills all over China, the discharge of waste water and waste residue caused by serious pollution of major rivers and lakes. Therefore, the dioxin industry in China's pollution must not be ignored.

(1) dioxin into the body of the way

The body can be exposed to dioxin by different means, including food, air, and drinking water. Among them, 90% from the diet, and animal food is its main source. In theory, the meat to cut fat, the use of low-fat milk powder, increase the intake of vegetables, fruits and cereals can effectively prevent dioxin on human harm.

(2) the way of food contamination

Due to the fat solubility of dioxin and its high stability in the environment, from the production and use of chlorine chemicals, fixed waste incineration, paper bleaching process caused by environmental pollution, mostly in the water through the aquatic plants, zooplankton - herbivorous fish - fish and fish and geese, ducks and other poultry food chain process, in the fish and poultry and its protein accumulation. **At the same time, due to the flow of atmospheric atmosphere, dioxin in the dust settling on the ground plants, pollution of vegetables, food and feed. Animal consumption of ontaminated feed also causes dioxin accumulation. Therefore, fish, poultry and their eggs, meat and other major pollution of food.**

(3) Carcinogenicity

2,3,7,8-tetrachlorodibenzo-p-dioxins were highly carcinogenic to animals and were studied in four animal species (rats, mice, hamsters and fish) Positive results. Continuous administration of 2,3,7,8-tetrachlorodibenzo-p-dioxins to rodents, both sexes can induce multi-site tumors, the lowest dose of liver cancer in mice as low as 10 pg / g (body weight). Epidemiological studies suggest that exposure to 2,3,7,8-tetrachlorodibenzo-p-dioxins and their homologues in the population is associated with an increased overall risk of all cancers, **according to which the International Cancer Research Center It is judged as carcinogenic to human carcinogenic class I.**

Dioxin is a carcinogen that can induce cancer alone with dioxin alone. Based on the results of animal experiments and epidemiological studies, dioxin can be considered as a human carcinogen.

The International Cancer Research Center classifies it as a definite human carcinogen (class I).

(4) dioxin control measures

In the face of the harm caused by the pollution of dioxin, the world's major industrialized countries on the basis of investigation and study, have developed measures to prevent dioxin pollution, **combined with China's special national conditions, China's dioxin control the following recommendations:**

① **to strengthen the disposal of waste incineration, control emissions**

By the State Environmental Protection Agency to develop control measures to reduce the large incineration plant dioxin emissions.

② **improve the production process, reduce the production of dioxin substances**

Control the production of chemical products in the process of dioxin, to prevent environmental pollution.

③ **to expand the publicity of environmental protection and food hygiene**

As the bulk of dioxin exposed to human contact from the diet, so the security of food supply system is essential. In theory, pay attention to dietary structure, reduce the intake of animal fat, can reduce dioxin intake. Fiber foods and chlorophyll help to eliminate long-term accumulation of dioxins in the body.

However, to completely solve the problem, we must improve the overall level of human awareness and production capacity, pay attention to ecological construction, reduce environmental pollution to achieve the goal of modernization in order to ensure the sustainable, stable and healthy development of human society.

Second, how to overcome cancer and how to prevent cancer I see two

(A) From the follow-up results it found the problems and asked questions (hint: the study of the prevention and control of the postoperative recurrence and metastasis is the key to improve the long-term postoperative effect)

↓

Find a way(to tackle cancer, where is the way?)

↓

Find Path and footprint (anti-cancer, anti-cancer metastasis scientific research, scientific and technological innovation series)

Published cancer monograph (3 Chinese version of the monograph on the national distribution, 4 full English english global release)

↓

Participated in the International Conference on Oncology (Participated in the AACR Academic Conference, Washington)

↓

Visit the Stoutin Cancer Institute in Houston, USA (2009)

↓

Walk out a new path of an immune regulation of molecular level in combination with traditional Chinese and Western medications

↓

- walk out of a new way to overcome cancer

- published English monograph "The Road to Overcome Cancer"

(To overcome the road of cancer)

It was worldwide published on December 6th, 2016 in Washington, USA.

(B) XZ-C proposed to attack the cancer launched a total attack

Xu Ze in its third book "new concept of cancer treatment and new methods" (published in Beijing in 2011) Chapter 38 proposed that this is the first time the international: "attack the cancer launched a total attack"

1, what is the total attack against cancer?

The total attack is to develop and go hand in hand the comprehensive work for the prevention of the cancer and cancer control and cancer treatment during the whole process of the occurrence and development of cancer cancer three stages of work in full swing, simultaneously and the prevention and treatment of cancer at the same time and level.

What are the prevention of cancer and cancer control and treatment of cancer?

Ie:

the prevention of cancer - before the formation of cancer

Cancer control- has malignant transformation of precancerous lesions

Cancer treatment - has formed a foci or metastases

Change the current setting up hospital mode

Change the current treatment pattern

Namely:

to change the current hospital model which is only focusing on treatment.

to change the current treatment models which is only focusing on the middle and late stage.

To change only treatment without the prevention into the prevention and control and treatment of cancer at the same level and attention

How to implement this new unification model?

It should be established the hospital with the prevention and control and treatment of cancer during the whole process of the occurrence and development of cancer

2, the way-out of the treatment is in the "three early" (early detection, early diagnosis, early treatment)

The aarly cancer treatment is effective and can be cured, especially precancerous lesions and can be well handled and can be cured.

(C) XZ-C proposed to overcome cancer and launch a total attack to create the Science City of conquering caner which is the first time in the international

To overcome the cancer it must create "the science city of capturing the cancer and launching a total attack"

How to overcome the cancer I see 1 - 5

1, how to overcome cancer? To overcome cancer, it must create "innovative molecular cancer medical school"

(1) why to set up "innovative molecular cancer medical school"?

(2) how to set up "innovative molecular cancer medical school"?

2, how to overcome cancer? To overcome the cancer, we must create "the innovative molecular tumor hospital of the prevention and treatment during the whole process of occurrence and development of cancer" (the global demonstration hospital with the prevention and treatment during the whole process of occurrence and development of cancer)

(1) Why should we start? (2) how to start?

3, how to overcome cancer? To overcome cancer, we must create "the Innovative Molecular Cancer Institute"

(1) Why should we start? (2) how to start?

4, how to overcome cancer? To overcome cancer, it must create "the experimental medicine cancer animal experimental center"

(1) Why should we start? (2) how to start?

5, how to overcome cancer? To overcome the cancer, we must create "the innovative molecular tumor nano-pharmaceutical factory" and "to create the analysis research group and laboratory of anti-cancer transfer active ingredients, molecular weight, structural formula and immunopharmacology of anti-cancer chinese medications at the molecular level"

(1) Why should we start?

Because conquering cancer must be studied and he development of anti-cancer, anti-cancer metastasis of the effective drugs, XZ-C considers that captures cancer must have two wheels:

One is the life sciences, biopharmaceutical (modern medicine) A wheel.

One is the clinical basis, immune regulation, anti-cancer bolt (Chinese herbal medicine) B wheels.

Its purpose is: in-depth development of Chinese herbal medications of anti-cancer, anti-transfer which is indeed effective drugs; to remove the coarse and to storage fine; the natural medications become as the resources and conduct the modern research and make it to become precision medicine.

To further study the molecular regulation of anti - cancer Chinese medication cells by immunoregulation.

To further explore the prevention and treatment of anti-cancer, anti-cancer Chinese herbal medication on early carcinoma in situ and precancerous lesions.

(D) XZ-C proposed to attack the cancer and to launch a total attack, it must establish anti-cancer research institute and anti-cancer system engineering, which is the first international

To do the anti-cancer research, to find carcinogenic factors, and to detect the carcinogenic or carcinogenic factors and to try to prevent these carcinogenic factors on the human body damage, the anti-cancer research institute should carry out anti-cancer research and the urgent need is that the research contents are rich and very broad.

Track the source of carcinogens or carcinogenic factors.

While Human beings searches for cancer etiology and conditions of the process, the most prominent is that more than 90% of the cancer are caused by environmental factors.

1, the relationship between air pollution and cancer

Humans have developed tens of millions of tons of coal, oil and natural gas as fuel and energy. Such as fire power, smelting steel, cars, aircraft and other means of transport and household life fuel and other production and life process, **day and night kept a lot of tar, bituminous coal, dust and other harmful substances being discharged into the atmosphere, causing air pollution.**

Air pollution can cause many diseases, especially respiratory diseases, the most serious is lung cancer.

2, water pollution and cancer

Water pollution is mainly caused by industrial and agricultural production and urban sewage. There are many types of pollutants in the water; the farm drugs and pesticides are one of the important pollutants in water; the neutral detergent in the surfactant also is promote cancer.

3, the soil pollution and cancer

A large number of industrial waste water and pesticide fertilizer pour into the soil so that it deteriorates the soil quality; the poison continues the accumulation which threatens the human health and is also carcinogenic factors.

4, chemistry and cancer

5, physical factors and cancer

6, biological factors and cancer

7, diet and cancer

8, lifestyle and cancer

9, clothing, food, live, line, house decoration and cancer

It should study the method of the effect of so many carcinogens or carcinogenic factors.

It is to study these sources of pollution and to try to stop at the source.

It is to study these carcinogenic mechanisms, its carcinogenic effects.

It is to study how to reduce or prevent the prevention of these carcinogens.

Because cancer patients cover the whole world and the industrial and agricultural waste water and the waste residue and waste gas pollution are also covered the world, therefore, it must be the whole world to attack cancer and to launch a total attack.

Professor Xu Ze suggested: ① various countries, provinces, all states should establish anti-cancer research institute (or institutions) and carry out anti-cancer system engineering for their own country, the province, the city to carry out anti-cancer work.

② the countries to establish anti-cancer regulations and to carry out (some should be legislation)

③ I will recommend this project to the World Health Organization to launch anti-cancer action, the goal is to try to reduce the incidence of cancer. To overcome cancer is the forefront of science, is a worldwide problem, cancer is a human disaster covering the whole world, people around the world are eager to one day to overcome cancer, for the benefit of mankind.

Cancer is a disaster of all mankind and must be struggling with the whole world

The people of the world work together

To overcome the cancer, to launch a total attack, this is an unprecedented event

For the benefit of mankind

Fifth, anti-cancer research work cannot walk slowly and should run forward to save the dying and heal the wound

Why did I propose to tackle cancer and launch a total attack? Because of the series of ideas and design studies that have taken care of cancer, I have been working for five to six years and we have made a whole set of basic ideas and design, planning and blueprints to tackle cancer. And published in 2011, monographs, "new concepts and new methods of cancer treatment," Chapter 38 with a chapter of the length of "the strategic thinking and recommendations to overcome cancer," it was proposed "to attack the cancer and to launch a total attack."

And then in 2013 it was put forward "to build the total design of the science city to overcome cancer." In August 2013 for the first time in the international community it was put forward: "the XZ-C research program of attacking cancer and launching a total attack." In July 2015 it was proposed and named the "dawn of the C-type plan" and put forward "to attack the cancer and launch a total attack" and "to build a science park to overcome cancer," this work is being reported and asking for implementation.

To overcome the cancer and to launch a total attack are unprecedented in human work and it must personally create experience and the personally practice.

China's daily about 8550 people were diagnosed with cancer, 6 is diagnosed with cancer per minute . Therefore, the research work of conquering cancer and launching the total offensive can not walk slowly and should run forward to save the dying.

2017.2.5 reference message:

The World Health Organization (WHO) today reported that 8.8 million people die from cancer each year in the world, with the highest number of cancer deaths in the respiratory system, according to data released by the World Health Organization on February 4, World Cancer Day, Up to 169.5 million per year.

The latest data are based on 2015 statistics, raising the number of people who die from cancer each year from 8.1 million in 2010 to $ 8.8 million.

The most deadly cancer, which is second only to respiratory cancer, is liver cancer (788,000 deaths per year), colorectal cancer (774,000), gastric cancer (753,600) and breast cancer (571,000).

Esophageal cancer (41.5 million), pancreatic cancer (358,000), prostate cancer (343,800), lymphoma (343,500) and other cancer worldwide are also high mortality rates.

From the gender point of view, 8.8 million cancer deaths in nearly 5 million men. For men, the highest incidence of cancer is respiratory cancer and liver cancer.

For women, the highest incidence of cancer is breast cancer and respiratory cancer.

Distribution from the regional point of view, the largest case of cancer in the Western Pacific region, including respiratory cancer and liver cancer accounted for the highest proportion.

After the West Pacific is the Southeast Asian region, including respiratory cancer, oral cancer and throat cancer accounted for the highest proportion.

In Europe, the most common cancer is also respiratory cancer, followed by colorectal cancer.

Cancer is covered by the global disaster, the global people are eager to one day to overcome cancer, eager to state, government, experts, scholars, scientists can find anti-cancer measures, so that people can stay away from cancer.

Professor Xu Ze has been engaged in clinical surgery for 60 years and uses "to overcome the cancer" as the research direction of animal experiments and clinical validation; the basic work has been 30 years, deeply appreciate that about cancer it not only should pay attention to treatment, but also should pay attention to prevention in order to stop at the source, therefore it was put forward: it should launch the total attack and conquer cancer and the prevention and treatment of cancer should be at the same level and attention.

1, how to overcome cancer?

The purpose should be:

(1) ① reduce the incidence of cancer

② improve cancer cure rate, extend the survival of cancer patients, improve the quality of life

(2) up to 1/3 can be prevented

1/3 can be cured

1/3 through treatment can extend life

2, how to improve the cure rate?

How to treat?

<u>It should walk out of a new path of cancer:</u>

(1) to overcome the cancer and to launch a total attack

① the general attack is to develop the work in full swing, simultaneously of the prevention and control and treatment three stages during of the occurrence and the development of cancer during the whole process of cancer. Troika, go hand in hand, keep pace with each other.

② change the current hospital mode - that is, to change the current governance as the focus of the hospital model.

Change the current treatment model - that is, to change the current treatment, the focus of the treatment model, the only cure, to prevent, control, governance both.

(2) how to implement this new hospital model?

It should be established the hospital with the prevention and control and treatment of cancer during the whole process of the occurrence and development of cancer.

(3) the way our of cancer treatment is in the "three early" (early detection, early diagnosis, early treatment), early cancer treatment effect is good, can be cured, especially cancer lesions can be well handled and can be cured.

3, how to reduce the incidence of cancer?

How to prevent?

It should walk out of a new way to prevent cancer:

(1) XZ-C that: how to prevent cancer? It should create anti-cancer research institute, and create anti-cancer system engineering.

To study carcinogenic factors and their sources and to study ways to prevent or avoid.

(2) what can be treated?

A, what are the carcinogenic factors?

B, what are the sources of carcinogenic factors?

How to prevent?

A, How to reduce its source?

B, how to stop its source?

The prevention of cancer work should be blocked at the source and should stop the source of carcinogenic factors.

The prevention of cancer is active and is attack.

Cancer is passive and is to keep.

How to prevent? What should it prevent? How to prevent? It should be in-depth study and the evaluation objectives are: to reduce the incidence.

How to treat? What should it treat? How to treat? It should be in-depth study and the evaluation objectives are: to improve the cure rate.

1. **How to improve the cure rate of cancer? How to extend the survival term of cancer patients, improve the quality of life and reduce complications?**

<u>How to treat?</u>

<u>After more than 30 years of experimental and clinical validation study, we have walked out of a new way to overcome cancer</u>

<u>(1) through experimental research and anti-cancer research of Chinese medication immunopharmacology and the combination of Chinese and Western medication at the molecular level, we walked out of the new path which is the traditional Chinese medication with immune regulation, regulation of immune activity, to prevent thymus atrophy, promote thymic hyperplasia, protect bone marrow hematopoietic function, improve immune surveillance.</u>

<u>We have walked out of a new path with XZ-C immune regulation and the combination of chinese and western medication at the molecular level to overcome cancer ---- the "Chinese-style anti-cancer" new road.</u>

A), I am a clinical surgeon, for chest, general work, why did I study the cancer? This is caused by the results after the petition from a number of cancer patients:

Since 1985, I have done the petition for more than 3,000 patients with thoracic and abdominal cancer patients, the results were found that most patients had the recurrence or metastasis within 2-3 years after the surgery, from the follow-up results it was found: postoperative recurrence and metastasis are the key for the postoperative long-term effect. And therefore we have raised an important question: that clinicians must pay attention to and study the prevention and control measures of the postoperative recurrence and metastasis to improve postoperative long-term efficacy.

So we established the Experimental Surgery Laboratory to do the experimental tumor research: the implementation of cancer cell transplantation, the establishment of tumor animal model and it was carried out a series of experimental tumor research.

B), we conducted a full 4 years of laboratory experiments in the laboratory was the clinical basis of research.

From the experimental results it was found that: the thymus in the host inoculated cancer cells was acute atrophy and the cell proliferation blocked and the volume was significantly reduced. From the above experimental study it was found that: thymic atrophy and immune dysfunction may be one of the causes of cancer and pathogenesis. Therefore, the (cancer) treatment principle must be to try to prevent thymic atrophy, promote thymocyte proliferation, increase immune function.

In order to try to prevent thymic atrophy, promote thymocyte hyperplasia, increased immune function, it was to find this medication form both the traditional Chinese medication and Western medication . In Western medication it is rare which can improve the immune drugs, promote thymus hyperplasia drugs so that we changed from the Chinese herbal medicine to find.

Why were the medications which can promote thymus hyperplasia, prevent thymus atrophy, enhance immune drugs searched from the Chinese medications?

Because polysaccharide traditional Chinese medication and tonic medication have many roles of immune regulation.

Chinese medication polysaccharide anti-cancer immune function research progresses quickly and have conducted a large number of immunopharmacological studies from the molecular level and polysaccharides can improve the body immune surveillance system.

Our laboratory conducted a series of experimental studies from natural medications looking for new anti-cancer, anti-metastatic, anti-thymic atrophy, and increased immune function immunoregulatory anti-cancer Chinese medications.

C), the exclusive research and the development of XZ-C immune regulation anti-cancer Chinese medication products

The experimental study + clinical application + typical case + case list

(Xu Ze - China) immunoregulatory anti-cancer series of traditional Chinese medication preparation and from experimental research to clinical validation, on the basis of the successful animal experiments, then applied to the clinical practice, after 30 years of 12000 cases of clinical validation, it has the significant effect for independent innovation.

XZ-C immunocompromised anti-cancer traditional Chinese medications are from China's more than 200 kinds of traditional Chinese herbal medications to screen out 48 kinds of the good anti-tumor rate of Chinese herbal in vivo tumor inhibition test medications in the tumor-bearing mice and after it is composed of the compound and the was tested in vivo tumor inhibition test in the mice and the compound tumor inhibition rate is much greater than the single herbicide inhibition rate. XZ-C1 has 100% inhibition of cancer cells and 100% does not kill normal cells with Fuzheng Guben to improve the role of human immune function.

From our experiments on XZ-C pharmacodynamics study it shows that: in the Ehrlich ascites cancer, S180, H22 hepatocellular carcinoma it has a good tumor inhibition rate.

Acute toxicity test in mice shows there is no obvious side effects. In the clinical long-term oral years (2-6-8 years) there is also no obvious side effects.

The Middle and advanced cancer patients are mostly weak and weak, fatigue, loss of appetite; after XZ-C immune regulation of anti-cancer Chinese medication for 4-8-12 weeks, it can significantly improve appetite, sleep, relieve pain, gradually restore physical.

2.Why should we prevent cancer?

Professor Xu Ze proposed that to overcome the cancer must pay attention to the cancer prevention research because the treatment of the disease should first treat the etiology; to treat the cause of the disease can be effective. The prevention of cancer is also the first study of carcinogenic factors and their sources and it is for cancer-causing factors to be stopped in order to be effective.

That is not only to rely on the existing anti-cancer science publicity knowledge, but should be macro, micro, ultra-micro, high-tech research.

How to conduct the cancer prevention research? Professor Xu Ze proposed: to create cancer preventin research institute, to create cancer prevention research system engineering, the establishment of graduate school, "the Science City of attacking the cancer and launch a total attack," the academic committee, experts, scholars will lead 100 doctoral and graduate students to prevent cancer, Research on the prevention cancer research. I will develop a large number of in-depth study of research topics, based on the known science, to explore the future of science, the development of science.

It is now the fourth stage of our research work. After 2011, we are conducting and conducting research work, step by step, positioning the research goal or "target" to reduce the incidence of cancer, improve the cure rate and prolong the survival period.

We have 28 years of cancer research work: the first three stages of experimental research and clinical research work, mainly in the treatment of new drugs, new methods of diagnosis, new technologies, new concepts of treatment, new methods. The experimental study was mainly for the establishment of a variety of cancer model, to explore the regulation and mechanism of the incidence of cancer and invasion and recurrence and metastasis to find the effective control of metastasis and recurrence of the effective measures. It was the experimental Study on Experimental Screening of Anti - cancer Chinese Herbal Medications.

But today is the 21st century, the second 10 years and the cancer incidence continues to rise and is still rampant and has the high mortality rate. I have been engaged in clinical cancer surgery for 60 years, the more patients and the more treated and the incidence of cancer continues to rise so that I deeply appreciate the cancer not only pay attention to treatment, but also to pay attention to prevention in order to stop at the source.

Therefore, I am deeply aware of that the work of cancer does not not only focus on the treatment, research new drugs, new methods, new technologies, but also must focus on how to reduce the incidence of cancer? How to prevent the incidence of cancer continues to rise in the momentum?

The current tumor hospital or oncology mode is to go all out to focus on treatment, for patients with advanced disease and has the poor efficacy, exhaustes human and financial resources, and fails to achieve lower morbidity, the more treatment and the more patients. <u>The status quo is: for a century the road is focusing on the heavy treatment and having light defense, or only treatment . Over the years we have just been working on cancer. But in the prevention of cancer the work is done very little, and almost did not do so that the incidence of cancer continues to rise.</u>

For the Review, reflection, cliché anti-cancer of the prevention of cancer work in a century, we have done in the cancer prevention research or work? What has it been done?

The medical school textbooks teaching content does not attach importance to the cancer prevention knowledge.

The medical school mode does not attach importance to anti-cancer science set up work.

Medical school or hospital research projects do not attach importance to anti-cancer research projects.

Journal of Oncology has not paid attention to cancer prevention work papers.

In short, the prevention of cancer is not attached importance and the prevention is not paid attention. Cliché prevention is as main which is not to be concerned about the implementation.

How to do? How to reduce the incidence of cancer? How to improve cancer cure rate? How to reduce cancer mortality? How do I extend my life? How to improve the quality of life?

It should be launched to overcome the general attack of cancer and work with both the prevention and the treatment of cancer.

The goal of cancer should be: to reduce morbidity, improve the cure rate, reduce mortality, prolong survival, improve quality of life, reduce complications.

The current global hospitals and the hospitals in China are going all out to engage in treatment, pay attention to the treatment and ignore defense, or only treatmet without the prevention.

XZ-C thinks of that this hospital model or cancer treatment model can not overcome the cancer and can not reduce the incidence. The global hospitals and our hospital must be on the overall strategy of cancer treatment to change from the focusing on treatment into the focusing on prevention and treatment.

Therefore, we propose to launch a total attack and design of cancer, XZ-C (Xu Ze-China) proposed to launch a total attack, that is, the three-stage work of the prevention cancer and cancer control and cancer treatment is carried out simultaneously.

It was put forward the "the necessity and feasibility report for attacking on cancer to start the general attack on".

It was proposed "the XZ-C research program to overcome the cancer and launch a total attack of".

Our 28 years of cancer research in the fourth phase of the research focus: after 2011 -

Cancer research work, step by step

- focus on research and focus on the overall strategic reform of cancer treatment to focus on the treatment of prevention and treatment
- We propose to launch the general attack on cancer, that is, cancer prevention and cancer control and treatment cancer three stages of work in full swing, simultaneously during the whole process of the occurrence and the development of cancer . That is:

Prevention cancer - before the formation of cancer

Control Cancer - malignant transformation of precancerous lesions

Treatment Cancer - has formed a foci or metastases

- total attack target: to reduce the incidence of cancer, reduce cancer mortality, improve the cure rate, prolong survival, improve quality of life, reduce complications.
- the need to attack the general attack of cancer

Why should I raise the total attack? Look at the present situation:

- the incidence of cancer is the status quo of the more patients treated more and more, our average daily 8550 cases of new cancer patients, the country every minute 6 people are diagnosed with cancer

- the status of cancer mortality is high, has been the first cause of death in urban and rural areas in China, the average daily 7,500 people died of cancer

- the status of treatment, despite the application of the traditional three treatment for nearly a hundred years, tens of thousands of cancer patients to bear the radiotherapy and chemotherapy, but how are the results? So far the cancer is still the first cause of death.

- the current tumor hospital or oncology Department of the status of the hospital model: heavy treatment and light defense, or only treatment, the more treatment and the more patients.

● the feasibility of attacking the total attack of cancer

Has whether it have the scientific basis or not about now it is proposed to attack the total attack of cancer? Is there a medical foundation? Is it possible to win the favorable conditions? Although nearly a century, the traditional therapy failed to conquer cancer, traditional therapy; the radiotherapy and chemotherapy can not overcome cancer, because it can only alleviate, can not be cured. Now it is proposed to launch a total attack, which has a scientific basis and medical basis, and is feasible.

Third, how to overcome cancer, how to prevent cancer I see three

(一) why put forward to overcome cancer, need to launch a total attack?

1, because the goal of cancer should be:

(1) reduce the incidence of cancer

Improve cancer cure rate, prolong the survival of patients, improve the quality of life

(2) up to 1/3 can be prevented

1/3 can be cured

1/3 through treatment can extend life

2, then, how can we reduce the incidence of cancer?

It should be that the defense and control are as the main and the prevention is as the main and is the based.

But for decades, we have gone through the road is to pay attention to the treatment and ignore the prevention or only the treatment .

I have been working on clinical cancer surgery for 60 years, reviewing decades of reflection on the failure of the lesson is only treatment, so the incidence of cancer is increasing, the more treatment and the more patients.

How to do? It should be as the main prevention and the main control; and carry out the prevention of health-oriented approach; It is only attaining the importance of anti-cancer in order to reduce the incidence of cancer. The prevention of cancer and cancer control and how to prevent cancer should be the most important.

How to carry out the implementation of anti-cancer, cancer prevention, prevention of health-oriented approach, how to reform and correct the current re-treatment, light defense, or just cure the hospital model, hospital policy? It must challenge the treatment of cancer Hospital policy and the reform can develop.

Xu Ze (Xu Ze) Professor proposed to launch a total attack, in fact, is the prevention and the control and the treatment at the same level; to prevent cancer and to cancer control are put into the important parts. Its essence is to implement and to carry out the health work policy of the "the prevention of the cancer and anti-cancer", "the prevention is the main". Our medical predecessors, the world's medical sages put forward "the prevention of the cancer and anti-cancer" and "the prevention"; this policy is very correct, but unfortunately we do not pay attention to the younger generation, are not understood.

In particular, our cancer researchers and the health workers did not recognize this; for a century it neglected prevention and cancer prevention does not attach importance; to prevention of the cancer was not paid attention to and ignored which led to such a high incidence of cancer today. China has 8550 new daily cancer, 6 people per minute was diagnosed with cancer, such a staggering data; it should be national affairs and livelihood issues.

The health work should be the "disease prevention and treatment", "the prevention is as the main", the health is to defend life, to defend health, and it should be implemented the "the prevention is as the main." To Launch the overall attack, its essence is to put the prevent cancer work to an important position as the main and important point of the prevention of the cancer and anti-cancer, in an attempt to reduce the incidence of cancer.

Therefore, XZ-C proposed to attack the cancer and launch a total attack.

What is the total attack? The total attack is the prevention of the cancer and cancer control and cancer treatment three at the same time to carry out, three carriages go hand in hand, in fact, is prevention and control and treatment at the same lever . It is to put the prevention of cancer and cancer control as the important parts; its essence is to implement cancer prevention and anti-cancer and the prevention as the main health work policy, is to regain the light defense or only cure mode reform, only reform can develop.

So how to prevent cancer? What is it to prevent? How to prevent? How to implement?

While Human beings is searching for the cause of cancer and the conditions of cancer occurrence, the most prominent discovery is that more than 90% of the cancer are caused by environmental factors. Therefore, XZ-C proposed to establish anti-cancer research institute and anti-cancer system engineering, carry out anti-cancer research, to find carcinogenic factors, to detect carcinogenic factors, and try to prevent these carcinogenic factors on human damage, and the anti-cancer research institution should carry out anti-cancer research and it is the urgent need to study a lot of content, very broad.

To track the source of carcinogens or carcinogenic factors, which way should it be carried out from?

At present, with the improvement of people's living standards, a variety of high-tech products to bring us a better life at the same time, it may also bring many negative effects. The carcinogens of a variety of chemical, physical, biological environment largely emerge; a variety of carcinogenic substances come into our human body or a variety of carcinogenic factors affect our body, leading to an increasing incidence of cancer.

Because cancer is thought to be mainly caused by factors such as the environment, diet, hobby and so on, people will attach great importance to the carcinogenic factors in the environment and strive to clear them.

In order to carry out the prevention of cancer and cancer control work, Professor Xu Ze proposed: it should prevent cancer from the clothing, food, live, walking and from the big environment and the small environment.

How to prevent cancer from clothing, food, live and walking? First, it should master and understand the situation of containing carcinogens in the clothing, food, live, and other crops and whether there will be carcinogens? It should be qualitative, quantitative, monitoring, and then set the standard, set the bottom line to discuss, put forward anti-cancer measures.

(二) cancer is a disaster of all mankind, must fight with it in the world, the people of the world struggle

1, the catastrophe of cancer covers the whole world

Cancer incidence in world range:

"The Five continents cancer incidence" publications in 2002 edition of the publication was published by the International Agency for Research on Cancer (IARC) and the International Association for the Registration of Cancer, which contains data from 50 of the 55 countries and 215 populations.

The IARC thematic report brings together the results of a retrospective analysis of different potential carcinogenic risk factors from interdisciplinary group of experts from different regions of the world. These panelists evaluated a number of factors (including chemical factors, complex mixtures, occupational exposure factors, physical and biological factors, and lifestyle) to increase the risk of cancer.

Since 1971, the panel has evaluated more than 900 factors, of which nearly 400 have been identified as carcinogenic factors or potential carcinogenic factors. The complete catalogs and categories of these factors are regularly updated and can be found at http://monographs.iarc.fr/. This catalog is a scientific basis for public health, other disciplines, and national health authorities to take measures to avoid exposure to potential carcinogenic factors.

World cancer incidence

There is a large regional difference in the incidence and mortality of cancer in the world as a whole and in some special organs. The WHO Cancer Mortality Database and the GLOBOCAN 2002 database provide data on the incidence and prevalence and mortality of 27 different carcinomas in various countries in 2002.

In 2002, an estimated 10.9 million new cases of cancer (53% of men and 47% of women), of which 5.1 million occurred in developed countries and 5.8 million cases occurred in less developed countries.

The number of cancer deaths was 6.7 million (57% for men, 43% for women), 2.7 million in developed countries and 4 million in less developed countries. An estimated 24.5 million patients survived with various cancers (5 years after diagnosis, excluding non-melanoma of the skin).

According to population standardization, cancer incidence and mortality in different regions of the world are shown.

2, the situation of the world's cancer patients mortality, the status quo

2017.2.5 reference message

The World Health Organization (WHO) today reported that 8.8 million people die from cancer each year in the world, with the highest number of cancer deaths in the respiratory system, according to data released by the World Health Organization on February 4, World Cancer Day, Up to 169.5 million per year.

The latest figures are based on 2015 statistics, raising the number of people who die each year from 8.1 million in 2010 to 8.8 million.

The most deadly cancer, which is second only to respiratory cancer, is liver cancer (788,000 deaths per year), colorectal cancer (774,000), gastric cancer (753,600) and breast cancer (571,000).

Esophageal cancer (41.5 million), pancreatic cancer (358,000), prostate cancer (343,800), lymphoma (343,500) and other cancer worldwide are also high mortality rates.

From the gender point of view, 8.8 million cancer deaths in nearly 5 million men. For men, the highest incidence of cancer is respiratory cancer and liver cancer.

For women, the highest incidence of cancer is breast cancer and respiratory cancer.

Distribution from the regional point of view, the largest case of cancer in the Western Pacific region, including respiratory cancer and liver cancer accounted for the highest proportion.

After the West Pacific is the Southeast Asian region, including respiratory cancer, oral cancer and throat cancer accounted for the highest proportion.

In Europe, the most deadly cancer is also respiratory cancer, followed by colorectal cancer.

Cancer is covered by the global disaster, the global people are eager to one day to overcome cancer, eager to state, government, experts, scholars, scientists can find anti-cancer measures, so that people can stay away from cancer.

3, at the current the status quo of the global cancer 5-year survival rate

Today, the current 5-year survival rate of global cancer is still hovering at a low level

It can be said that today's clinicians in the clinical treatment of cancer options and methods available more and more. But we have to face a reality, a large number of clinical epidemiological analysis shows that the diagnosis and treatment of the ability and means of maturation and development, and the overall effect of tumor improvement seems not fully synchronized. **According to the American Cancer Society (The American Cancer Society) data (Figure), nearly a decade, a variety of malignancy diagnosis and treatment level than in the past has been greatly improved, but its 5-year survival rate is still hovering in a Lower level.** Such as the 2004 global colon cancer 5-year survival rate of 62%, although the colon cancer diagnostic techniques and surgical treatment has made considerable progress, but only increased to 65%, did not make a breakthrough. Liver cancer etiology, epidemiological studies and a variety of treatment techniques have been greatly improved, but the current 5-year survival rate of only 18%, 10 years ago, only increased by 11 percentage points, how to improve the prognosis of patients is still troubled Hepatobiliary surgeon's problem. The mortality rate of gastric cancer has been high, although the level of surgical technology continues to improve, but the 5-year survival rate of gastric cancer from only 10 years ago, 23% to 29%. In addition, the 5-year survival rate of pancreatic cancer than 10 years ago little change in the 5% up and down; esophageal cancer 5-year survival rate has been maintained at 14%; breast cancer 5-year survival rate from 10 years ago, 87% Down to the current 79%, cervical cancer from 71% to 69%, lung cancer 5-year survival rate from 15% to the current 14%.

XZ-C proposed the advice and suggestions of that to attack the cancer and launch a total attack must establish anti-cancer research institute and anti-cancer system engineering.

To do Anti-cancer research, to find carcinogenic factors and to detect the source of carcinogens or carcinogenic factors, and try to prevent these carcinogenic factors on the human body damage, anti-cancer research institute should carry out anti-cancer research. It is the urgent need to study a lot of content, very broad.

Track the source of carcinogens or carcinogenic factors.

While Human beings is in the process of the search for cancer etiology and conditions, the most prominent discovery is that more than 90% of the cancer is caused by environmental factors.

How to implement the creation of this anti-cancer research institute?

Professor Xu Ze XZ-C proposed anti-cancer design, proposed anti-cancer system engineering:

It should study the action way of so many carcinogens or carcinogenic factors.

It is to study these sources of pollution and try to stop at the source.

IT is to study these carcinogenic mechanisms and its carcinogenic effects.

It is to study how to reduce or prevent the prevention of these carcinogens.

It is because cancer patients cover the whole world and the industrial and agricultural waste water and waste residue and waste gas pollution also cover the world, therefore, it must be the whole world to attack the cancer and launch a total attack.

Professor Xu Ze suggested: ① various countries, provinces, all states should establish anti-cancer research institute (or institutions), carry out anti-cancer system engineering, for their own country, the province, the city to carry out anti-cancer work.

② each country establishes anti-cancer regulations and carry out (some should be legislation)

③ I will recommend this project to the World Health Organization to launch anti-cancer action, the goal is to try to reduce the incidence of cancer. To overcome cancer, is the forefront of science, is a worldwide problem, cancer is a human disaster, covering the whole world, people around the world are eager to one day to overcome cancer, for the benefit of mankind.

④ to promote scientific research ethics, medicine is benevolence, legislation for the first first

Scientific research ethics: products should have moral standards

Standard: it should not harm human health as the standard and as the bottom line

The basic ethics: all products should be harmless to people, do not harm people's health, especially for children

(To be beautiful, the flowers of the living environment, living environment)

⑤ the health administrative departments defend life and protect health, it should lead, hold, support and to guide anti-cancer measures and anti-cancer engineering and anti-cancer testing and anti-cancer monitoring.

Cancer is a disaster of all mankind, it must struggle with the world, the people of the world struggle, human beings should not sit still, physicians should not do nothing, health administration should not do nothing, should lead and guide the series of anti-cancer research project, common forward and work together, complementary advantages, the leadership and the guidance to overcome cancer and to launch a total attack.

XZ-C proposed to attack the cancer and to launch a total attack, is an unprecedented work of mankind, it must create their own experience and must practice in person. This is a new cement road, every step will leave the eternal scientific footprints.

The reform of the model of setting up the hospital: it should be changed to the prevention of cancer and control cancer and cancer treatment at the same level; or the prevention of cancer and cancer treatment at the same attention.

The way out of Cancer treatment is in the "three early": it must study the new technologies and the new methods of the diagnosis and treatment of the "three early".

How do a country to carry out and to build the "Science City" to conquer cancer and to attack a comprehensive attack to the cancer? I am initially envisioned and designed:

It is the recommendation: set the "National Cancer Working Group"(the detail will be discussed in the future).

So that each country's cancer research group must be flourishing,fruitful,benefit the people,beneficial to a well-off society,everyone is healthy, stay away from cancer.

Fourth, how to overcome cancer, how to prevent cancer I see four

How to prevent cancer from "the two types of society"?

(A) the construction of "two-oriented society" has a great relevance with the prevention cancer and controlling cancer

(1) Why should we build a "two-oriented society"?

Because industrial development has made great contributions to economic development, however, the environmental pollution brought about by industrial development is also very serious and must be strictly controlled by pollution control. why? The reason is that the environmental pollution will damage people's health.

The Status of industrial pollution emissions:

① Wastewater and water pollutants.

Chemical and papermaking and ferrous metal smelting are the main source of wastewater discharge.

② exhaust gas.

Industry is the main body of air pollutant emissions.

Energy production and consumption are the main source of air pollutant emissions in China, and have high pollution and did not bring the corresponding high yield.

China's environmental policy is a summary of the environmental policy of the history of social development at home and abroad, and the principles, principles, regulations, standards, systems and other policies formulated and implemented for the effective protection and improvement of the environment., Is China's environmental protection and management of the actual code of conducts.

China's existing environmental policy framework is shown in the figure

The Constitution and the basic national policy

Basic policy Basic strategy Sustainable development strategy "Double type" society

What is "the two-way society"?

That is the resource-level and environment-friendly, that is, "dual-type society."

Building a saving resource society put the prominent position of the development strategy on the industrialization and the modernization and implemented to each unit, each family. Building an environment-friendly society, is to highlight the important action of environmental protection, is to curb the deterioration of the environment imperative, it is also one of the important measures to prevent cancer.

At present, we are carrying out resource-saving and environment-friendly society, building comprehensive supporting test for energy-saving emission reduction, sewage treatment. This policy and work, and cancer prevention and control work is closely related, but also one of the important measures to prevent cancer.

Through energy-saving emission reduction, pollution prevention, pollution control, construction of "two-oriented society", people improve their health knowledge, environmental pollution and other carcinogenic factors for effective intervention, will reduce the incidence of cancer.

(B) environmental pollution can increase the incidence of cancer

I deeply understand: why is it to reduce the engage in "two-oriented society" of energy-saving emission and environment-friendly?

Because with the development of modern industrialization, a large number of energy consumption, a large number of production and life during the day and night kept a lot of tar, soot, dust and other harmful gases into the atmosphere, and causes the atmospheric pollution and water pollution and soil pollution and food contamination and occupational carcinogen surge.

In recent decades, the incidence and mortality of lung cancer in Western developed countries has increased rapidly such as the British lung cancer mortality in 1930 to 100 million, up to 1975 up to 120.3 / 10 million, 45 years, an increase of 12 times.

United States 1934 - 1974 male lung cancer mortality increased from 3.0 / 10 to 54.5 / 10 million, an increase of 17 times. The above data is amazing. If not energy-saving emission reduction, it will be a lot of emissions of pollution, greatly damage human health, promote cancer incidence and mortality rate of rapid growth.

According to the World Health Organization on February 4, "World Cancer Day," the date of the release of data, said: At present the world every year 8.8 million people died of cancer, including respiratory cancer death The highest number of up to 169.5 million per year.

From the gender point of view, 8.8 million cancer deaths in nearly 5 million men. For men, the highest incidence of cancer is respiratory cancer and liver cancer.

For women, the highest incidence of cancer is breast cancer and respiratory cancer.

Distribution from the regional point of view, the largest cancer case is the Western Pacific region, including respiratory cancer and liver cancer accounted for the highest ratio.

The most deadly cancer in Europe is also the cancer of the respiratory system, followed by colorectal cancer.

Cancer is covered by the world, the people of the world are eager to one day to overcome cancer, eager to all countries, governments, experts, scholars, scientists can find anti-cancer measures, so that people can stay away from cancer.

(C) why should we build a environment-friendly society with "two-oriented society"?

Because of environmental pollution is harmful to society, harmful to human life; to improve the environment, to prevent and control the pollution, to defend health are conducive to building a healthy, happy, harmonious, environment-friendly society, community.

So, what is the environmental pollution?

① the most frightening is that environmental pollutants contain many carcinogens, causing people to increase the incidence of cancer. Such as damage to the Japanese nuclear power plant, resulting in the surrounding air, water, soil, food, nuclear radiation material concentration greatly increased, to promote leukemia, cancer and other morbidity increased, not only to harm the contemporary and endanger generations.

(2) damage people's life and health, radiation, nuclear radiation, bacteria, viruses, harmful chemical poisoning, air pollution, water pollution, soil pollution, food pollution, not only harm people's life and health, but also lead to an increasing incidence of human cancer.

③ a large number of pollution of chemical substances, harmful gases, harmful water, fertilizer, pesticides can lead to cancer, gene mutation, causing high risk of cancer, high incidence.

Therefore, to reduce the incidence of cancer, we must improve the environment, prevention and control pollution, building an environment-friendly society, a harmonious society, a harmonious society.

(D) I think about the current energy-saving emission reduction, pollution prevention and pollution, to create a "two-oriented society" is to prevent cancer and I level prevention of cancer prevention. Its purpose and effect can achieve Class I prevention.

Anti-cancer strategy should be the prevention of cancer, cancer control, the use of I-level prevention, II-level prevention, III-level prevention. I deeply think that the current pollution reduction, pollution control is a class I prevention, in fact, from the fundament of the prevention of cancer measures, in fact, it is the prevention of cancer measures which the masses participate under the government mobilization.

Cancer is not only a serious threat to human health, but also an important factor in rising medical costs. China's annual costs of the direct use of cancer treatment is nearly 100 billion yuan so that patients and the whole society bear a huge financial burden. Many patients spent tens of thousands or even hundreds of thousands; however there is no the corresponding effect and the eventually the results are that both the human and financial are empty; the cancer mortality is still the first, how should I do? It is worthy of the analysis, reflection for our clinicians and it should be studied. How is the road of the study to go? It is sure to understand the current problems in the treatment.

Although countries have invested heavily in the treatment of cancer patients, the 5-year survival rate of some common cancers has not improved significantly over the past 20 years.

How to do? The way out of cancer is prevention; the prevention and intervention are the most important in the field of public health.

In recent years, it has been recognized that more than 90% of the cancer is caused by environmental factors, to protect and restore a good environment, is an important part of the prevention of cancer. 1/3 of the cancer can be prevented.

The relationship of the environment and cancer is very close; the environmental pollution can cause a variety of carcinogenic substances into the human body or a variety of carcinogenic factors which affect the human body. How to prove the relationship between environmental pollution and cancer? In the history, there are many examples confirmed.

The environmental pollution in the air pollution can increase the incidence of lung cancer. In the Industrial developed countries, the harmful gases from the power generation, steel, automobile, aircraft, fuel, energy, a large number of soot and other come into the atmosphere and causes polluting the air, leading to lung cancer morbidity and mortality is increasing.

The environmental pollution in the water pollution and cancer: water pollution is mainly caused by industrial and agricultural production and urban sewage. Water pollution can induce or promote the occurrence of cancer.

Chemical pollution in environmental pollution is also closely related to the incidence of human cancer; more than 90% of the human cancer have the relation to the environmental factors which is mainly chemical factors.

The research on the source of environmental pollution carcinogens and how to eliminate this pollution are a very important issue in the prevention of cancer; the prevention of cancer must be pollution prevention and treatment.

I think the energy-saving emission reduction, pollution prevention and treatment of cancer are the I-level prevention to stop the occurrence of cancer

resistance at the source. And that this is a good time to help "capture cancer", I am convinced that building a well-off society will also achieve the prevention of cancer and cancer control and get a good effect so that people are healthy, away from cancer.

(E) So far there is no practical solution to carry out the prevention of cancer and cancer control; it is not only from the technical and tactical to proceed, but from the strategic focus, it should be implemented by people-oriented, fundamentally stresses the people and the environment harmony. The scientific research must be carried out to explore innovation.

Science is an endless frontier, and research is endless.

With the development of the eyes, eyes forward, for energy-saving emission reduction, pollution prevention, pollution control and anti-cancer, cancer prevention of cancer incidence of related scientific research, will produce a lot of new knowledge is not yet known, and even the original innovation The results of scientific research and the emergence of new disciplines, new industries.

I deeply appreciate this policy and work, energy-saving emission reduction, pollution prevention, pollution control construction "two-oriented society", which itself contains the prevention of cancer and cancer control and have the significance effect. But I did not make it clear. Therefore, I would like to make a suggestion to introduce some prevention of cancer and cancer control programs and measures to make anti-cancer work into the community and raise people's awareness of cancer prevention while building a "two-oriented society". To carry out the planning and measures of the prevention of cancer and control cancer and the group control of the prevention of cancer measures will receive a significant reduction in the incidence of cancer effect.

Volume IV

Table of Contents

First, The proposal of the "Reform, Innovation and Development of Cancer Treatment"

I have been engaged in clinical surgery for 60 years. In 1991 I suddenly had acute myocardial infarction. I was recovered and rehabilitated after I was rescued and hospitalized for six months. I cannot go to the operation room to do the power surgery, calmed down my heart and mind, hid in a small building, concentrated on the basis of cancer and clinical study. After 28 years of cold and heat hard work and hard work, carried out a series of experimental research and clinical validation work, has made a series of scientific and technological innovation and scientific research results.

I am a clinical surgeon, why do you study cancer? This is due to a result of letter petitions and surveys from a group of cancer patients.

In 1985 I will conduct the letter petitions and surveys from more than 3000 cases of the cancer patients which I did the chest and abdominal surgery by my own, and the results are: it was found that most patients had the recurrence or metastasis after 2-3 years, and some had the recurrence and metastasis even after a few months, 1 year. From the results of follow-up it was found: postoperative recurrence and metastasis are the keys to long-term effect of surgery. And therefore we have raised an important question: that clinicians must pay attention to and study the prevention and treatment methods of postoperative recurrence and metastasis so as to improve postoperative long-term efficacy. Therefore, it is necessary to carry out the experimental research of clinical basis. So we established the Animal Experimental Surgery Laboratory (later in 1991 set up the Hubei Institute of Experimental Surgery, Research direction for the capture of cancer). We spent 20 years from the following three aspects, conducted a series of experimental research and clinical validation.

1, Carried out a series of experimental tumor research: the implementation of cancer cell transplantation, the establishment of He cancer animal model. To explore the mechanism and the law of pathogenesis, invasion, metastasis,

recurrence of cancer, and to look for the effective measures of the regulation and control of cancer invasion, metastasis and recurrence.

We conducted a full four years of cancer laboratory experiments in the laboratory which was the research of clinical basis, and the research project topics which had been chosen are clinical problems, with a view or an expectation to experimental research to explain or solve these clinical problems.

In our laboratory from the experimental tumor study it was found:

(1) The cancer-bearing animal models can be produced on the removal of thymus in mice (30 Kunming mice); the injection of immunosuppressive agents can also contribute to the establishment of animal model in our laboratory.

The study was concluded as that: the occurrence and development of cancer have a clear relationship with the host immune organ thymus and its function

(2) Does the inferior immune lead to the cancer or the cancer lead to the inferior immune at all? Our experimental results: the inferior immune leads to the occurrence and development of the cancer, without the descent of immunologic function, it is not easy to realize the successful inoculation. It is suggested by the experimental results: improving and maintaining the good immunologic function and protecting the good thymus of the central immune organ are the important measures for preventing the occurrence of cancer.

Whether it is low immune first and then easy to get cancer, or first get cancer and then causes low immune?

The experimental results are: first it has the low immunization and then cancer occurs; if there is no the development of low immune function, it is not easy to have the successful inoculation. The results of this experiment suggest that improving and maintaining good immune function is one of the important measures to prevent cancer.

(3) When making experiments to probe into the effects of tumor on immune organ, this lab finds that the thymus meets with progressive atrophy with the advance of the cancer (600 cancer-bearing animal model mice). The thymus of the host meets with the acute progressive atrophy after the cancer cells are inoculated,

(4) it is proven by the above-mentioned experimental results: the advance of the tumor makes the thymus meet with progressive atrophy, then, can we take some measures to prevent the atrophy of the thymus of the host? Therefore, we further perfect the design to seek for the method or drug to prevent the atrophy of the thymus of the cancer-bearing mice through the experimental study on animal. So we make the experimental study to recover the function of the immune organ through cell transplantation of the immune organ. We discuss the atrophy of the thymus of the immune organ in preventing the advance of tumor, seek for the method to recover the functions of the thymus and reconstruct the immune, carry out the cell transplantation of foetal liver, spleen and thymus with the mice and establish the immunologic function through adoptive immunity. It is shown by the results: through the joint transplantation of three groups of cells, namely S, T and L (200 experimental mice), the entire extinction rate of the tumor in the long term is 46.67% and the one with the entire extinction of the tumor get a long survival life.

Based on the above experimental study, in the third monograph "new concepts and new methods of cancer treatment," the second chapter it was put forward to: "thymus atrophy, immune dysfunction is one of the pathogenesis of cancer", in Chapter 3: Theoretical basis and experimental basis of "XZ-C immunoregulation therapy". And reported at the International Conference on Oncology in Washington, DC, in September 2013, which attracted wide attention and attention.

2, the experimental research from the Chinese medicine to find, to screen anti-cancer, anti-cancer metastasis drug new

In our laboratory through tumor inhibition experiments in the tumor-bearing mice in vivo model, from traditional Chinese medications to find the traditional

Chinese medication which only inhibit cancer cells without affecting the normal cells of and can inhibit the metastasis of cancer cells, we spent a full three years and tested and screened each of the traditional anti-cancer prescriptions and anti-cancer prescription reported in the use of Chinese herbal medicine in vivo tumor suppression tumor screening experiments. The results showed that there were 48 kinds of traditional Chinese medicine which had inhibitory effect on cancer cells. There were 26 kinds of Chinese medicine which had the effect of increasing immune regulation (elimination of 152 kinds of Chinese medications which do not have inhibition to cancer cells). By optimizing the combination, and then by the animal model of tumor in vivo tumor inhibition test, it was observed the effects of thymus, spleen, liver, kidney and others and composed of XZ-C1-10 anti-cancer traditional Chinese medicine preparations, XZ-C1 could significantly inhibit cancer cells without affecting the normal cells; XZ-C4 can promote thymic hyperplasia, increased immune function; XZ-C8 can protect the marrow to protect bone marrow hematopoietic function; XZ-C immunomodulation of traditional Chinese medications can improve the quality of life of patients with advanced cancer, Increase immune functions, enhance the body's anti-cancer ability, enhance physical fitness, improve appetite, significantly improve the symptoms.

3, clinical validation work

Through the above four years of the basic experimental study to explore the recurrence and metastasis mechanism, and after 3 years of the experimental study from the natural medicine herbal screening to find a group of XZ-C1-10 immunomodulation of anti-cancer medications, and then 16 years of clinical validation of 12000 cases of patients in late or postoperative metastatic cancer in the cancer specialist clinic, the application of XZ-C immunomodulation anti-cancer traditional Chinese medications achieved good results, can improve the quality of life of patients, improve patient symptoms, significantly prolong the survival of patients.

4, outlined anti-cancer research course

(1) After the rehabilitation of my heart mycardiac infarctions, I should be a good rest, why have I done a series of cancer basic and clinical research?

In April 1991, the author put forward the application of the key scientific and technological project to the National Science and Technology Commission. The project name was "the experimental and clinical research to further explore the effects of Chinese medications of the prevention and treatment of cancer on gastric cancer, hepatocellular carcinoma and precancerous lesions of gastric cancer". In June Hubei Provincial Science and Technology Director of the Office of the province formed a group of three project leaders (Tongji Medical College 1, Hubei Medical College 1, Hubei College of Traditional Chinese Medicine 1) applying for the State Science and Technology Commission project to Beijing to report the Ministry of Health Chinese medicine . 2 months later the provincial governor and director with the head of the three subjects to Beijing to the Ministry of Health to further report the subject design and acceptance task tasks. 2 months later, the project task was issued, and it is about to sign special contract of a national science and technology research project, and Professor Xu Ze sudden had acute myocardial infarction with anterolateral wall and high lateral wall myocardial infarction. After rescued, treated and hospitalized for six months, then after discharge Professor Xu had been resting for six months, then was gradually improved recovery. The National Science and Technology Commission also tackled the subject, suspended.

In 1993, Professor Xu Ze's physical health gradually recovered, and he would like to continue to carry out the idea of the content of the idea, because the author had a large number of patients with cancer follow-up after radical surgery, the results were found that cancer recurrence and metastasis were the key factors which had the impact of cancer Postoperative long-term efficacy it must study the relevant clinical basis and effective methods of preventing postoperative recurrence and metastasis so that it was determined to do research work in this regard which it should do and can do, but there are ideas but no scientific research funding, then began to find ways to self-funded research funding. In 1993 the author's wife retired, she applied for a clinic, its meager income as the starting point for research funding. Kunming mice were purchased from the Animal Center of the Academy of Medical Sciences to carry out animal experiments, preparation of animal cages and related equipment, equipment, start animal experiments. The meager income of the clinic is used to support Professor Xu Ze animal experiment scientific research, careful planning to save the application. The 6 rooms on the second floor are used for animal experiments. In 1996, Professor Xu Ze was 63 years old, also apply for retirement. Since then, with the support of this meager income, a series of experimental research and clinical validation work were done. After 20 years of hard work and hard work, and finally basically completed the subject of the National Science and Technology Commission, summarized and the experimental data and clinical research data into three monographs which had been published since 2011.

(2) Several Experiences

In the past, the author carried out scientific research work in medical colleges and universities, had the help of supervisors and colleagues, and had excellent conditions in the laboratory, undertook the subject of the National Natural Science Foundation, the subject matter of the State Science and Technology Commission, and had the two achievements of the scientific research achievements: one term was for the domestic advanced level, one was for the international advanced level, won the second prize of scientific and technological achievements twice in Hubei Province, won the first prize of health science and technology achievements once in Hubei Province.

But now different, in this special case, in a clinic or outpatient department, one thing is that there was no condition, the second thing that there was no equipment. Under the conditions, how can we carry out and complete the national project tasks? I have the following superficial experience.

① self-reliance, self-financing. For patients to see clinics, outpatient income as research funding.

② to stay or remain outpatient medical records, full follow-up.

③ to establish a special scientific research collaboration, according to scientific research cooperation and cooperation.

④ to establish detailed medical records (including the patient's epidemiological data), in-depth analysis of each case after the successful experience of treatment, failure of the lessons and the particularity of the disease.

⑤ with the cooperation strategy of the instrument sharing, equipment sharing and sharing the results of scientific research which do not add large-scale equipment, therefore sharing with medical institutions and the hospital, and the sophisticated equipment inspection tests were done in the affiliated medical school.

⑥ The optional front-line science issues failed to declare the subject (due to nearly a century); after getting the results, it was only to report the scientific research to the Ministry, provinces and municipalities .

⑦ The old professors can also be complete research subject in a private outpatient department, through research cooperation with sharing equipment in the tertiary institutions and the results of sharing strategies, the full use of advanced equipment conditions and combined with their decades of clinical experience,.

After 20 years of cold and hot hard work, it was carried out a series of experimental research and clinical validation work, and finally basically completed the "Eighth Five" research topics which was applied from the National Science and Technology Commission, and the experimental and clinical research materials and data, and the conclusion were summed up the collection, and was written more than 100 research papers. Because there was no research funding, they can not be published according to the magazine, was published according to the new books which had been published as three monographs.

5, Outline anti-cancer research and research results

(1) published monographs on cancer research -

After 20 years of hard work and hard work, it was carried out a series of experimental research and clinical validation work, the experimental and clinical validation data collation which was my more than 50 years of clinical case review, analysis, reflection, experience and my own more than a decade of cancer experimental results and discoveries from the experimental to clinical, but also from clinical to experimental was summed up the collection and published as three monographs: 1, "new understanding of cancer treatment and new model", Hubei Science and Technology Publishing House, Xu Ze In January 2001. 2, "new concept and new methods of cancer metastasis ", published by the Beijing People's Medical Publishing House, Xu Ze, January 2006. In April 2007 issued by the People's Republic of China issued a "three hundred" original book certificate. 3, "new concepts and new methods of cancer treatment", published by the Beijing People's Medical Publishing House, Xu Ze / Xu Jie, October 2011. Followed by American physician Dr. Bin Wu translated into English. The English version was published in Washington on March 26, 2013 and was issued internationally.

These three monographs are our difficult trek, hard climbing, step by step in the three different scientific research stages of scientific research, three different levels of achievement. (The first monograph at the age of 67, the second monograph at the age of 73, the third monograph at the age of 78, the English version of the third monograph at the age of 80, the English edition, the Washington issue, the international distribution)

(2) Brief description of anti-cancer, anti-cancer metastasis research results

We have 28 years (1985-----) cancer research work in animal experiments, clinical basic research, clinical validation work has made a series of scientific and technological innovation scientific and technological achievements. As the contents are more, here is only directory, research topics and belongs to the original innovation or independent innovation.

① "thymus atrophy, immune dysfunction is one of the causes of cancer and pathogenesis"

- Advances the new discovery in the study of the etiology and pathogenesis of cancer

[Scientific research] • [Science and technology innovation A]

② "The theoretical basis and experimental basis of protection of thymus and increasing immune function of XZ-C immunomodulation therapy,"

- put forward the theoretical basis and experimental basis of immunoregulation therapy for cancer

[Scientific research] • [Science and technology innovation A]

③ "cancer treatment should change the concept and the establishment of a comprehensive treatment concept"

- put forward the new concept of cancer treatment principles

[Scientific research] • [Science and technology innovation B]

④ "The assembling new model of cancer multidisciplinary comprehensive treatment"

- proposing a new concept of cancer treatment portfolio model [scientific research] • [science and technology innovation B]

⑤ "the analysis, evaluation and questioning of solid tumor systemic intravenous chemotherapy"

- questioned the traditional drug administration approach, the dose calculation and the efficacy evaluation of the treatment of systemic cancer therapy for systemic intravenous chemotherapy

[Scientific research] • [Science and technology innovation B]

⑥ "the initiative to change the solid body tumor intravenous chemotherapy into the target organ intravascular chemotherapy"

- Advocacy for traditional cancer therapy

[Scientific research] • [Science and technology innovation B]

⑦ "the initiative of the improvement measures on postoperative cancer adjuvant chemotherapy"

- Advocacy for traditional cancer chemotherapy

[Scientific research] • [Science and technology innovation B]

⑧ "there are three main existing forms of cancer in the human body"

Advice on the new concept of cancer metastasis therapy

- The third form is the group of cancer cells that are being metastasis

[Scientific research] • [Science and technology innovation A]

⑨ "the whole process of cancer development," two points and one line"

Advice on the therapy innovation of cancer metastasis therapy

[Scientific research] • [Science and technology innovation B]

⑩ "the three steps of anti-cancer treatment"

- Propose the theoretical innovation of the new concept of cancer metastasis therapy

- The "eight steps" of the metastasis of cancer cells are summarized as "three stages" and try to break each step

[Scientific research] • [Science and technology innovation A]

(11) "open up the third field of anti-cancer metastasis therapy"

- put forward the theory innovation of the new concept of cancer metastasis therapy, it was discovered and put forward the third field of human anti-cancer metastasis therapy

- The circulatory system has a large number of immune surveillance cells, annihilating the transit of cancer cells in the "main battlefield" is in the blood circulation

[Scientific research] • [Science and technology innovation A]

(12) "The research overview of XZ-C immunocompromised anti-cancer traditional Chinese medications"

In vitro culture of cancer cells, the screening experimental study of the cancer inhibition rate of Chinese herbal medication on of

The experimental study on the effect of Chinese herbal medication on the tumor inhibition rate of in tumor-bearing animals

[Scientific research] • [Science and technology innovation B]

(13) "the experimental study and clinical efficacy observation of XZ-C immunomodulatory anti-cancer traditional Chinese medication treatment of malignant tumors"

Animal Experiment research and Clinical Application

- XZ-C immunoregulation anti-cancer traditional Chinese medication is the result of the modernization of traditional Chinese medication

[Scientific research] • [Science and technology innovation A]

(14) "the case lists and some typical cases of XZ-C immunoregulation anti-cancer traditional Chinese medication treatment"

[Scientific research] • [Science and technology innovation B]

(15) "cancer treatment reform and innovation research"

Adhere to the road of scientific research and innovation of anti - cancer metastasis with Chinese characteristics

Research on cancer treatment reform and innovation

[Scientific research] • [Science and technology innovation B]

(16) "walking out of a new way to overcome cancer"

- it has initially formed the theoretical system of XZ-C immune regulation, is experiencing clinical application, observation and verification

- has had an exclusive research and development products: XZ-C immunoregulation anti-cancer traditional Chinese medication series, has a large number of clinical validation cases

- 20 years has initially walked out of a new way to overcome cancer

[Scientific research] • [Science and technology innovation B]

6. The next step in cancer research work

(1) our research journey of the ideological understanding and scientific thinking

The journey of ideological awareness and scientific thinking during 28 years of cancer research work research can be divided into four stages. Its brief introduction **is that:**

The first stage of 1985 - 1999

- Identify the problem from the follow-up results → ask questions → research questions; to target the study or to target "in the study of cancer prevention and treatment of postoperative recurrence and metastasis method is the key to improve the long-term efficacy."

- From the review and the analysis and the reflection, it was found that the current cancer traditional therapies exist the questions, which need to be further studied and improved;

- Recognize the current problems with traditional cancer therapies, and it should change their minds and change the observation;

- the summary of information and the collation and the collection were published the first monograph "new understanding of cancer treatment and new model" in January 2001 Hubei Science and Technology Publishing House.

② the second stage after 2001 -

- Targeting the target of the study and the "target" of cancer therapy is targeted for anti-metastasis and pointing out that the key to cancer treatment is anti-metastasis;

- Conducted a series of new methods of anti - cancer metastasis, recurrence, clinical research and clinical basis and clinical validation, and then ascended into theoretical innovation so that it was propoed the new thinking and new method of ant-cancer metastasis;

- Summary of information, collation, collection, published the second monograph "new concepts and new methods of cancer metastasis therapy" in January 2006 published by the People's Medical Publishing House, Xinhua Bookstore, in April 2007 received the "three one hundred" original book award and certificate issued by the People's Republic of China Press and Publication General.

③ the third stage after 2006 -

- The research aim and main point are the whole process of prevention and treatment of cancer occurrence and development;
- Closely combined with clinical practice, reform and innovation, research and development for the problems and malpractices of current clinical traditional therapies;
- Recognize the strategy of cancer prevention and treatment must move forward, the way out of cancer treatment is in the "three early", anti-cancer out of the way is in the prevention;

I have been engaged in tumor surgery for 60 years, more and more patients, the incidence of cancer is also rising, high mortality rate, so I deeply appreciate that cancer should not only pay attention to treatment, but also pay attention to prevention, in order to stop at the source, Was carried out a series of research, summarize the information, organize, collect, publish the third monograph "new concept and new method of cancer treatment" in October 2011 published by the People's Medical Publishing House, Xinhua Bookstore. Followed by American physician Dr. Bin Wu translated into English. The English version of this book was published in Washington on March 26, 2013, with international distribution.

④ the fourth stage after 2011 -

Now it is the fourth stage of our research work and is being carried out and developed. The research work is step by step and the study of the target or "target" is located in reducing the incidence of cancer and improving the cure rate and prolonging the survival time.

We have 28 years of cancer research work: the first three stages of the experimental research and clinical research work is mainly the research of the new drugs in the treatment and the new methods of diagnosis and the new technologies and the new concepts and new methods of treatment. The experimental study is mainly for the establishment of a variety of animal models of cancer to explore the incidence of cancer, invasion and recurrence and metastasis mechanism and the regulation, to find the effective regulation and the effective measures of the metastasis and the recurrence and to do the experimental Study on Experimental Screening of Anti - cancer Chinese Herbal Medication.

But until today the second 10 years of the 21st century, cancer is still rampant, the incidence continues to rise with the high mortality rate. I have been engaged in clinical cancer surgery for 60 years. The more treated and the more patients; the incidence of cancer continues to rise so that I deeply appreciate that in order to stop at the source it not only pays attention to treatment, but also pays attention to prevention.

Therefore, I am deeply aware of that the research work of cancer not only focused on the treatment, researching the new drugs and the new methods and the new technologies, but also must focus on how to reduce the incidence of cancer and how to prevent the incidence of cancer from continuing to rise in the momentum?

The current tumor hospital or oncology mode is to go all out to focus on treatment; for patients with advanced disease, it has poor efficacy and it exhausts human and financial resources, and fails to achieve lower morbidity; the more treatment the more patients. The status quo is: through the road in a century it is a focusing on the treatment and ignoring the defense, or there is only treatment but no prevention. Over the years we have just been working and researching cancer treatment. But in prevention of cancer work it did very little and it almost did not do so that the incidence of cancer continues to rise.

From the Review and the reflection of the cliché prevention of cancer and the anti-cancer work what have we done in the prevention of cancer research or work since a century? What has the achievement had?

In the medical school textbooks teaching content does not attach importance to the knowledge of prevention of cancer

In hospital mode it does not attach importance to science research program of cancer prevention.

In Journal of Cancer Medical Science there is no paper of paying attention to prevention

In short, the prevention of cancer does not attach importance; the prevention of cancer does not pay attention. Cliché prevention is the main, which did not pay attention to and did not implemented.

How to do? How to reduce the incidence of cancer? How to improve cancer cure rate? How to reduce cancer mortality? How do I extend my life? How to improve the quality of life?

It should launch the total attack of overcoming cancer and both the prevention and the treatment are at the equal attention.

The goal of conquering cancer should be: reduce morbidity, improve the cure rate, reduce mortality, prolong survival, improve quality of life, and reduce complications.

The current global hospitals and the hospitals in China are going all out to engage in treatment and pay attention to the treatment of cancer and ignore the defense, or only treatment with the prevention.

XZ-C thinks of that this hospital model or cancer treatment model can not overcome the cancer, can not reduce the incidence. The global hospitals and our hospital must change the overall strategy of cancer treatment from focusing on cancer treatment into focusing on both the prevention and the treatment.

Therefore, we propose the design and the plans of conquering cancer to launch a total attack . XZ-C proposed to launch a total attack, that is, the prevention of cancer and cancer control and cancer treatment of these three-phase work were developed comprehensively and carried out simultaneously.

(2) It was put forward to the "the need and the feasibility of the report to overcome cancer and to launch the general attack on cancer"

It was put forward to "XZ-C research program to overcome cancer and to launch the total attack of cancer"

The research focus of our 28 years of cancer research in the fourth phase: after 2011 -

Cancer research work gets deeply step by step

The study objectives and the focuses of the overall strategics of cancer treatment can be changed from focusing on treatment into the prevention and treatment of cancer at the equal attention we proposed to launch the general attack on cancer, that is, the work during three stages of cancer prevention, cancer control, cancer treatment during the whole process of the occurrence and the development of cancer should be developed comprehensive in full swing, simultaneously. That is:

Prevention of cancer - before the formation of cancer

Cancer control - malignant transformation of precancerous lesions

Cancer treatment - has formed a foci or metastases

the general offensive target: to reduce the incidence of cancer, and to reduce cancer mortality, to improve the cure rate, to prolong survival and to improve quality of life and to reduce complications.

the need to launch the general attack of cancer

Why should I make a general attack? Look at the present situation:

- the incidence of cancer is the status quo of the more treated the more patients, the new cancer patients of our daily average are 8550 cases, 6 people per minute are diagnosed with cancer in the country

- the status of cancer death is high, has been the first cause of death in urban and rural areas in China, the average daily 7,500 people died of cancer

- the status of treatment, despite the application of the traditional three treatment for nearly a hundred years, tens of thousands of cancer patients bear radiotherapy and chemotherapy, but how are the results? So far the cancer is still the first cause of death.

- the status quo of the current tumor hospital or oncology department of hospital model: pay attention to the treatment and ignore the defense, or only have the treatment. the more treatment the more patients.

the feasibility of launching attack and capturing cancer

Now is there scientific basis of proposing to launch the total attack of conquering cancer? Is there a medical foundation? Is it possible to win the favorable conditions? Although nearly a century, the traditional therapy failed to conquer cancer, the radiotherapy and the chemotherapy of the traditional therapy can not overcome cancer because it can only alleviate, and can not be cured. But it also made a lot of achievements and experience, and it should further research on the medical basis and expand the results. It is should be feasible and should be timely.

Now it is proposed to launch a total attack has the following scientific basis and medical basis and it is feasible.

Because the United States surrendered cancer has achieved initial results, because now some of the cancer have found a preventive method, screening can treat some of the cancer, immunocompetent drug have great prospects, molecular targeting drug has much attention, the advanced cancer has been seen as chronic disease, and the application of vaccine treatment of cancer becomes possible; to launch a total offensive and both the prevention and the treatment are the same attention; it must change the status quo; the prevention and control of hepatitis B also become prevention and treatment of liver cancer.

Therefore, the current is the best time is conducive to propose to launch a total attack on conquering cancer .

In October 2011 Xu Ze published "cancer treatment of new concepts and new methods" and proposed the "strategy to overcome cancer and ideas."

June 2013 Xu Ze also proposed "to overcome the cancer to start the general idea and design" in an attempt to reduce the incidence of cancer, reduce mortality, improve the cure rate, prolong survival and the total attack is the prevention of cancer + control cancer + the treatment of the cancer ; the carriage comes in hand.

In August 2013 for the first time in the international community Xu Ze proposed: "to overcome the cancer and to launch a total attack of the XZ-C research program" - the overall strategic reform and development of China's cancer treatment.

This research program was the original innovation and it put forward: the "declared war on cancer" is the time, and it should launch the total attack. To avoid talk and to pay attention to the heavy hard work; no matter how far the path of overcoming cancer is, it should always start to go.

Our dreams are to overcome cancer and to build a well-off society, and everyone is healthy far away from cancer.

- **how to launch the total attack on cancer?**

XZ-C put forward the idea,strategy, planning diagram of tackling the total attack of cancer and pointed out that the total attack is the work of three stages of the cancer prevention and the cancer control and the cancer treatment which can be developed comprehensively in full swing, simultaneously.

As we all know "how to reduce cancer mortality? How to improve the cure rate? How to extend the survival period?

- the out-way of cancer treatment is in the "three early" (early detection, early diagnosis, early treatment);the early cancer treatment effect is good and can be cured, especially the precancerous lesions are handled well, and can be cured.

It is now recognized that the occurrence of 90% of cancer has a great relationship with the environmental pollution, although our medical staff go all out in the treatment of cancer; it is still that the more treatment and the more patient and the incidence is indeed rising and it must be blocked at the source. To prevent the occurrence of cancer it must try to reduce the incidence rate of cancer.

The occurrence of cancer is closely related to people's clothing, food, shelter and living habits. Therefore, I deeply think that it can not rely on medical staff, and it must rely on the government's major policy; cancer treatment should dependent on medical staff and researchers to study the new drugs and the new diagnostic methods and the new treatment techniques and the new concepts and the new method and new theory of the treatment.

The prevention of cancer and anti-cancer work must rely on the efforts of the government-led and leadership and the experts and the scholars and the the masses are involved and the thousands of households participates in order to do.

There are three problems with the current medical profession:

- **First, the more treatment the more patients, the incidence is on the rise, which 90% is related to the environment. We have 28 years of cancer research work (1985 -----)**

After the review and reflect of experimental research and clinical work it is deeply appreciated that it is not only paid attention to treatment, but also paid attention to prevention in order to stop at the source, and it must be the prevention and the treatment of cancer at the equal attention . A century ago, the medical pioneers have put forward "prevention of cancer, anti-cancer", but since a century people did not pay attention to the research and measures

of cancer prevention. In 1971 only President Nixon put forward the "cancer prevention slogan" to declare war on cancer.

Second, the current diagnostic methods are behind; B ultrasound, CT, BMI are currently the most advanced diagnostic methods, but once diagnosed, it mostly was in the late stage and the effect is very poor. It must seek to the study and to seek the new methods and the new reagents and the new technology of early diagnosis; if it can be diagnosed in the early and precancerous lesions, then early cancer can be cured.

Third, currently some of the patients have the phenomenon of over-diagnosis and over-treatment which the patient has been damaged as so to prompt to reduce immune function of the patients, resulting in disease progression, such as too much CT numbers and too much chemotherapy, it must be paid attention to and be attached the importance to .

① After we experience 28 years of the basis of cancer and clinical research of cancer, it deeply appreciates: to achieve the purpose of cancer prevention and control:

② It must start the total attack. That is, three stages of work: the cancer prevention and the cancer control and the cancer treatment work together and simultaneously, troika, go hand in hand in order to achieve lower morbidity, improve the cure rate, reduce mortality and prolong survival. If only treatment without the defense, it will never be able to overcome cancer because it cannot reduce the incidence and the more treatment the more patients.

It must be that the government leads and that the experts and the scholars put the efforts and that the masses participate in the mobilization of all and thousands of households participate in order to do. At present, China is building two types of society: the ecological civilization, the energy saving and emission reduction, the pollution prevention and the correction of the pollution prevention; building a well-off society and building an innovation-oriented country are the government-led and the mass participation and the mobilization of the whole people and the thousands of households involved in the work . It has vigorous development and carrying out and it is a good time, if missed, it will no longer come, if it can conduct the "ride research", it will be able to improve the awareness of anti-cancer in all people to reach the results of preventing cancer and controlling cancer. It gets the effect of decreasing the cancer occurrence rate in our country and our province and the city.

As a result, Prof. Xu Ze presented the following feasibility report and proposal in August 2015.

(1) It was put forward for the first time in the international community:

"the necessity and feasibility report of overcoming cancer and launching the total attack on cancer"

The overall strategic reform of cancer treatment in China should shift the focus of treatment into prevention and treatment at the equal attention

(2) for the first time in the international community it is put forward:

"To build prevention and treatment hospital during whole process of cancer occurrence and development

(Global demonstration of cancer prevention and treatment hospital)

"to build the imagination and feasibility report of the prevention and treatment hospital during the anti-cancer whole process"

- Describe the necessity and feasibility of establishing a complete prevention and cure hospital

(3) for the first time in the international community it was put forward:

"To build the imagine of the total attack of conquering cancer and the basic design and feasibility report of the science city"

- is equivalent to design the whole framework with a chinese characteristic design of conquering cancer

(4) for the first time in the international community it was put forward:

"In building a moderately society at the same time, the proposed" ride research "-----conduct the medical science research of the prevention and the control cancer and the necessity and feasibility report of cancer prevention and treatment"

- Adhere to the new path of anti - cancer, cancer prevention with the Chinese characteristics of well-off society

These four research projects are the first proposal in the international and is the international initiative and the international leader which opened up a new field of anti-cancer research.

To open up a new field of research will open up a new era of anti-cancer research and will play an epoch-making significance in the course of human anti-cancer research, from the emphasis on the cancer treatment and ignoring the defense into both the prevention and treatment at the same attention in an attempt to reduce cancer incidence rate and to improve the cancer cure rateat the same time.

To open up a new field of research, it is possible to conquer cancer, and even overcome cancer because for a century, in cancer treatment people are based on the treatment, and treatment is based on killing cancer cells. But the chemotherapy is a first-class kinetics and can not kill cancer cells and can only kill a certain number of cancer cells, there will still have the cancer cells continue to produce, therefore, its efficacy is set to "ease", and the relief time is only 4 weeks or more. It will still recur and metastasis so chemotherapy cannot cure cancer, although it was used more than half a century, cancer is still the first cause of death of urban and rural residents.

To propose to conquer cancer and to launch a total attack needs for courage and for wisdom and strength and for scientific basis.

- Cancer is the enemy of all classes. Cancer complex is beyond human imagination, which is the most fiery positions in the field of biomedical and gathers the world's largest and elite research team and the scientific research elite.

- Human beings should not sit still, physicians should not do nothing, I think we should put forward the general idea and basic design of attacking cancer and launching the total attack, avoid empty talking, hard work, building a good laboratory, strengthening the experimental research and the basic research and clinical research.

We have two tasks on the shoulder of the physician: one is to treat the patient, one is the development of medication; we should overcome the cancer in this strategic high-tech field to achieve leapfrog development and to take our characteristics of the technology innovation road of the anti-cancer, anti-transfer and to innovate the achievement and rusults.

What should I do next?

This is in need for the government leadership and the government-led and the experts and scholars efforts and the masses involved.

The next step is to work hard and to implement the XZ-C research program; from scratch and from the small to the large, the professional group go hand in hand to carry out, to avoid empty talk, and to do the hard work and to follow the concept of the scientific development with having a plan and having a focus on hard work

The general imagination and design of conquering cancer of how the next step of the work to carry out and achieve the above:

I tentatively envisaged:

How to implement the cancer prevention and treatment of the new ideas and innovative content? It should be built to build a new type of cancer prevention and treatment of the hospital, according to the prevention and treatment of cancer, the development of the whole process of strategic thinking of the anti-hospital. First it creates the model and the demonstration of the Global Prevention and Treatment Hospital.

To overcome the cancer must cultivate multidisciplinary senior personnel. From a clinical point of view the following disciplines are related to the research of cancer research: the immunology and cancer related group; the virus and cancer related group; the endocrine and cancer related group; fungi and cancer related group; Chronic inflammation and cancer related group; molecular biology and cancer related group; gene and cancer related group; environment and cancer related group; Chinese medication and cancer related group.

We must cultivate high-level professionals and intermediate professionals with the prevention and the control and thet treatment of cancer. The education must train the personnel for attacking the total offensive of cancer. It is applied their knowledge. It must cultivate more than high-level talent, and the talent must have this professional theoretical knowledge and professional skills, the talent must be real learning, the talent must be both ability and political integrity and the medicine is benevolence and the legislation is for the first.

It is recommended to create "to overcome the Cancer Science City" test;

It is recommended to overcome the cancer to set up a number of the related groups of the research group;

It is recommended to create a global demonstration or model of the prevention and treatment hospital first;

It is suggested that it must pay attention to the construction of the laboratory. With a good laboratory, it can produce the scientific research results of the original innovation or independent innovation and will help to overcome cancer.

Here, we put forward: "a number of suggestions of the personnel training of the scientific and technological innovation and the laboratory construction, the conversion of the results for the construction of innovative countries". With innovative talent and with a good laboratory the scientific research work in cancer prevention and cancer control and cancer treatment will certainly achieve fruitful results, and strive to achieve the new results of the prevention and treatment of cancer in China's medical care and strive to achieve a major breakthrough in originality of overcoming cancer in the key areas of the scientific research.

With the continuous improvement of people's living standards, a variety of chemical, physical, biological environment, a large number of carcinogens, a variety of carcinogenic substances come into our body or a variety of carcinogens affect our body so the environment and cancer research, the environmental protection Cancer research will open up the new research areas and the new research industries.

(1) the treatment of malignant tumors appeared twice leap since the last two centuries

Looking back over the past 100 years, the human was suffering from cancer, and so far the formation of cancer is still the lack of the most essential understanding, that is, the normal cell proliferation is subject to what factors control, how they lost control of proliferation and become malignant cells.

In the last two centuries the treatment of malignant tumors has experienced two leaps:

The first time was in 1890, Halstad proposed the concept of tumor rooting.

The second is in the 1970s, Fish integrated chemotherapy in radical surgery (adjuvant chemotherapy or neoadjuvant chemotherapy)

After that the treatment of malignant tumors was wandering before and did not move forward.

Fish was a systemic route of intravenous administration, after half a century, so far it failed to reduce mortality, also failed to prevent recurrence and metastasis; the mortality is still the first.

(2) President Nixon issued the Anti-Cancer Declaration in 1971 and raised the anti-cancer slogan in the United Nations.

In 1971 the United States Congress passed a "National Cancer Regulations", and by President Nixon issued "anti-cancer declaration." So it put a considerable amount of manpower and financial resources in order to overcome cancer in one fell swoop.

In December 1971, President Richard Nixon presented the anti-cancer slogan in the United Nations.

42 years have passed, and now Nixon has also been ancient, in cancer research has also made many significant progress, such as the discovery of tumor suppressor genes, the advent of monoclonal antibodies, the application of CT and magnetic resonance imaging, the improvement of the ultrasound and endoscopy and the innovation of the various treatment methods.

However, in the first two 10 years in the current 2 1 century the mortality rate of the lung cancer, colon cancer and others of the largest threatening for the human is basically the same as 50 years ago. Cancer deaths are still the first cause of death of urban and rural residents in China.

So the experts in medicine, biology and related disciplines began to reflect. The most scientists believe that the prevention and treatment of the tumor just can get the most effects from the most basic issues, that is, from the nature of cancer cells, pathogenesis, cancer cell metabolic characteristics and signal transduction etc to understand the cancer "Lushan true face", only like this way in order to have the cancer prevention and treatment.

It should carry out the interdisciplinary research and to promote the basic research and the clinical research cooperation, attention to clinical research.

It must be carried out the clinical basic research and if there is no breakthrough in basic research, the clinical efficacy is difficult to improve.

My third book, "New Concepts and New Methods of Cancer Therapy," is a new concept, innovative content that combines the experimental research and a new concept of clinically proven cancer therapies. It should be implemented in the majority of cancer patients benefit.

Second, XZ-C proposed the research program of conquering cancer and launching a total offensive

The overall strategic reform and development of cancer treatment

How to overcome the cancer? I see:

To avoid empty talking, to focus on hard work, no matter how far the path of overcoming cancer it is, it should always start to go

(one)

- it is time to declare war on cancer, and should start the total attack.

The goal of capturing cancer is to reduce morbidity, reduce mortality, improve cure rate, prolong survival, improve quality of life and reduce complications.

To avoid empty talk, to focus on heavy work, no matter how far away the road of capturing cancer it is, it shuld start to go, Wanli Long March always go, thousands of miles began with a single step.

- What should I do next? Now it was proposed to overcome cancer and to launch a total attack. I hope to get leadership support at all levels. I know that to achieve the purpose of cancer prevention, control cancer, cancer treatment must be government leadership, government-led, experts, scholars efforts, the masses to participate in the mobilization of all, thousands of households to participate in order to do.
- Recognize that more than 80% of the cancer is caused by or closely related to environmental factors. Building a well-off society and anti-cancer, cancer control has a great relevance, therefore, we propose to prevent the cancer and to launch a total attack, adhere to the Chinese characteristics of anti-cancer, cancer prevention path.

At present, China's country is implementing the spirit of the 18th Party Congress and comprehensively building a well-off society to ensure the goal of achieving a well-off society in 2020. Our dreams, to overcome cancer, to build a well-off society, everyone is healthy and away from cancer.

(two)

Why did I propose to launch a total attack? Why is it urgent? Look at the current situation: (according to the National Cancer Registration Center released the "2012 China Cancer Registration Annual Report"

- the status quo of the incidence of cancer is that the more treatment the more patients, our average daily new cancer patients is for the 8550 cases, 6 persons per minute are confirmed as cancer in the national.

- the status of cancer mortality is high, has been the first cause of death in urban and rural areas, 7,500 people died of cancer in the average daily.

- the status of treatment, despite the application of the traditional three treatment for nearly a hundred years, tens of thousands of cancer patients bear the chemotherapy and chemotherapy, but what are the results? So far the cancer is still the first cause of death.

- the current situation of the hospital mode is to regain the light defense, or only treatment, the more treatment the more patients.

The status quo is: a century through the road is a heavy treatment and light defense, or only treatment . Anti-cancer is the cause of mankind, but over the years we have just studied on cancer treatment, but do little work on cancer prevention, almost did not do.

- Therefore, XZ-C suggests that the general idea and overall design of the cancer should be launched, as well as the overall planning, route, and blueprint.

On the treatment of cancer it must have a whole strategic reform from light defense into for both of the prevention and treatment.

It should update their minds, update their knowledge, move forward in reform, innovate in reform, and develop in reform.

(three)

- Cancer is the enemy of all mankind and should arouse the common struggle of mankind around the world. The complexity of cancer is beyond human imagination, which is the hottest position in biomedicine, gathering the world's largest, elite research team and research elite.

- To tackle cancer as the main direction of the study, experimental and clinical anti-cancer research should be a key area of scientific research, should achieve an original breakthrough.

- There are 2.7 million cases of cancer deaths each year, with an average of 7,500 deaths per day in cancer. Such amazing data should be included as scientific research in key areas of scientific and technological innovation.

- Human beings should not sit still, physicians should not do nothing, I think we should propose to the general idea and basic design of capturing cancer, "declared war on cancer" and launch a total attack. To avoid the empty talk, to pay attention to heavy hard work, building a good laboratory, to strengthen experimental research, basic research and clinical research.

We have two tasks on the shoulder of the physician, one is to treat the patient, one is the development of medicine, we should overcome the cancer in this strategic high-tech field to achieve leapfrog development, take our characteristics of anti-cancer, anti-transfer technology innovation Road, innovation, and strive to enter the forefront of the world.

- Because cancer patients are getting more and more, the morbidity is on the rise, the mortality rate is high, recognizing that cancer should not only pay attention to treatment, but also pay attention to prevention, in order to stop at the source, is the research goal and focus on the occurrence of cancer, Development of the whole process of prevention and control of the study.

Xu ZE in October 2011 published in Beijing, "new concepts and new methods of cancer treatment," Chapter 38 of the proposed "to overcome the strategic thinking of cancer and suggestions." The book was later published by the American medical scientist Dr. Bin Wu and other English, the English version published in March 26, 2013 in Washington, the international distribution.

In June 2013 Xu Ze also put forward the "the general idea and design to conquer cancer and launch the total attacka" in an attempt to reduce the incidence of cancer, reduce mortality, improve the cure rate, prolong survival.

"XZ-C proposed the research program to conquer the cancer and to launch a total offensive"

The overall strategic reform and development of cancer treatment

Prof. Xu ZE, Honorary President of Wuhan Anti-Cancer Research Association, **presented the following feasibility report and proposal in July 2015.**

(1) It was put forward for the first time in the international community:

"the necessity and feasibility report of overcoming cancer and launching the total attack on cancer"

The overall strategic reform of cancer treatment in China should shift the focus of treatment into prevention and treatment at the equal attention

(2) for the first time in the international community it is put forward:

"To build prevention and treatment hospital during whole process of cancer occurrence and development

(Global demonstration of cancer prevention and treatment hospital)

"to build the imagination and feasibility report of the prevention and treatment hospital during the anti-cancer whole process"

- Describe the necessity and feasibility of establishing a complete prevention and cure hospital

(3) for the first time in the international community it was put forward:

"To build the imagine of the total attack of conquering cancer and the basic design and feasibility report of the science city"

- is equivalent to design the whole framework with a chinese characteristic design of conquering cancer

(4) for the first time in the international community it was put forward:

"In building a moderately society at the same time, the proposed" ride research "-----conduct the medical science research of the prevention and the control cancer and the necessity and feasibility report of cancer prevention and treatment"

- Adhere to the new path of anti - cancer, cancer prevention with the Chinese characteristics of well-off society

These four research projects are the first proposal in the international and is the international initiative and the international leader which opened up a new field of anti-cancer research.

To shift from paying attention to cancer treatment and ignoring prevention into paying attention to both the treatment and prevention, try to decrease the cancer incidence rate, to increase the cancer cure rate.

To open up a new field of research is possible to conquer cancer, and even overcome cancer.

Third, the report of the necessity and the feasibility for conquering and attaching cancer

- the overall strategic reform of china's cancer treatment from focusing on treatment to focusing on both cancer prevention and treatment at the equal attention

Cancer is a common enemy of all mankind, should mobilize the world's scientists, leaders, the masses involved in research to overcome cancer, should call the global mobilization to capture cancer, the current is the time, it is urgent.

The goal of conquering cancer is to reduce morbidity, reduce mortality, improve cure rate, prolong survival, improve quality of life and reduce complications.

The current treatment of cancer hospital or cancer cancer mainly concentrated in the late stage, the treatment effect is poor.

The way-out of Cancer treatment is in the "three early", early detection, early diagnosis, early treatment. Early treatment of patients has good results and improves the treatment effect so that it is necessary to reduce the mortality rate of cancer, improve the cure rate.

If we can do cancer treatment very well in the precancerous lesions or early stage, then the patients who progress to the invasion and metastasis and the late stages will be reduced, which is to reduce the incidence of cancer.

If you ignore the precancerous lesions, early patients, it is impossible to reduce the incidence of cancer cancer. The key to cancer treatment is in the "three early", and how to deal with precancerous lesions, it is a critical stage of cancer prevention and treatment.

I have been engaged in clinical cancer surgery for 60 years, the more treatment and the more patients, the incidence of cancer is also rising, so I deeply appreciate that cancer should not only pay attention to treatment, but also pay attention to prevention, in order to stop at the source.

Cancer is not only a serious threat to human health, but also an important factor in the rapid rise in medical costs. China's annual cancer treatment with the direct cost of nearly 100 billion yuan, so that patients and the whole society to bear a huge financial burden.

Although countries spend a lot of money on the treatment of cancer patients, but the past 20 years, some of the common 5-year survival of cancer has not improved significantly. For example, in the United States from 1974 to 1990, the 5-year survival rate of esophageal cancer rose from only 7% to 9%, gastric cancer from 16% to 19%, liver cancer from 3% to 6%, lung cancer from 12% to 15% Pancreatic cancer is basically no change is still 3%.

How to do? The way out of cancer is prevention.

For malignant tumors, prevention is better than cure. Through the adjustment of public health resources and strategies, strategic shift, the focus shifted from treatment to prevention, both cancer prevention and treatment at the equal attention, to carry out active and effective early warning, early diagnosis and intervention study to reduce the incidence of cancer and improve the cure rate, has become a global cancer research The consensus of the workers.

How to fight cancer? How to overcome cancer

XZ-C proposed the overall design and overall attack design, as well as the overall attack planning, route, blueprint of attacking the cancer and launch the attack.

What is So-called total attack? That is the prevention of cancer and cancer control and cancer treatment three carriages, keep pace, prevention and treatment of both at the same level.

The overall strategic reform of focusing on cancer treatment and light defense into the emphasis on the prevention and treatment at the same level and attention; both the prevention and anti-cancer should be updated thinking and updated awareness; it is to progress in the reform and to be the innovation in the reform and to be the development in the reform.

1, XZ-C proposed to the general idea and design of conquering cancer

(1) What is the total attack on the capture of cancer?

The total attack is to develop the comprehensive work of the prevention and treatment of cancer during the three stages of the whole process of the occurrence and development of cancer in full swing, simultaneously. That is: the prevention of cancer---- before the formation of cancer ; the control of Cancer ----- malignant transformation of precancerous lesions; the treatment of Cancer - has formed a foci or metastases

The main goal: to reduce the incidence of cancer, reduce cancer death, improve the cure rate, prolong survival, improve quality of life, reduce complications.

Xu Ze (XU ZE) Professor proposed the general offensive ideas, strategies, planning of overcoming cancer and launch a total attach as follows:

How to overcome cancer

Where is the road?

Our ideas, strategies, planning should be divided into three parts (or three stages)

Aiming for the whole process of the occurrence and the development of cancer to do prevention and treatment

Before the formation of cancer ------ for the prevention part------ anti-mutation

There may be malignant tendencies of precancerous lesions ----for the intervention part

There may be malignant tendencies of precancerous lesions -----for the intervention part

The treatment of primary cancer that has foci is treated with anti-metastatic treatment

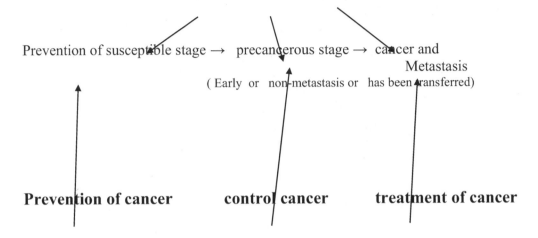

Prevention of susceptible stage → precancerous stage → cancer and
Metastasis
(Early or non-metastasis or has been transferred)

Prevention of cancer   **control cancer**   **treatment of cancer**

(2) why did I put forward to the total attack?

The current tumor hospital or oncology departments all pay attention to heavy treatment and light prevention or only treatment.

I entered the Zhongnan Tongji Medical College in 1951, so far 65 years, experienced and witnessed the whole process of the prevention and treatment of cancer in China for a century. Review of the 20th century, China and the global hospitals, although it also mentioned to prevent cancer and anti-cancer work, but in fact the focus has been formed in the primary cancer treatment and anti-metastatic treatment of cancer, which are in the invasion period, the middle and the late stages ; the treatment effect is poor.

So far to the second decade of the 21st century, the world's hospitals, China's provincial cancer hospital, the hospital affiliated hospital oncology, the three level hospitals are cancer treatment hospital, tumor hospital are clinical treatment. The modes of building the hospitals are all for the treatment of hospitals, oncology academic journals are also clinically diagnosis or clinically based, although there are several for the cancer prevention magazine, but very few anti-cancer work articles. In short, the 20th century, the tumor hospital and the university affiliated hospital of the tumor are heavy treatment, or only treatment.

Review, reflection, cliché anti-cancer, anti-cancer work, for a century what have we done in the prevention-cancer research or work? What achievement did you have?

The status quo is: a century through the road is to pay attention to treatment and light prevention, or only treatment. Prevention of cancer, anti-cancer is the undertaking or cause of mankind, but over the years we do only in the anti-cancer and cancer treatment research work. But in prevention of cancer work was done very little, almost did not do.

Medical school textbooks teaching content does not attach importance to prevention of cancer knowledge.

The hospital mode of building hospital does not attach importance to set up work of prevention of cancer science.

Medical school or hospital research projects do not attach importance to prevention of cancer research projects. Journal of Oncology has not paid attention to prevention of cancer work papers. In short, prevention of cancer does not attach importance; the prevention of cancer was not pay attention to.

Cliché anti-cancer, anti-cancer work, cliché prevention of cancer is as the main point, which was not paid attention to and not implemented.

(3) how to launch the total attack on cancer?

XZ-C (Xu Ze-China) proposed to launch the total attack, that is, three stages of work: prevention of cancer, cancer control, and cancer treatment are carried out comprehensively and implemented simultaneously.

As we all know: how to reduce cancer mortality rate? How to improve the cure rate? How to extend life?

- the way out of cancer treatment is in the "three early" (early detection, early diagnosis, early treatment); the effect of the early cancer treatment is good, can be cured completely, especially if cancer lesions are handled well, all of them can be cured completely.

How to overcome the cancer I see:

2, The necessity of launching the total attack to capture cancer

Why should I raise the total attack? Why is it urgent? Status: see the present situation:

(1) the incidence of cancer incidence of the disease is more treatment and more patients, the current incidence of cancer in China is the annual incidence of cancer cases of 312 million cases, the average daily new cancer patients 8550 cases, 6 per minute diagnosed as cancer.

(2) the status quo of cancer mortality is high, has been the first cause of death in urban and rural areas in China, the annual death of cancer cases, 2.7 million people, an average of 7,500 people died of cancer every day, every 7 dead 1 person died of cancer.

(3) the status of treatment

Although the application of the traditional three treatments has been for nearly a hundred years, tens of thousands of cancer patients used the radiotherapy and chemotherapy, but how are the results? So far the cancer is still the first cause of death, although the patient used the formal, systematic radiotherapy and / or chemotherapy, or radiotherapy and chemotherapy, it still failed to prevent cancer metastasis, recurrence,

(4) the current tumor hospital or oncology mode of the status quo

① go all out to focus on treatment, for the late and poor efficacy, exhausted human and financial resources, and failed to achieve lower mortality, improve the cure rate, reduce morbidity.

② only treatment, or heavy treatment with light defense, the more treatment and the more patients.

③ ignored the "three early", ignoring the precancerous lesions.

④ neglected prevention.

⑤ people: while talking about cancer, the skin color changes

Patient, family members: helpless or no hope

Doctors and nurses: powerless, medical treatment stay in the three treatments, the effect is wandering and doesn't move forward.

the attitude of people understanding: a variety of chemical, physical, biological environment carcinogens appears in a large number, a variety of carcinogenic substances into the human body or a variety of carcinogens affect the human body, people seem to be shrouded in the environment of carcinogens in the ocean; while some people talk about cancer, the skin color changes. It seems that all of the vegetation are soldiers, some people are insensitive, goes its own way in the life of their own way. Cancer is not terrible, terrible is that we do not have this simple knowledge. With this basic knowledge, most of the cancer can be avoided and can be prevented.

⑥ many large hospitals, university affiliated hospitals have not established a laboratory, can not carry out basic research or basic clinical research of cancer, because if no basic research breakthrough, the clinical efficacy is difficult to improve. "Oncology" is still the most backward in the current medical disciplines, why? Because the etiology, pathogenesis, pathophysiology of "oncology" are not yet clear. The pathogenesis and cancer cell metastasis mechanism are still lack of understanding and the complex biological behavior of cancer cells is still lack of sufficient understanding, and therefore the current treatment program is still quite blind, it must establish a laboratory for basic research and clinical basis the study.

3, the feasibility of overcoming cancer and launching the total attack

Does it have no scientific basis about now it is proposed to attack the total attack of cancer? Is there a medical foundation? Is it possible to win the favorable conditions? Although nearly a century, the traditional therapy failed to conquer cancer, traditional therapy such as radiotherapy and chemotherapy can not rely on to overcome cancer, because it can only alleviate, can not be cured, even if it has also made a lot of achievements and experience therefore, it should be based on this medical research to expand the results.

(1) human beings in the surrender of cancer has made great achievements

Since December 1971, when the then president of the United States Nongsong signed the "National Cancer Act", is considered a human war on cancer officially declared.

Fortunately, 42 years have passed, reviewing its achievements, shows that humans have made great achievements in surrendering cancer: statistics show that the incidence of cancer in the United States since 1996 began to decline significantly, cancer mortality since 1990 Has fallen by 17%, cancer 5-year survival rate increased by 18%, made significant new results, indicating that cancer is likely to be gradually surrendered.

(2) Now some of the cancer found a prevention method

① study found that chronic inflammation is the leading cause of cervical cancer, liver cancer, gastric cancer, the main reason for cervical cancer is based on chronic cervicitis; liver cancer is based on chronic hepatitis, cirrhosis, gastric cancer and more is based on chronic gastritis, gastric ulcer. Prevention of these parts of the inflammation or eradication of cancer pathogenic factors (such as stomach, colon cancer treatment of Helicobacter pylori) may prevent the occurrence of cancer.

② As we all know, lifestyle is one of the key factors in the pathogenesis of cancer, especially tobacco. Advocacy for smoking and healthy eating habits can prevent the occurrence of lung cancer and other cancers. To promote anti-cancer lifestyle is: smoking, limit alcohol, weight loss.

(3) screening can prevent or treat part of the cancer

① colorectal cancer is the basis of polyp, remove the polyps can prevent the occurrence of cancer, and colonoscopy screening can reduce the incidence of colorectal cancer and mortality. Where there are intestinal symptoms or blood in the stool it should have colonoscopy.

② cervical smears can be effectively found in cervical precancerous lesions, through the treatment of precancerous lesions it can prevent cancer.

③ The mammography can be screened early breast cancer.

The above three kinds of cancer, if which can be as early detection, the vast majority can be cured.

(4). The immune control drug prospects gratifying

No matter how complex the mechanism behind cancer, the body immunosuppression is the key to cancer progression. Removal of immunosuppressive factors, recovery system cells on the identification of cancer cells, can effectively resist cancer. More and more research evidence shows that by regulating the body's immune system, it is possible to achieve the purpose of cancer control. Through the activation of the body's anti-tumor immune system to treat the tumor, is currently the majority of researchers excited areas, the next major breakthrough in cancer is likely to come from this.

In order to explore the etiology, pathogenesis and pathophysiology of cancer, we have carried out a series of animal experimental studies. From the experimental results, we have obtained new findings and new revelation: thymus atrophy and immune function are one of the causes and pathogenesis of cancer so Xu Ze (Xu Ze) professor proposed at the international conference that one of the pathogenesis and etiology may be thymus atrophy, central immune sensory dysfunction, immune dysfunction, immune surveillance capacity decline and immune escape.

As a result of laboratory study it was found that: in the cancer-bearing mice thymus was atrophic atrophy, central immune sensory function damage, decreased immune function, immune surveillance is low, so the treatment principle must be to prevent thymus atrophy, promote thymus Hyperplasia, protection of bone marrow hematopoietic function to improve immune surveillance, for the immune regulation of cancer provides a theoretical basis and experimental basis.

Based on the above research on the cause and pathogenesis of cancer, the new idea and new method of XZ-C immunoregulation therapy are put forward. After 30 years of cancer specialist outpatient clinic more than 12,000 cases of advanced cancer patients with clinical validation, it was confirmed that the principle of treatment of chest care is reasonable, the effect is satisfactory. Application of immune regulation of traditional Chinese medicine, and achieved good results, improve the quality of life, significantly extending the survival period.

XZ-C (XU ZE-China) immunoassay is presented by Professor Xu Ze for the first time in his book "New Concepts and Methods of Cancer Metastasis in 2006" in 2006, and he thinks that under normal circumstances, cancer and body defense Between the dynamic balance, the occurrence of cancer is caused by dynamic imbalance. If the state has been adjusted to a normal level, you can control the growth of cancer and make it subside.

It is well known that the occurrence, progression and prognosis of cancer is determined by a combination of two factors, that is, the biological characteristics of cancer cells and the host organism itself, the ability to control cancer cells, such as it is the balance between the two, the cancer can be controlled, if both Imbalance, cancer will develop.

Under normal circumstances, the host of the body itself has a certain ability to control cancer cells, but in the presence of cancer, these control defensive ability to varying degrees of inhibition and damage, resulting in cancer cells lost immune surveillance, the occurrence of cancer immune escape, Making cancer cells further development, metastasis.

Through the above four years to explore the recurrence and metastasis mechanism of the basic experimental study, and after 3 years from the natural medicine herbal experiments in vivo through the tumor in vivo tumor inhibition test, from the herbal medicine to screen out a number of good tumor inhibition rate of traditional Chinese medications. They were composed of XZ-C1-10 anti-cancer immune regulation of traditional Chinese medications .

(5) The molecular targeted drug therapy is eye-catching

In 1960, Philadelphia researchers found that there was a chromosomal abnormality in patients with chronic myeloid leukemia (CML). Years later, the researchers found that this was the results of a chromosome 9 and 22 chromosome long-arm translocation. **Since this chromosomal abnormality was first found at the expense (Philadelphia), it was named the Philadelphia (ph) chromosome**. The chromosome has also become a target for CML targeted therapy for 40 years. In 2001 the first confirmed to be against Philadelphia chromosome molecular defects - imatinib.

Followed by the human epidermal growth factor receptor 2 (HER2) as the target targeting drug Quartin monoclonal antibody, the treatment of HER2-positive breast cancer, VEGF as the target of paclitaxel and EGFR as the target Cetuximab treatment of colorectal cancer. The targets of EGFR are as gefitinib and erlotinib for non - small cell lung cancer treatment.

Molecular targeted drugs are cell stabilizers, most patients can not achieve CR, PR, but the condition is stable and improve the quality of life. Removal of foritidine, erlotinib, imatinib, the need to use in combination with chemotherapy drugs.

Molecular targeting drugs represent a new class of anti-cancer drugs, and imatinib (Gleevec) is a typical example that can control cancer by inhibiting abnormal molecules that cause cancer, without damaging other normal nuclei. There have been a growing number of molecular targeted drugs for the treatment of cancer, such as B cell lymphoma of rituximab (Rituximab) treatment of breast cancer trastuzumab (Trastuzumab) and the treatment of lung cancer Nepal (Gifitinib) erlotinib (Erlotinib) and so on. Targeted therapy brings anti-tumor hope.

(6) The advanced cancer has been considered as the chronic diseases

Like high bloodness, coronary heart disease, advanced cancer has a variety of drug options, there are many kinds of molecular targeted drugs as a candidate, as well as biological therapy, immunotherapy, immunomodulation therapy, integrated traditional Chinese and Western medicine treatment, through the above joint treatment, it can survive with the tumor, some patients with advanced cancer can also survive for many years.

(7) to make the application of vaccine treatment of cancer as possible, human papillomavirus (HPV) can cause cervical cancer and HPV vaccine was found

In 1983, Professor Hausen found a new HPVDNA in the cervical cancer biopsy to find the new HPV16 virus. In 1984, HPV16 and HPV18 were cloned from cervical cancer patients, and later proved worldwide About 70% of cervical cancer patients are carrying both viruses.

In 1991, a large epidemiology confirmed that HPV was a causative agent for cervical cancer. HPV vaccine research started, and into clinical research.

In June 2006, preventive vaccines for cervical cancer were approved by the US Food and Drug Administration (FDA).

HPV vaccine is divided into two kinds of preventive vaccines and therapeutic vaccines, the current success of the study is a preventive vaccine.

HPV infection caused by cervical cancer can be vaccinated to prevent, which makes people finally realize the dream of having cancer vaccine.

(8) To launched the total attack and the prevention and treatment of cancer at the same attention which will change the status quo

Cancer has been beyond the cardiovascular and cerebrovascular diseases, become the primary cause of death of urban and rural people, which is mainly due to heavy treatment and the light defense, and even only treatment ; census is not a wide range of promotion, the proportion of early diagnosis of cancer is low and it did not attach importance to the three early, to the treatment of precancerous lesions. As well as the effectiveness of the ban on smoking and the growing environmental pollution are getting worse. It can be expected, China's cancer prevention and control situation in the future for a long time is still grim. In view of this situation, it should be proposed to attack the cancer and launch a total attack, that is, the prevention of cancer, cancer control, treatment, Troika go hand in hand, prevention and treatment at the same attention will gradually change the status quo.

(9) hepatitis B prevention and control, that is, is to do the prevention and treatment of primary liver cancer and the primary liver cancer in China occurred on the basis of liver cirrhosis lesions

Hepatitis B →chronic active liver → liver stiffness → portal hypertension →Enlarged spleen or/ and Ascites or/and Jaundice or/and Hepatic encephalopathy

To prevent and treat primary liver cancer should be appropriate to prevent hepatitis B.

Hepatitis B (hepatitis B) not only seriously affects the health of patients, but also the family and the community which caused a heavy economic burden, is harmful to the health of the people of the important public health problems. China is a high incidence of hepatitis B in 1992, the national epidemiological survey of hepatitis B showed that the population of chronic hepatitis B virus (HBV) carrying rate of 9.75%, that is, every one of 10 people for hepatitis B.

Prevention of the occurrence of primary liver cancer s necessary to prevent liver cirrhosis caused by hepatitis B. Hepatitis B and cirrhosis of the patients are high-risk groups and should be actively treated to prevent its malignant.

The newborns vaccination of hepatitis B vaccine is an important measure to control hepatitis B, through the implementation of neonatal hepatitis B vaccination, effectively protect the children infected with HBV, hepatitis B prevention and control significantly.

Prevention and control of hepatitis B also prevention and treatment of liver cancer caused by hepatitis B cirrhosis.

4, the current is the best time and is conducive to put forward the capture of cancer and launching a total attack.

(1) At present, China is building an innovative country, is the prosperity of scientific and technological innovation, the National Science and Technology Innovation

Conference deepened the reform of science and technology system, decided to enter the ranks of innovative countries in 2020, its goal for key areas of scientific research achieves a major breakthrough. Strategic high-tech fields achieve leapfrog development; a number of areas of new achievements went into the forefront of the world; universal scientific quality generally improved, into the ranks of innovative countries.

How to build an innovative country? Innovative countries should not only prosper their own innovation, but also prosperity of the original innovation, not only catch the international advanced level, but also reach the international leading level.

Cancer is the enemy of all mankind, the complexity of cancer beyond human imagination, which is the hottest field of biomedical position, gathered the world's largest elite research team and research elites.

Cancer is not a disease, but a similar feature of a wide range of diseases, although cancer treatment has been more than a century, now it entered the first two decades of the 21st century, but "oncology" is still the most backward of a discipline in the current medical subjects, why? Because the etiology, pathogenesis, pathophysiology of the "oncology" of are not yet clear. Oncology for scientific research, is a virgin land and need to conduct a lot of basic scientific research and clinical basic research.

To overcome the cancer as the main direction of the study and to do the experimental and clinical anti-cancer research should be the key areas of scientific research to achieve the original breakthrough.

According to the National Cancer Registration Center released the "2012 China Cancer Registration Annual Report", the annual number of new cases of cancer is about 312 million cases, an average of 8550 people a day, the country every 6 people diagnosed with cancer.

There are 2.7 million cases of cancer deaths per year, with an average of 7,500 deaths per day. Such amazing data should be included as scientific research in key areas of scientific and technological innovation.

Human beings should not sit still, physicians should not do nothing, I think we should put forward the general idea of conception of cancer and basic design of "declared war on cancer" which is the time and it should launch the total attack.

We have two tasks on the shoulder of the physician, one is to treat the patient, one is the development of medication, we should overcome the cancer in this strategic high-tech field to achieve leapfrog development, take our characteristics of anti-cancer anti-transfer technology innovation path, Innovation, and strive to enter the forefront of the world.

My second book "new concepts and new methods of cancer metastasis therapy", was published in January 2006, Beijing People's Medical Publishing House, Xu Ze with. In April 2007 a "three hundred" original book certificate was issued by the People's Republic of China .

My third book "new concept and new method of cancer treatment" was published in October 2011 Beijing. By People's Medical Publishing House, Xu Ze, Xu Jie. It was Followed by that American medical doctor Dr. Bin Wu translated into English, the English version in March 26, 2013 published in Washington, the international distribution.

(2) the current province and the city are in accelerating the realization of Wuhan city circle "two-oriented society" construction of a new breakthrough and the Wuhan is built as a national center city. In this excellent situation, we should grasp the national implementation of the strategy to promote the rise of the central region and the Wuhan city circle "two-oriented society" comprehensive reform of the sincere construction of new areas of great opportunity to blaze new trails. I deeply think that: in this excellent situation, great opportunity, it also creates a good opportunity for cancer prevention and cancer control research work,. Therefore, I suggest: you can engage in "ride research", never missed; if missed, the time will no longer come.

What is "riding car research"? This is what I think, no one mentioned in the literature. The current rise of the central strategy and the construction of "two-oriented society", is a historic great initiative: is the great initiative of the great country and the people ; is the power in the current and the benefits are in the future; it is the greatness of welfare for the health benefits of hundreds of millions of people. I would like to take a "research train" under this great historical wheel to engage in the prevention of cancer, anti-cancer research work done up will receive fruitful results and may even get "two-oriented society" new breakthrough.

I think the current energy-saving emission reduction and pollution prevention and control and "build two-type society" are I-level prevention to prevent cancer prevention. Its purpose and effect can reach the level of prevention of cancer I level. This is a golden opportunity, it must lap this golden opportunity; if missed, it will no longer come. I have been engaged in the experimental study of tumor surgery and clinical practice for half a century. It is deeply to realize that in order to reache the purpose of cancer prevention and control it must be government-led, experts, scholars efforts, the masses to participate in the mobilization of all, thousands of households to participate in order to do. And now the province and the city are the risc of the central strategy of the in-depth implementation of the national central city and the "two-oriented society" construction, it is government-led, the masses to participate in the mobilization of all the thousands of households involved in the work; it must improve the cancer awareness to achieve the effects of the prevention of cancer and cancer control and to receive to the effect of significantly reducing cancer incidence rate, which is the Chinese characteristics of "two types of society" anti-cancer, cancer prevention path.

Therefore, the current is the most time, is conducive for us to attack the cancer and to launch a total attack.

(3) At present, China is implementing the spirit of the 18th National Congress and meeting the well-off society to ensure the goal of building a well-off society in an all-round way in 2020.

The main contents are "the significant progress in resource-saving and environment-friendly society construction and the total discharge of major pollutants is significantly reduced and the stability of the ecosystem is enhanced and the people's environment has improved obviously."

Strengthen the natural ecosystem and environmental protection efforts, adhere to the prevention of the main, comprehensive management, to address the environmental health of the people seriously focus on the focus.

Building a well-off society and people improve their health knowledge and the environmental pollution and other pathogenic factors have the effective intervention will reduce the incidence of cancer-related.

Recognize that more than 90% of the cancer are caused or closely related to the environmental factors. Building a well-off society has a great relevance to the prevention of cancer and cancer control, therefore, we propose to attack the cancer and launch a total attack, to adhere to the Chinese characteristics of anti-cancer and cancer prevention path.

In the building of a moderately prosperous society, rural urbanization work, it is to develop the prevention of cancer and anti-cancer outline and it is put forward and develop the prevention of cancer and anti-cancer measures. It is to develop the cancer prevention and control planning and measures in the new towns, new rural.

Recognize the building of a well-off society should be everyone healthy, away from cancer, anti-cancer out of the way lies in the prevention; in the rural urbanization in China it is to carry out the prevention of cancer, anti-cancer work and to adhere to the path of Chinese characteristics of the prevention of cancer, anti-cancer. It is put forward the necessity of launching the total attack.

Our dreams are to o overcome cancer, build a well-off society, everyone healthy, away from cancer.

5, to avoid empty talking about, to pay attention to heavy hard work, no matter how far away the road to attack cancer it is, it should always start to go

What should I do next? Now it is proposed to overcome cancer and launch a total attack. Hope to get leadership support at all levels. We must know how to achieve the purpose of cancer prevention and control, we must be government leaders, government-led, experts, scholars efforts, the masses to participate in the mobilization of all nations, thousands of households to participate in order to do so.

(1) regardless of the way to overcome the cancer how far, how long it is, it should always start to go, always go to the long march, thousands of miles begins with a single step. Miles long march, it should start the start, as long as the forward, the grass will always come out of a way, the focus is to avoid empty talking about and to keep the hard work, hard work can be a result and the hard work is to act. The current status quo is to focus on treatment an light defense, or only treatment; To overcome the cancer should be launched a total attack and the prevention of cancer, cancer control, cancer treatment three carriages go hand in hand; go hand in hand - vigorously experiment, vigorously practice, hard work.

How to work? "Conducting scientific research on cancer control and prevention to develop plans and measures for cancer control" (see another article)

(2) the current situation is difficult to focus, but it should also start

To promote research and experiment and to call for mobilization of the whole people, to promote the capture of cancer, to launch a total attack, to launch the prevention of cancer, cancer control, cancer treatment, three carriages go hand in hand to launch the total attack. The whole people appeal to improve the prevention of cancer, cancer control knowledge, related to the real interests of each person, in order to achieve awareness of conquering cancer, it must mobilize the whole people, the whole people work, I know that to achieve this goal, we must arouse the people; to overcome the cancer, we must mobilize all the people to mobilize, a mighty force, government leadership, government-led, expert efforts, the masses to participate in order to do.

(3) why is it today to launch a total attack? No time to wait, have to propose to launch a total attack ; and the opportunity can not be missed and it have to propose to launch the total attack.

The original hope that in the modern oncology, the traditional three treatment can conquer and even overcome cancer; now it appears that is can not rely on chemotherapy to overcome cancer, after 30 years of clinical practice gradually believe that radiotherapy and chemotherapy can not overcome cancer, because it exists Many problems and drawbacks, it can only alleviate, that is, short-term improvement, can not be cured. It can only be used as adjuvant therapy, can not cure, can only palliative (may be shortened some).

That is being the case, it should find another way, launch a total attack, take a new road. The whole treatment = surgery + biotherapy + immunoregulation therapy + Chinese and Western combination therapy + targeted therapy. The short-term treatment = radiotherapy +chemotherapy as the supplemented (not long-range, not excessive)

The way-out of Cancer treatment is in the "three early", the way out of anti-cancer is in the prevention.

1/3 of the cancer can be prevented. It should pay attention to the basis of precancerous lesions and clinical diagnosis and treatment technology research. The road of scientific research is to carry out multidisciplinary research, special in-depth basis and clinical disciplines, and it should be woven with the specialist group which is closely related to a number of cancer, special in-depth basis and clinical research.

6, The total and general idea of how to carry out and achieve the above capture of cancer

① Professor Xu Ze proposed the proposal of "the establishment of the National Cancer Working Group,", and "province, city attack cancer work group (station)" first pilot experiment (see another article).

IT was Proposed to create "to overcome the Cancer Science City" test (see another article).

The recommendations to conquer cancer is to set up several research group (see another article)

It is First create a global model of the hospital for prevention and treatment (see another article).

"Declaring war on cancer" is the time, should start the total attack. That is, the prevention of cancer, cancer control, cancer treatment three carriages go hand in hand, at the same time to carry out prevention and treatment both. The prevention of cancer and cancer control goal are to reduce the incidence of cancer ; the prevention goal is to reduce mortality, improve the cure rate, prolong survival, live long, good quality of life.

② to capture cancer and to launch a total attack, personnel training is the key (see another article)

It is necessary to cultivate high-level professionals and intermediate professionals with prevention, control and governance. Personnel must have this specialist knowledge and technology. At present, multidisciplinary comprehensive treatment is necessary. Talent must be true to learn, talent must both ability and political integrity. Training personnel must pay attention to the construction of the laboratory; with a good laboratory, it is to have the main innovation or the original innovation of scientific research. With the laboratory, it can have the talent and have the scientific research results.

With the results of scientific and technological innovation, we must promptly transform into clinical medicine to improve the level of medical care, so that patients benefit. The following disciplines are related to the research of cancer research: immunology and cancer related group; virus and cancer related group; endocrine and cancer related group; fungi and cancer related group; Chronic inflammation related group; molecular biology and cancer related group; gene and cancer related group; environment and cancer related group. (See another article)

The existing oncology talent, mostly for the radiotherapy and chemotherapy, education must be launched to capture the cancer total attack to train the personnel, apply their knowledge. Education is used for the construction of innovative countries, apply their knowledge, and it can be innovative results.

7, the past and the future of oncology development

(1) twice leaps which treatment of malignant tumors appeared in the two centuries

Looking back over the past 100 years, human being is contempt by cancer, so far the formation of cancer is still the lack of the most essential understanding, the normal cell proliferation is subject to what factors control, and how they lost control of proliferation and become malignant cells.

In the last two centuries, the treatment of malignant tumors has experienced two leaps:

The first time was 1890, Halstad proposed the concept of tumor rooting.

The second is the 1970s, Fish will be integrated chemotherapy in radical surgery (adjuvant chemotherapy or neoadjuvant chemotherapy)

After then, treatment of malignant tumors are wandering without moving forward.

Fish is a systemic route of intravenous administration, after half a century, so far failed to reduce mortality, also failed to prevent recurrence and metastasis, and mortality is still the first.

Now we question and reform this traditional doctrine and the way of the administration of the traditional method, and to have innovative views, to target the organ intravascular administration, and combined with the establishment of XZ-C comprehensive treatment and XZ-C immunomodulation therapy (ie immune Chemotherapy), will likely help to promote the current state of hovering.

(2) President Nixon issued the Anti-Cancer Declaration in 1971 and filed an anti-cancer slogan in his joint speech.

In 1971 the United States Congress passed a "National Cancer Regulations", and by President Nixon issued "anti-cancer declaration", then put a considerable human and financial resources, with a view to overcome cancer in one fell swoop.

In December 1971, President Richard Nixon presented the anti-cancer slogan in the United Nations.

42 years have passed, and now Nixon has also been ancient, in cancer research it has also made many significant progress, such as the discovery of tumor suppressor genes, the advent of monoclonal antibodies, CT and magnetic resonance imaging, ultrasound and endoscopy and the improvement of various treatment methods of innovation.

However, in the current 21 years of the 21st century, the first 10 years, the largest human association of lung cancer, colon cancer and other mortality rate is still basically the same as 50 years ago, cancer deaths are still the first cause of death of urban and rural residents in China.

So the experts in medicine, biology and related disciplines began to reflect, most scientists believe that the prevention and treatment of the tumor should start from the most basic issues, that is, from the nature of cancer cells, pathogenesis, cancer cell metabolic characteristics and signal transduction to understand the cancer "Lushan true face", only as this, it is to have the most effective prevention and treatment of cancer.

To carry out interdisciplinary research, to promote basic research and clinical research cooperation, attention to clinical research.

It must be carried out clinical basic research and if there is no breakthrough in basic research, the clinical efficacy is difficult to improve.

(3) In 1982, Oldham founded the theory of biological response regulation, on the basis of which he proposed in 1984, the fourth mode of cancer treatment (four modatity of camcer treatment) biological therapy. According to the theory of biological response, under normal circumstances, tumor and body defense are in a dynamic balance between the occurrence of tumor and even invasion, metastasis, is entirely caused by this dynamic imbalance. The state of the imbalance has been artificially adjusted to the normal level, you can control the growth of the tumor and make it subside.

Biotherapy is to adjust this biological response by supplementing, inducing, or activating the cellular viable, biological, and / or cytokines that are inherent in the inherent bioreaction regulatory system.

Biological therapy is different from the previous three other treatment modes, namely, surgery, radiation therapy and chemotherapy, to directly attack the tumor as the goal. The scope of biotherapy is significantly beyond the traditional concept of immunotherapy, because the dynamic balance between the body and the tumor is not limited to the immune response, but also related to a variety of tumor-related regulatory genes and cytokines.

Biological response regulator (BRM) has opened up a new field of tumor biotherapy, at present, BRM is as the fourth program of the tumor by the medical profession attention.

(4) As cancer patients become more and more, the incidence rate is rising, the mortality rate is high, recognizing that cancer should not only pay attention to treatment, but also pay attention to prevention, to prevent the source. Is the study of the objectives and focus on the occurrence of cancer, the development of the whole process of prevention and treatment of the study.

In October 2011 Xu Ze published "new concept of cancer treatment and new methods" in the "the strategy of the way-out and suggestions to overcome the cancer." In June 2013 XZ-C also proposed "the general idea and design to overcome the cancer and launch" in an attempt to reduce the incidence of cancer, reduce mortality, improve the cure rate, prolong survival.

The total attack that is the three carriages of prevention of cancer + control cancer + cancer treatment go hand in hand

The prevention of cancer: can achieve cancer I level prevention through the construction of "two-oriented society" and building a moderately society "ride research".

Control cancer: through the "three early" outpatient, the management of the precancerous lesions, screening.

Treatment of cancer: surgery + immune regulation + biological therapy + differentiation induction therapy + integrated traditional Chinese and Western medicine treatment are as the main methods and the radiotherapy and chemotherapy are as a supplement.

Recent goals: to curb the development of cancer frenzy, reduce its incidence, and gradually improve the cure rate, and gradually reality three 1/3.

- One third of the cancer can be prevented
- One third of the cancer can be cured by early treatment
- One third of the patients can relieve pain through effective treatment

To be victory over cancer, where is the road?

How do I see cancer?

The author (XU ZE) thinks of that the road is in the scientific research, the road is the scientific research of the prevention and treatment of cancer;

The road is the scientific experimental research of exploring he cause of cancer, pathogenesis, pathophysiology;

The road is in the scientific experimental research of the whole process of the occurrence and development of cancer;

The road is the study of the reform and development of traditional therapy;

The road is to carry out multidisciplinary research, the formation of the relevant specialist group, special in-depth basis and clinical disciplines;

The road is the study of animal experimental research and basic and clinical research of cancer metastasis, recurrence prevention and treatment ;

The road is the study on the diagnosis and treatment techology of "three early" and precancerous lesions.

Through the scientific research of cancer prevention and treatment, mankind will overcome cancer, and ultimately will overcome cancer.

Fourth, "the construction of the hospital of cancer prevention and treatment of the whole process of cancer occurrence and development"

(The global demonstration hospital of cancer prevention and treatment)

"The envisage and feasibility To build Wuhan anti-cancer hospital throughout the prevention and treatment"

- Explain the necessity and feasibility of establishing a full-scale hospital for prevention and treatment

The current cancer has become the main disease of becoming a serious threat to human health, the incidence of an average annual rate is increasing by the 3% -5%

of the rate; the number of the incidence and death compared with 10 years ago, respectively is increasing 24.7% and 19.2%, and the traditional three treatment methods have been nearly a hundred years of history, cancer mortality is still the first, how to do? How should the road go? It is worthy of our review, reflection, analysis, summing up success and failure and both positive and negative experiences and lessons, thinking about why traditional therapy did not significantly reduce mortality, why did not control relapse and transfer? What is the problems of the traditional therapy and the traditional concept? It should be in-depth study.

What is the path of conquering cancer?

How to overcome the cancer? I believe that the road is in the scientific research, the road is the scientific research on the prevention and treatment of cancer; the road is the scientific research of the whole process of cancer occurrence and development, the road is to reform and have innovation of the traditional therapy ; the road is the study of "Three Early".

Through the scientific research of cancer prevention and treatment, mankind will overcome cancer, and ultimately will overcome cancer.

It should set up the hospital of the whole process of cancer prevention and cancer control, to carry out the medical practice and hard work of the whole process of prevention and treatment. Under the guidance of the concept of scientific development, with the development of the eyes, with the spirit of innovation, eyes forward, facing the future, the development of medicine, developing the medicine of cancer prevention and treatment in practice ; practice produces a real knowledge, work produces the achievement and the results in order to help with overcoming cancer.

1, the urgent need of the current oncology discipline is to carry out the cancer scientific research

(1) It must be aware of the current problems of oncology

① the basic problem is that the three traditional treatment has been applied for nearly a hundred years, the cancer mortality rate is still the first urban and rural areas. What should we do? It is should be analyzed, reflected and researched.

② postoperative recurrence is still very serious; the patients and their families are afraid of recurrence; some patients fears or are anxious for all day long after surgery. How should the surgeon prevent recurrence, prevent postoperative metastasis? It is to deserve our study.

③ metastasis is the core of cancer, is the key to survival, everyone is afraid of cancer metastasis. How effective anti-cancer metastasis, control cancer cell metastasis? should it be carried out basic and clinical research?

④ It must recognize the status of the existence of tumor disciplines. what are the problems? how can it be done? Although cancer treatment has been more than a century, it has now entered the second decade of the 21st century, but "oncology" is still the most backward of the current medical disciplines, why? It is because the etiology, pathogenesis, pathophysiology of "oncology" are not yet clear. Oncology of the scientific research is a virgin land and need to have a lot of basic scientific research and clinical basic research. Conducting cancer science research is an urgent need for current oncology disciplines.

⑤ Although countries invest a lot of money for the treatment of cancer patients, although the traditional three treatment for nearly a hundred years, but the cancer mortality rate is still the first reason for the death of urban and rural residents in China, the main reasons are the following:

A, the etiology of cancer is not entirely clear, the pathogenesis of cancer cell metastasis mechanism is still lack of understanding.

B, it is lack of adequate understanding of the complex biological behavior of cancer.

C, the treatment program is still quite blind.

D, the diagnostic means are behind, once found, that is late, so the result of the treatment is poor.

E, many large hospitals have not established a laboratory, can not carry out the basic research of cancer, anti-cancer metastasis, recurrence, must be involved in cancer animal model of basic research, because if no basic research breakthrough, the clinical efficacy is difficult to improve.

(2) It must be aware of the current problems of treatment

① chemotherapy needs to be further research and improvement

Whether postoperative adjuvant chemotherapy prevents recurrence, whether it prevents metastasis, and how it can help prevent postoperative recurrence and metastasis or not are worthy of our study, we should come up with their own data and experience to conduct further research and refinement.

Through the clinical medical practice case review, analysis, and reflection, it was found:

A, some patients with adjuvant chemotherapy failed to prevent recurrence;

B, some patients postoperative adjuvant chemotherapy failed to prevent metastasis;

C, some patients postoperative adjuvant chemotherapy to promote immune failure.

Through the review, analysis, and reflection of the current status of tumor chemotherapy in China, it was found:

A, traditional chemotherapy to suppress immune function, inhibition of bone marrow hematopoietic function, immune decline can promote tumor development.

B, white blood cell (WBC) reduction is one of the common toxicity of chemotherapy, WBC decline can lead to serious infection → a large number of antibiotics → double infection (fungal infection) → immune failure.

C, the traditional chemotherapy damage to the host, because the chemotherapy cell poison as a "double-edged sword", that is, killing cells and kill normal cells (chemotherapy drugs about 99.6%, kill normal cells, especially bone marrow hematopoietic cells and immune cells, only about 0.4% Drug cancer cells)

D, the traditional intravenous chemotherapy for intermittent treatment, intermittent cannot be treated, that is, there is the role of killing cancer cells only 3-5 days of intravenous administration, then no killing cancer cells (Figure 1), it is only a short time to kill (3-5), can not once and for all, after 3-5 days the cancer cells continue to proliferate, split (Figure 2), so it can only alleviate in a short time.

so it can only alleviate in a short time.

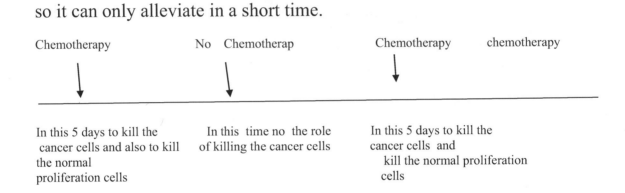

Figure 1 The time to kill cancer cells

E, the traditional therapy target only focus on chemotherapy can kill cancer cells, while ignoring the host itself on cancer resistance and control, because the tumor occurs, the development depends on the level of host immune function and the biological characteristics of the tumor itself, that decision The biological characteristics of the tumor cells and the host of the constraints on the two factors than the potential, if the balance is controlled, if the two imbalance is progress. Traditional radiotherapy and chemotherapy are to promote the decline in immune function, it is possible to make the two more unbalanced.

F, whether is the solid tumor (stomach, colorectal, liver, gallbladder, pancreas, spleen, abdominal, pelvic and other tumors) systemic intravenous chemotherapy route scientific and reasonable or not? It should be questioned.

a This route of administration, through the heart pump to chemotherapy cells to the body distribution of toxic drugs, killing the body organs of the organs, it is unreasonable.

Now many solid malignancies, postoperative adjuvant chemotherapy were used intravenous intravenous infusion, the elbow vein infusion → superior vena cava → right heart → through the pulmonary artery into the lungs → via the pulmonary vein into the left heart → through the aortic flow distribution in the body The (About 0.4%), and the vast majority (about 99.6%) of the chemotherapy cells are distributed in the body organs and kill normal cells, especially immune cells, bone marrow hematopoietic cells, resulting in The patient was severely damaged, serious side effects, and the solid foci did not play a significant role. Therefore, the above-mentioned solid tumor intravenous chemotherapy route of administration is unreasonable, unscientific, the cytotoxic system is distributed, is damaged in the patient.

b This route of administration can not be directly reached the portal vein system, vena cava system and the portal vein system is generally not connected by the superior vena cava is difficult to reach the portal vein.

Chemotherapy is to use cytotoxic cancer cells, must first study clear where the cancer cells are? it is to be targeted, clear objectives. Along the line of cancer cell line transfer, the cancer cells to track and kill, and along the tumor vein flow, chemotherapy drugs can follow this path to kill the cancer cells are being transferred. So, stomach, colorectal, liver, gallbladder, pancreas, spleen, abdomen and other cancer cells in there? It is mainly in the hepatic portal vein system. But the vena cava system and the portal vein system is generally not connected by the elbow vein → vena cava route of administration can not enter the portal vein system, so the abdominal tumor of the systemic intravenous chemotherapy route of administration is unreasonable, unscientific, Detrimental to the patient. It is because it cannot enter the portal vein system where cancer cells exist.

For half a century, tens of thousands of cancer patients around the world have suffered from the huge pain of widespread killing of normal cells by chemotherapy. Clinicians should seriously think, analyze, reflect, evaluate. For the solid tumor should not be administered by the elbow vein, but should try to target the tube tube intravascular administration, should try to correct the current irrational route of administration, and to reform, innovation and development.

③ the current chemotherapy is often a certain blindness, postoperative adjuvant chemotherapy, the surgical specimens were not for cancer cell culture, and thus can not be the patient's cancer chemotherapy drug susceptibility test. The current courtyard alone experience patients with blind chemotherapy. It has a chemotherapy and do not know whether to kill cancer cells and it can only be said to have completed a chemotherapy work. It may be beneficial to some patients, but may be harmful to a considerable number of patients, if the patient is resistant to the drug, it is not only beneficial, but harmful.

(3) the main contradiction of current chemotherapy

So far, the purpose of tumor chemotherapy is still mainly to kill cancer cells, the drugs used are mostly cytotoxic, no selectivity, regardless of cancer cells or normal cells will be damaged. Through the case review, analysis, reflection, I realized that the existence of the following several major contradictions in chemotherapy.

① the contradiction between the chemotherapeutic drug poison and the damaged host

The purpose of the treatment of cancer is to eliminate the tumor, to protect the body, to restore health, and the current chemotherapy is to kill both the tumor and the normal cells and hurt the host and lose everything.

② persistent and intermittent contradictions

Cancer cells continue to split, and the contradiction between intermittent chemotherapy, cancer cell proliferation and division of cell cycle proliferation is continuous, and because of its inhibition of bone marrow hematopoietic function and peripheral white blood cells, chemotherapy drugs can only be used intermittently; there is a contradiction between cell division and intermittent chemotherapy. Even in the 3-5 days of chemotherapy to kill most of the cancer cells, but after a few days, the efficacy disappeared, the remaining cancer stem cells will continue to split, proliferation, cloning, recurrence, metastasis. Therefore, simply kill cancer cells do not meet the biological characteristics of cancer cells and biological behavior.

③ The contradiction of rising immune function and falling immune function

The use of chemotherapy drugs tends to reduce the immune function of patients, and there is a contradiction with cancer treatment must improve the immune function. Chemotherapy drugs are leading to decreased immune function; the longer the course of treatment, the more the decline in immune function, or even lose immune surveillance, cancer cells spread further.

(4) radiotherapy need to be further studied and improved

Radiotherapy is for local treatment and the transfer is systemic problems. How to play its role in anti-metastatic therapy? how to protect the patient's organs from nuclear radiation damage? It is to be further studied and improved.

(5)The "radical surgery" design need to be further studied and improved to reduce postoperative recurrence and metastasis. Since it is "radical surgery", why does not it achieve the purpose of radical treatment? Since doing lymph node dissection, why transfer? These are required for further study. How to reduce the intraoperative tumor-free technology? how to reduce and to prevent intraoperative cancer cell shedding?how to reduce the intraoperative promotion of cancer cell metastasis? how to reduce the spread from the tumor vein? All of these are things which clinicians should pay attention to the problems in the practices. Surgical operation should be light, stable and accurate. Surgery is the primary methods to prevent the transfer, to prevent postoperative recurrence and metastasis and it must be done from the surgery and should prevent the operation of cancer cells to protect the shedding, planting, spread.

2, the existing problems of the current building tumor hospital model

(1) the current status of the tumor hospital

① background and sub-division

General provincial tumor hospital with tumor surgery, cancer gynecology, oncology, radiotherapy, chemotherapy, comprehensive … … and other subjects

Department of Oncology Hospital and the top three hospital of the tumor only have oncology, radiotherapy, chemotherapy, comprehensive … … and other subjects

Surgical cancer surgery is performed in surgery

Gynecological cancer surgery are in gynecology

Orthopedic cancer surgery in orthopedics

ENT cancer treatment in the ENT

② tasks and objects

The task is mainly treatment, the object is mainly in the late, transfer, relapse of patients with poor efficacy.

③ treatment: mainly kill cancer cells

Radiotherapy, chemotherapy, chemotherapy + radiotherapy

④ treatment results: the mortality rate is still the first, the incidence is still rising

(2) the existence problems of the hospital model

① focus on the focus of treatment, for the late, metastasis, recurrence of advanced cancer patients with poor efficacy, exhausted human and financial resources, and failed to achieve lower mortality, improve the cure rate, reduce morbidity.

② only treatment, or heavy treatment with light defense, the more treatment and the more patients.

③ ignored the commitment to "three early", early detection, early diagnosis, early treatment. The Early patients have the good curative effect and the high cure rate.

④ ignore the precancerous state, precancerous lesions of the treatment

⑤ ignored the prevention

(3) it should be reformed, innovated and developed for the problems existing in the unification mode

① solve the hospital model, and gradually solve the prevention and treatment at the same attention and the focus shifted to the left.

To solve the problem of prevention and treatment, prevention and control strategy, prevention and treatment strategy, the goal is to reduce morbidity, reduce mortality and improve the cure rate.

In order to improve the therapeutic effect, improve the cure rate and reduce the mortality rate, we must pay attention to the above: "it must understand the current problems in the treatment", to further study and improve, for the above problems to be reform, innovation and development. So as to improve the quality of medical care, reduce mortality and improve the cure rate.

③ in order to control cancer → fight cancer → capture cancer, the goal must be to reduce morbidity, reduce mortality, improve the cure rate, it should be both treatment and control. Building hospitals should be the hospital with cancer prevention and treatment at the same attention .

Building journals should be a magazine on tumor prevention and control, and should be both important for prevention and treatment. Both medical and educational and scientific research must be both important for prevention and control.

Medical school teaching work curriculum must be the prevention and treatment at the same level.

Scientific research project set up must be both the prevention and treatment at the same level.

Tumor and Environmental Science and Life Sciences and Ecological Sciences must be multidisciplinary to infiltrate, create new disciplines, discipline disciplines, and develop new industries.

So, it will be to overcome cancer → conquest cancer → capture cancer, will improve cancer prevention, control, treatment .

3, The status quo of the current incidence of cancer in China

The current cancer has become a major threat to human health, the main disease, the incidence of an average annual rate of 3% -5% increase. According to the National Cancer Registration Center released the "2012 China Cancer Registration Annual Report." New cases of cancer each year are about 312 million cases, an average of 8550 per day, the country every minute there are six people diagnosed with cancer.

Malignant tumor disease rate of 35 to 39 years of age were 87.07 / 10 million.

In 40 to 44 years old age it was 154.53 / 10 million.

In More than 50 years of age it accounted for more than 80% of the total incidence of the disease.

More than 1% of the incidence of cancer over 60 years of age.

In 80 years of age it is to reach the peak.

National cancer mortality rate was 180.54 / 10 million, each year due to cancer deaths it is 2.7 million cases. The probability of cancer deaths among Chinese residents is 13%, that is, one in every seven to eight people is killed by cancer. Tumor mortality was higher in men than in women, 1.68: 1.

From the disease, the first place in the national malignant tumor is lung cancer, followed by gastric cancer, colorectal cancer, liver cancer and esophageal cancer. Ranking first in the national malignant tumor is still lung cancer, followed by liver cancer, stomach cancer, esophageal cancer and colorectal cancer. The highest mortality rate, both men and women are lung cancer.

Although cancer treatment has been more than a century, now it is to enter the 21st century and the second 10 years, the Beijing Municipal Health Bureau statistics show that in 2010 the number of lung cancer in Beijing population male malignancy incidence was the first and in women it is the second place, second only to breast cancer. From 2001 to 2010, the incidence of lung cancer in the city was increased by 56%, one-fifth of the city's new cancer are lung cancer patients.

In China's urban population, the incidence of lung cancer is close to the level of developed countries.

Hubei Province Cancer Center Director Wei Shaozhong introduced that in Wuhan City in 2009 it was registered 12590 cancer patients, 6961 deaths, and was equivalent to 1049 people per month suffering from cancer, 580 people died of cancer.

From 2003 to 2009, the incidence of cancer was in Wuhan from 165.82 / 10 million to 257.89 / 10 million, increased year by year.

It is Consistent with the national situation and the incidence of lung cancer in Wuhan is the highest mortality rate; from the genders, the highest rate of female is the breast cancer.

The first five cancers in male in Wuhan are lung cancer, liver cancer, colorectal cancer, gastric cancer, urogenital cancer, the first five women is breast cancer, lung cancer, reproductive system cancer, colon cancer, gastric cancer.

The incidence of female breast cancer is high, but the mortality rate is much lower than lung cancer, indicating early diagnosis and treatment of breast cancer early results. As early as early detection, early treatment, it can achieve better treatment, and even cured.

4, how can it be to reduce the incidence of cancer? How can we improve cancer cure rate? It must be the prevention of the cancer and control of the cancer and treatment of cancer and change the hospital building mode.

So how to prevent? How to control? How to trea?

How can it be to be improved the cure rate?

- the way out of cancer treatment is in the "three early".

How to reduce morbidity?

The way out of cancer is prevention.

In the current cancer hospital the treatment of cancer mainly is concentrated in the late stage, the treatment effect is poor.

(1), how to improve cancer cure rate? the way-out of Cancer treatment is in the "three early"

Cancer's production and growth will go through stage of susceptibility, precancerous lesion and invasive stage. All the present tumor hospitals or tumor departments mainly focus on the cancer treatment in middle or advanced stage. The Therapeutic effects are poor. If patients in middle or advanced stage can accept surgical operation, then they will be treated surgically. But if not, they will only receive palliative treatment. Therefore, cancer treatment lies in "early detection, early diagnosis and early treatment". Generally, patients in the early stage will get a better therapeutic effect. The increase of therapeutic effect will certainly reduce the fatality rate of cancer. Consequently, we must put much emphasis on the study of early-stage diagnostic and therapeutic methods, and on the treatment of precancerous lesion for lessening medium-term or terminal patients in the invasive stage.

stage of susceptibility	precancerous lesion	early stage	no metastasis	have metastasized	
				local position	amphi position
①	②	③	④	⑤	⑥

① Cancer prevention

② Outpatient service of "three kinds of earliness"

③ Surgical operation

④ Place surgical operation first, radiotherapy, chemotherapy and biological TCM second

⑤ Possible to undergo surgical operation

⑥ To give treatment as carcinomatous metastasis

If patients have been treated well in the stage of precancerous lesion or early stage, then the number of patients in middle or advanced stage of invasion and metastasis will fall off. Thus, the cancer incidence rate will also decline. Therefore, we hold that the present tumor hospitals in various places mainly focus on the cancer treatment in middle or advanced stage. Even though the therapeutic result is effective, it can only bring the reduction of cancer mortality rate. But if ignoring the stage of susceptibility, precancerous lesion or early stage, it will be impossible to reduce the cancer incidence rate. Therefore, we must put much emphasis on the whole process of cancer production and growth. After all this is the real global change of strategic importance.

The writer has engaged in surgical oncology for over sixty years. More and more patients suffer from cancer, and the cancer incidence rate also rises. The writer deeply feels that people should emphasize not only therapy but also prevention. Only in this way could the cancer be killed in the source. Cancer treatment lies in "three kinds of earliness" (early detection, early diagnosis and early treatment); anti-cancer method lies in prevention.

As stated above, the strategic center of gravity of tumor treatment and prevention moves forward. There are two aspects in its meaning. One is to prevent cancer by changing life style and improving environmental pollution; the other is to cure precancerous lesion for inhibiting cancer's development to the invasion stage, middle stage or advanced stage.

In 1990, our institute's specialist out-patient department of tumor surgery once opened the outpatient service of "three kinds of earliness" to carry out various endoscopies and biopsies, through which have found many atypical hyperplasia of stomach, intestinal metaplasia, atrophic gastritis and hyperplasia of mammary glands, etc. These "precancerous lesions" are difficult to treat. Then how to handle these precancerous lesions or precancerous conditions so as to prevent their cancerations urgently needs clinical researches to look for better treatment methods.

(2), Put emphasis on fundamental and clinical researches of precancerous lesions with diagnosis and treatment techniques.

"Three kinds of earliness" is the key to cancer treatment. While how to handle precancerous lesion is the key stage for cancer prevention and treatment.

The present cancer diagnosis mainly depends on image examinations of type-B ultrasonic, CT and MRI. But as soon as the cancer comes to light, it has reached the middle or advanced stage. Many patients have lost the chance of radical excision. Although the complex treatment has been done, the therapeutic effects are still poor. If the cancer is in the early stage or belongs to the carcinoma in situ, then the curative effect of operation will be better and the cancer can be cured. Therefore, the cancer treatment should strive for "three kinds of earliness", which refers to early detection, early diagnosis and early treatment.

Because cancer's pathogenic factors are not very clear, the primary prevention is still quite difficult.

Studies in recent years indicate that malignant tumor rarely has a direct carcinomatous change in normal tissues. Before the occurrence of tumor in clinical diagnosis, cancer often goes through quite a long evolution stage, which is the stage of precancerous lesion. Early identification and control of these precancerous lesions will bring positive significances for the secondary prevention of cancer.

What is precancerous lesion? The precancerous lesion is a histopathology concept, which refers to a kind of tissues with the dysplasia of cells. Precancerous lesion has the potential to become cancerous. If there is no cure in a long period, precancerous lesion will evolve into cancer. In other words, precancerous lesion just has the possibility of changing into cancer. But not all the precancerous lesions will eventually become cancer. Through proper treatments, precancerous lesions may return to their normal states or have a spontaneous regression.

Canceration is a developing process with several stages. There is a stage of precancerous lesion between normal cells and cancer. It is a slow process from precancerous lesion evolving into cancer, which needs many years or even more than ten years. The length of canceration course is closely related to the strength of carcinogenic factors, individual susceptibility and immunologic function. Therefore, the study of precancerous lesion is of great importance to cancer's prevention and control.

(3) More than one third of the cancer can be prevented

The tumor formation is a long process with several factors and stages. Precancerous lesion is of reversibility, so cancer is preventable.

The several factors, steps and stages of tumor formation have the following features.

The generation and growth of tumor can be roughly divided into several stages of initiation, promotion, metastasis and others. Cellular canceration induced by chemical carcinogen is a multistage process. The chemical carcinogenesis process of Experimental animals and the generating process of human tumors (such as colon cancer) have a series of changes, which are hyperplasia → pathological changes → benign tumor → malignant tumor → tumor metastasis, etc. The whole change process is complicated with multiple stages of initiation, promotion and evolution, etc. It often takes a long cytometaplasia time to change from normal cells to the tumor that can be detected clinically, which is a long cumulative process.

(1) Two-stage theory of tumor formation: In 1942, Beremblum carried out the experimental study of mouse's skin canceration induction, in which he used benzoapyrene to treat mice's skins for about one year, and only three out of one hundred and two mice suffered from skin tumors. If mice's skins were treated with benzoapyrene for several months and then treated with the tumor promoter-croton oil, thirty-six out of eighty-three mice suffered from skin cancers, whose incidence rate was ten times higher than that of using benzoapyrene alone. If mice's skins were first treated with croton oil for several months and then treated with a carcinogenic substance, there would be no induced tumor. If mice's skins were only treated with croton oil for a long time, whose incidence rate of tumor would be lower than that of using benzoapyrene alone (1/106).

On the basis of this study results, Beremblum and Subik have proposed that cancerous process contains two different but intimate stages. One is a specific provocation stage. Small dosages of carcinogenic substance induce normal cells to become potential cancer cells. The other is nonspecific promoting stage. Potential cancer cells are further promoted to suffer from mutation and evolve into tumor under the action of tumor promoters, such as croton oil and others.

People hold that provocation process refers to the process that normal cells change into potential cancer cells under the action of carcinogenic substances. The time of promoting process is fairly short and generally irreversible. While promoting process is the process that potential cancer cells change into cancer cells under the action of tumor promoters. The early promoting stage is reversible but the late stage is irreversible.

Carcinogenic substance is a kind of mutagen, which plays a decisive role in canceration process. While cancer promoters do not have the mutagenicity, which can only promote potential cancer cells to have a further proliferation change and gradually evolve into cancer cells. During these two processes of provocation and promoting stages, induced cells grow out of control, escape from the host's immune surveillance, gradually form tumor cells with malignant phenotype and then evolve into tumor cells with infiltration and metastasis. This theory recognizes that tumor generation is quite a long process (months, years and even more than ten years) and will be impossible through a single factor or stage, which is very important to cancer prevention and control. It prompts that people have enough time to build up cancer-fighting ability, strengthen immunity, change life style and improve environmental pollution to prevent cancer. Intervention measures should be emphasized to tackle the reversible stage of cancer promoting.

(4) how to reduce the incidence of cancer? - The way out for cancer is prevention

For almost half a century, human spectrum of disease has undergone a drastic change. Most communicable diseases have been effectively controlled. Chronic diseases, such as cardiovascular diseases and malignant tumors have been the most serious diseases threatening human health.

Cancer has become the most serious public health problem in the world. Compared with other chronic diseases, cancer's prevention and control face a greater challenge.

Over the last thirty years, the fatality rate of cancer in China is on an obvious rise, which has occupied the number one in causes of death of urban and rural residents. On average, one out of every four deceased persons dies from cancer.

Cancer not only seriously threatens human health but also causes the rapid rise of hospitalization costs. The direct costs of cancer treatment in China are about one hundred billion RMB every year, which makes patients and the whole society bear a huge economic burden.

Although each country inputs a large number of funds to treat cancer patients, the five-year survival rate of some common cancers has no obvious improvement in the recent twenty years. For instance, during the years from 1974 to 1990 in USA, the five-year survival rate of esophagus cancer only rose from 7% to 9%, stomach cancer from 16% to 19%, liver cancer from 3% to 6%, lung cancer from 12% to 15% and that of pancreatic cancer remained the same as 3%.

What's to be done? Anti-cancer method lies in prevention. Prevention and intervention is the most important thing in the field of public health.

As for the malignant cancer, prevention outweighs therapy. Worldwide tumor researchers have reached a consensus of adjusting public health resources and policies, shifting strategic focus from therapy to prevention, and carrying out positive and effective studies of pre-warning, early diagnosis and intervention to lower tumor incidence rate and raise curative rate.

The evidence in *Cancer Report* provided by World Health Organization proves that up to one thirds of cancers can be prevented. As long as every national government, medical workers and the common people actively take actions and shift the research emphasis of tumor prevention and treatment to tumor prevention, they can prevent above one thirds or even about half of the cancers.

5, the road of how to overcome cancer is to study the establishment of hospital of prevention and treatment of cancer during the whole process of cancer occurrence and development and change the current building hospital mode which focuses on treatment and ignores defense

XU ZE on the strategic thinking, planning sketches, of the prevention and treatment of cancer during the whole process of occurrence and development ; how to overcome of cancer? the road is to study the prevention and treatment of cancer during the whole process of cancer occurrence and development, practice a real knowledge, practice to product the results.

Xu ZE (Xu ZE) on the thought, strategy and program against cancer are shown in the following schematic drawing.

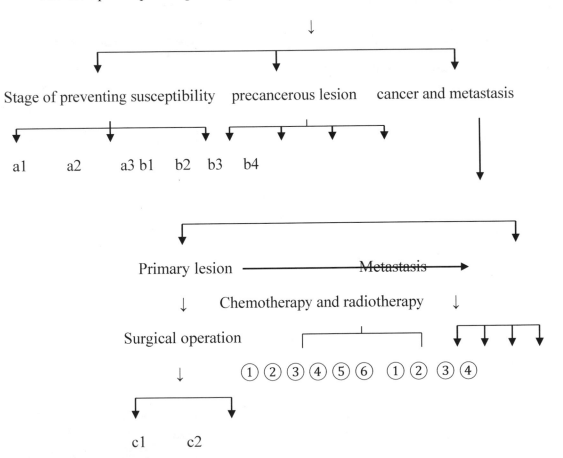

↓

Our thought, strategy and experience should be divided into three parts

↓

Before the formation of cancer——prevention part——anti- mutation

↓

Precancerous lesion with possible tendency of malignant change——intervention part

↓

The therapeutic part of primary cancer with the formation of focus and anti-metastasis

↓

Stage of preventing susceptibility   precancerous lesion   cancer and metastasis

a1   a2   a3 b1   b2   b3   b4

Primary lesion —————— ~~Metastasis~~ ——→

↓   Chemotherapy and radiotherapy   ↓

Surgical operation

① ② ③ ④ ⑤ ⑥   ① ② ③ ④

↓

c1   c2

a1. "Two-oriented society" contains essences and measures

a2. "Lift scientific research" makes plans and measures of cancer control

a3. Propaganda, education and study of popular science

b1. General investigation of physical examination

b2. Selective examination of high risk group

b3. Outpatient service of "early detection, early diagnosis and early treatment"

b4. Induced differentiation

c1. Improve free-tumor technique

c2. Prevent intraoperative implantation of cast-off cells

① with indication

② individuation

③ scientization

④ drug sensitive test

⑤ try to reduce untoward reaction

⑥ "intelligent resistance to cancer" of target administration

① targeted therapy

② anti-metastasis and anti-relapse therapies

③ BRM biological therapy

④ immunoregulation therapy

Figure. The diagram of the strategic thinking of prevention and treatment of cancer during the whole process of development and occurrence

I am going to apply for a new idea and a new approach to the occurrence and development of cancer, as shown in the plan diagram, according to my third book, "New Concepts and New Methods for the Treatment of Cancer", in Chapter 38, page 308 as the hospital of the prevention and treatment, unlike the current hospital mode is the invasion as the main.

This kind of innovative hospital mode is aimed at the prevention and treatment of the whole process of cancer occurrence and development. It is closely related to the clinical practice. In view of the existing problems and shortcomings of the traditional therapy, this paper puts forward a series of suggestions, development of.

Five, the basic design and feasibility to set up the total attach envisage of overcoming cancer and science city"

--- is equivalent to the design of the overall framework with a Chinese characteristics of capturing cancer

Why is it put forward the general imagination and design of overcoming cancer? How to attack? It should be a comprehensive planning and layout

<u>1, recognize the need to put forward the total attack</u>

(1) in the research journey it is gradually to recognize the need to put forward the total attack

This initiative is a review, reflection, analysis, summary of successful experiences and lessons of failure in a large number of clinical practice cases of long-term cancer specialist out-patient clinics for more than 30 years, and progressively and slowly recognized and put forward. These acquaintances mainly appear in my three monographs, I recovered after a serious illness, quietly to hide in the small building for 18 years with solitary military alone war, went it alone, summed up their own experimental research and clinical validation information, has published three monographs, in the first monograph "new understanding and new model of cancer treatment" was published in 2001, which in the book it was put forward to a new understanding and in the international community it was first proposed "chemotherapy to be further research and improvement." At that time people are afraid to agree, but some patients and doctors have feelings. In 2002 when participating in the Barcelona International Medical Association Conference and reporting it, it received an excellent paper certificate.

The second monograph "new concepts and new methods of cancer metastasis therapy" was published in 2006 and was based on the first book on the basis of scientific research, the "target" of the cancer treatment was located in the anti-metastasis, indicating that the key of cancer treatment is anti-metastasis.

It was conducted a series of the experimental research and clinical basic research and clinical validation research of anti - cancer metastasis and recurrence, and rose to the theoretical innovation, and it was put forward the new idea and the methods of anti – metastasis. In April 2007 it was received the "three hundred" original book award issued by the People's Republic of China Press and Publication Administration.

The third monograph "new concept and new method of cancer treatment" was published in 2011, is based on the second monograph research results on the basis of forward development, the research objectives focused on the study of prevention and treatment during the whole process of cancer occurrence and development; it is close to connect with the clinical reality, aimed at the existence problems and shortcomings of traditional treatment of the current clinical practice, it was put forward the reform and innovation and research and development; it is realized that cancer prevention and treatment strategy must move forward, the way out of treatment of cancer is in the "three early" and in the prevention. The book was published in April 2013, and was published in Washington and sold in globe such as UK Europe and America.

I have been engaged in tumor surgery for 57 years, more and more patients, the incidence of cancer is also rising, high mortality rate, so I deeply appreciate that cancer should not only pay attention to treatment, but also pay attention to prevention, in order to stop at the source.

Three monographs are three different stages, three different levels of height, three different understandings. In the different levels of height there is the different scenery and there are the different understanding, different eyes; a mountain is higher than a mountain and a mountain has better scenery than a mountain. (This is just three books comparing with their own)

Therefore, after the third monograph, I put forward the task, mission, opportunity and challenge of anti-cancer research, under the guidance of the scientific concept of development, take the Chinese characteristics of anti-cancer metastasis research and innovation, put forward the strategic thinking and suggestions of conquering cancer and put forward the need for total attack.

Under the situation of the current high incidence of cancer and high mortality rate it is realized the need to launch a total attack.

People have been fighting cancer for hundreds of years, but so far cancer is still rampant in the crowd and it is the effectiveness of the emblem and the incidence is still rising and the mortality rate is high.

According to statistics in 1995, the world's annual new cancer is 7 million people, the number of deaths each year is 500 million people. In China's cancer in 1996 the number is 1.8 million, the death toll is 1.28 million. In terms of mortality, the tumor is at the head of the disease and becomes the most serious disease that threatens human health.

"2012 China Cancer Registration Annual Report", the annual new cancer fell to 312 million cases, the average daily 8550 people, in the country every minute there are 6 people diagnosed with cancer. The current cancer is the first cause of the death of urban and rural residents in China, and every one of the seven deaths is cancer.

The current cancer has become a serious threat to human health and the main disease; the incidence of an average annual rate increases by 3% -5% of the incidence rate, the more treatment and the more patients, the mortality rate is high. People should not do nothing, humans should not sit still, I think we should put forward the general idea of conception and basic design of conquering cancer and it is the time to "declared war on cancer" and it should launch the total attack.

(2) to recognize the problems and drawbacks of radiotherapy and chemotherapy and it is difficult to rely on them to conquering cancer, under this condition it is to raise the need to launch a general attack

① Review of the traditional three therapies in the century and historical evaluation

Three treatments of Cancer traditional therapy: surgical treatment, radiotherapy, chemotherapy have been for nearly a hundred years, how are the results of its treatment? It should be reviewed and evaluated about the efficacy for a century, from theory to practice, to the efficacy. Can it be relied on three major treatments to conquer cancer in the future? How is its prospects assessment?the evaluation criteria arc: reduce morbidity, reduce mortality, prolong survival, improve quality of life, reduce complications.

We should stop and collate, analyze, review, reflect, sum up success and failure both positive and negative experience and lessons, what are the results? What lessons are there? Did the patient benefit? Whether to prolong life and reduce pain: you should carefully analyze the successful experience, conscientiously sum up the lessons of failure, find out the problems, find out the experience and lessons. It should think about why traditional therapy did not significantly reduce mortality? It should think about why traditional therapy does not control relapse, transfer? It should think about why the three treatments have been for nearly a hundred years, and now the cancer mortality rate is still the number one of the death rate in the city of China and township residents? I entered the Tongji Medical College medical school for 62 years, for clinical surgery of tumor surgery has been 57 years, experience and witness the traditional three treatment for half a century. It is deeply to think about how to evaluate the efficacy of the century.

What is the treatment of cancer patients? It is often considered to be: the patient's survival period is long, good quality of life, symptoms improved, fewer complications.

The three major means of the traditional treatment of cancer has made a brilliant contribution to human anti-cancer business. However, until the first two decades of the 21st century, cancer is still rampant, the more treatment and the more patients, the incidence of cancer continues to rise, high mortality, remains the first cause of urban and rural deaths in China.

Although the patient has undergone regular, systemic radiotherapy and / or chemotherapy after surgery, it has not been able to prevent the recurrence of cancer cells. Why traditional treatment did not significantly reduce mortality? Does it suggest that traditional therapies do not meet the biological characteristics of cancer cells? What is the problem with traditional radiotherapy and chemotherapy? What is the traditional concept of cancer therapies? What is theoretically or conceptual problem? How to correct its shortcomings on the concept or understanding so that it becomes the more perfect?

Through the review and analysis and evaluation and reflection of clinical practice cases and postoperative adjuvant chemotherapy cases, it was found that there are problems:

(1) in some patients the postoperative adjuvant chemotherapy failed to prevent recurrence;

(2) in some patients the postoperative adjuvant chemotherapy failed to prevent metastasis;

(3) in some patients the chemotherapy promotes immune failure.

From the clinical practice of case to analysis and reflect why the postoperative chemotherapy failed to prevent cancer recurrence, metastasis?

From the role of chemotherapy drugs in the cancer cell cycle to analyze and reflect; from the chemical drugs to suppress the overall immune function to analyze and reflect; from the drug resistance of chemotherapy to analyze and to reflect it was found:

(1) For the current chemotherapy there are some important errors;

(2) the current chemotherapy exists to a major contradiction.

Through the review, analysis, evaluation, reflection of the clinical medical practice case it was found the following problems:

"Analysis, evaluation and questioning of systemic intravenous chemotherapy for solid tumors"; (see another article)

"Review, analysis and commentary on the three major treatments for cancer"; (see another article)

"Chemotherapy needs to be further research and improvement." (See another article)

Update thinking, update awareness

Through the review, analysis, evaluation and self-reflection of 7 years of experimental experiments and 30 years of specialist outpatient clinics on more than 6,000 cases of diagnosis and treatment, it is summed up the success and failure of both positive and negative experience and lessons and it was thought of why the traditional therapy did not significantly reduce the death Rate? why did not it control relapse and transfer? What are the questions of the traditional concept of traditional therapy? So I gradually realize that the current cancer traditional therapies may still have some important errors. For example:

① the traditional chemotherapy suppresses the immune function and inhibit the bone marrow hematopoietic function;

② the conventional intravenous chemotherapy is the intermittent treatment; in the intermittent period cancer can not be treated and intermittent cancer cells continue to proliferate and divide;

③ traditional therapy damage the host, because the chemotherapy cell poison for the "double-edged sword", both kill cancer cells and kill normal cells;

④ traditional therapy goal only focuses on that chemotherapy can kill cancer cells, while ignoring the host itself on cancer resistance and control because the occurrence and development of the tumor depends on the level of host immune function and the biological characteristics of the tumor itself, that is determined by The biological characteristics of tumor cells and the host of the constraints on the impact of the two potential, if it is the balance, cancer is controlled; if the two are imbalance, cancer is progress. Traditional radiotherapy and chemotherapy are to promote the decline in immune function and it may make the two more potential imbalance;

5, the traditional therapy damages the central immune organs, cancer Thymus has been inhibited, and chemotherapy inhibits bone marrow, as "snow plus frogs or worse". So that the entire central immune organs were damaged and failed to effectively protect;

6, the traditional therapy is injury therapy and has a certain blow to the the entire central immune organs which can not be effectively protected;

7, Traditional therapy neglects the anti-cancer ability of the human body itself, ignores the role of anticancer cells (NK cell population, K cell population, LAK cell population, macrophage population, TK cell population) in the host cancer system and ignores the role of the host of the anti-cancer cytokine system IFN, IL-2, TNF, LT and ignores the role of the host of the tumor suppressor gene and tumor suppressor gene (the human body has oncogenes and tumor suppressor genes, but also cancer metastasis gene and tumor suppressor gene) and ignores the role of the neurohumoral system and endocrine hormone system in the body and ignores the role of anti-cancer agencies and their influencing factors in the human body, as well as its role of the regulation, balance and stabilization of the host mechanism itself and ignores the inherent factors of the human body's anti-cancer activity, Blindly kill cancer cellsy kill cancer cells;

8, traditional therapy goal is relatively simple, just kill cancer cells. And it is not consistent with the actual situation of the biological characteristics of cancer now known such as cancer cell invasion behavior; the metastasis is involved in the multiple steps; the incentives factors of the relapse can be the latent months or years and then have recurrence. It has been recognized that antineoplastic agents are not necessarily resistant to metastasis and the anti-metastatic drugs are not necessarily anti-tumor.

How to do? Both the above problems should be further research, and conduct the basis of experimental research and clinical research, deepen the reform, should update thinking, update awareness, update observation, in the reform forward, innovation. Innovation, there must be a challenge to the traditional concept, to overcome its shortcomings, to correct its shortcomings so that it become more perfect. Innovation must challenge the status quo and beyond the status quo. Innovation also searches another way to find a new way to overcome cancer.

Why do I come to the 21st century today, the second 10 years to put forward to attack the cancer to launch a total attack? It is no time to wait and it has to propose to launch the total attack. If it is the chance, it should not miss and it has to propose to launch a total attack.

② It is recognized

The original hope in modern oncology, the traditional three treatments such as the surgery and radiotherapy, and chemotherapy can overcome cancer, it seems unlikely to rely on traditional therapy in the radiotherapy, chemotherapy to overcome cancer. Why cannot radiotherapy and chemotherapy overcome cancer? It is because its treatment target is only the relief (CR, PR), remission is not cured, but it is just the short-term that is a few weeks of improvement, then it will progress, increase, transfer. How to do? It must be reformed and have the innovation and develop. Can not is it relied on to overcome cancer? should it have another way? Current treatment of the status quo is wandering before, how do? The way out is to reform.

Surgical treatment of traditional therapy is still the main treatment of solid tumors, is the main science and technology of conquering cancer in the future.

(1) Recognizing that more than 90% of the cancer is caused by environmental factors or closely related to; in our city, "two-oriented society" construction has a great relevance to the prevention of cancer cancer, cancer control and it is proposed to launch a total attack and to adhere to the road of the prevention of cancer and cancer control with Chinese characteristics "two-styles of the Society.

① building energy-saving emission reduction, environment-friendly "two-oriented society" has a great relevance to the prevention of cancer and controllingcancer

The current province, the city is ongoing energy-saving emission reduction, pollution reduction and building a "two-oriented society" is the governance of environmental pollution, people and social environment are harmony, will greatly reduce the air, water, food contaminants and carcinogenic substances, therefore, the construction of "two-oriented society" has a great relevance to the prevention of cancer and cancer control.

Human beings is in the search for cancer etiology and factors in the process and carried out extensive exploration and accumulated a wealth of knowledge and the most prominent of which it is found that more than 90% of the cancer are caused by environmental factors or closely related.

The United Nations Health Organization: 1/3 of the cancer can be prevented; 1/3 of the cancer can be cured by early treatment; 1/3 of the cancer can be effective treatment to alleviate the symptoms and prolong life. Therefore, it can be considered that cancer can be prevented.

It is important to be aware of the importance of cancer prevention, environmental factors and inappropriate social behavior are important pathogenic factors that may or may not be avoided by these external or human factors.

Through energy-saving emission reduction, pollution prevention, pollution control, construction of "two-oriented society", people improve their health knowledge, environmental pollution and other carcinogenic factors for effective intervention, it will reduce the incidence of cancer.

② adhere to the road of the prevention of cancer and cancer control with the Chinese characteristics "two types of society".

China's energy-saving emission reduction, the province's "two-oriented society", through efforts, will inevitably achieve the great results at the same time to reduce the incidence of cancer. This is the Chinese cancer prevention and cancer control characteristics, is the road of the prevention of cancer and cancer control with Chinese characteristics of "two-oriented society". After 3-5 years of obtaining the experience of successful work in the province and the city from building a "two-oriented society" combined with the path of the prevention of cancer and cancer control of the Chinese characteristics, it can be introduced to the country and the world.

It is a great opportunity to carry out the excellent situation of energy-saving emission reduction, it is a golden opportunity to carry out the prevention of cancer and anti-cancer work; if it is missed, it will no longer come, so I proposed the basic imagination and designs to overcome cancer and launch the attack and it was put forward a comprehensive planning and layout of the basic design of the framework.

(2) recognize and the building of a well-off society and everyone is healthy away from cancer and the way-out of the prevention of cancer and control cancer lies in prevention; in urbanization and rural areas, it is to adhere to the road of the Chinese characteristics of the prevention and anti-cancer and it is put forward the need for general attack.

By 2020, we will achieve a grand goal of building a well-off society in an all-round way. The people's living standard has been improved. The construction of resource-saving and environment-friendly society has made great progress.

We should build a well-off society in an all-round way. We should adhere to the "Cancer innovation path in rural urbanization anti-cancer work which goes into the community, seize the opportunity to deepen the reform of important areas, so that it is to make "two-oriented society" prevention of cancer and cancer control work go into the community. Everyone is healthy and away from cancer.

2, how to set up the basic idea and design of launching a total attack and conquering cancer

How to overcome the cancer and to launch a total attack? Xu Ze (Professor Xu Ze) proposed the following basic ideas:

(1) how to overcome cancer? It must establish a "cancer animal experimental center"

To overcome cancer → conquest cancer → capture cancer, we must first understand the basic understanding of cancer: the cause of cancer, pathogenesis, pathophysiology, immunopathology, cancer cell biological behavior? Transfer mechanism? Why grow? Recurrence mechanism? A series of oncology and tumor-related issues have not yet clear. The scientific research of oncology is a virgin land and need to have a lot of basic scientific research and clinical basic research; to carry out basic research in cancer science is the urgent needs of the current oncology.Therefore, we must establish a "cancer animal experimental center".

To carry out the basic research of oncology, a good laboratory is the key, scientific design, scientific vision, must be through laboratory experiments, in order to draw conclusions, the results.

To transform the research design into scientific research results must have a good laboratory.

We believe that the construction of a scientific base for the construction of a total attack on cancer (science city) must first vigorously build a laboratory so that many basic problems have experimental research, open up the basis of research on oncology and it should encourage the development of new areas of research and product Talent and the result to help capture cancer.

The basic research in medical science is very important to the progress made in the fight against cancer. If there is no breakthrough in basic research, the clinical efficacy is difficult to improve.

The government should open up new areas of research, fight cancer, develop new products, new industries, and realize the new knowledge of these tasks from basic science research.

The current "oncology" is the most backward of the medical disciplines of a discipline, why? Because the "tumor" the name of the disease are not defined, there are various names? Some people write "tumor", "malignant tumor", "new creature", "cancer lumps", "cancer", "canccr" ... ... and so on, to define a disease name, you must understand the cause, pathogenesis, pathology, But the etiology, pathogenesis, pathophysiology of "oncology" are not yet clear and need to have a lot of basic scientific research and clinical basic research. To carry out cancer experimental scientific research is the urgent need of the current oncology discipline.

How can we overcome cancer? How can we start the total attack? A good laboratory is the key. If there is no good laboratory, although there are talent, there are topics, there are projects, there are funds, if not the experiment, it can only be fantasy, empty talk, can not be a result, can not be accomplished.

Experimental surgery in the development of medical science is extremely important, it is to open a closed area of the key medicine, many diseases prevention and control methods are after many times the experimental study, and achieved a stable results before use in clinical and promote the development of medical career.

Why do we have an animal experimental study to establish the Cancer Animal Experimental Center?

The purpose of medical research is to study the disease, to understand the disease, to seek new methods, new technologies, new theories to improve the level of medicine, prevention and treatment of disease. However, the characteristics of medical research is characterized by its research object is the human body itself, and its research results and applied to the human body. Therefore, the results must be strict scientific, accurate and reliable, harmless to the human body. People are the most valuable, many experiments and observations do not allow the researchers in accordance with the wishes of the human body directly to the test, the need to use simulation methods, the establishment of animal models, experimental research. To be fully harmless to the human body after the success of animal experiments on the basis of success, can be applied to clinical, applied to the human body.

In order to overcome the cancer, start the total attack, we must establish a cancer animal experimental center, the laboratory must be related to good equipment, conditions, experimental personnel need to concentrate on, can calm downand carry out experimental research work, we must attach importance to the three bases and three stricts."

(2) how to overcome cancer? It must be the founder of "innovative molecular cancer medical school", training personnel, training the relevant personnel who can participate in the capture of cancer and launch the total attack and talent must be genuine talent.

Personnel must have knowledge of medical college, must also have life science knowledge, genetic engineering, molecular biology, environmental science, environmental science, Chinese medicine knowledge, medical multidisciplinary knowledge, immunology, endocrinology, virology, immunopharmacology ... ... and so on.

The current tumor hospital or the top three hospital cancer department most have the medical, radiotherapy, chemotherapy, comprehensive ... ... and other knowledge and the talent status is now mainly radiotherapy, chemotherapy and other professionals.

To overcome the cancer, talent is the key, how to cultivate talent is the key, the study of cancer requires a number of disciplines of knowledge and technology and genetic engineering, molecular biology, virological experimental personnel; to have knowledge must also have technology and it is to have the ability to operate; to have technology needs to have knowledge so that under the guidance of the theory it is to develop the high-end technology and it needs to have the first-class talent of conquering the tackle, we must concentrate on, calm down, concentrate on this work; where is talent from? it is based on our own training and the own machine hatchs talent.

In order to overcome the cancer, to launch a total attack, the people who future participation or commitment to the work must have the necessary knowledge and technology.

In view of the fact that more than 90% of the cancer is caused by environmental factors or closely related to; in the current we are ongoing resource-saving and environment-friendly society to build a comprehensive test of energy-saving emission reduction, sewage treatment, this policy and work have a great relevance with prevention of cancer and cancer control work, we must cultivate the relevant personnel.

Therefore, we must build innovative molecular cancer medical school and experimental secondary school talent. In the 21st century the modern high-tech knowledge was summarized as three aspects: life science knowledge; environmental science knowledge; information science knowledge.

The current educational content can not keep up with the development of the times. To overcome the total attack of cancer, we must develop modern high-tech disciplines, must have a good laboratory, but in the current it is lack of laboratory talent. In order to prevent cancer and cancer control and to construct the "two-oriented society" and to conquer cancer, it is not the lack of college graduates, graduate students, but the lack of modern high-tech middle-level specialist talents with the laboratory experiments experience who can go deep into the community to carry out the general attack and to prevent cancer and to control cancer.

Therefore, it is proposed that it must be founded:

① The founder of "innovative molecular cancer medical school", training modern high-tech senior cancer doctor (four years college).

② "innovative modern high-tech experimental life science and technology college" (secondary three-year system)

Foster the establishment of laboratory personnel for tertiary institutions. Modern life science and technology progresses rapidly, genetic engineering, molecular biology, cell inheritance rapid develop.

③ founder of "modern high-tech environmental science and technology college" (secondary school three years)

Environmental science has attracted the attention of the world, it will be emerging disciplines, new industries, the current energy-saving emission reduction, pollution control, building a "two-oriented society" must conduct a large number of research topics for the research, use modern high-tech talent in-depth community, to develop the work of combined with prevention of cancer and anti-cancer.

(3) how to overcome cancer? It must have the practice base of be implemented to overcome the cancer and launch a total attack, must "build the hospital of the prevention and treatment of cancer during the whole process of development and occurrence of cancer" - global demonstration of cancer prevention and treatment hospital.

Why is the global demonstration of cancer prevention and treatment research? It is because it was the first time in the world that the XZ-C had launched an initiative to attack the cancer, which was presented in his 38th chapter in the edition of the New Concept and New Approach to Cancer Therapy published in 2011.

Professor Xu Ze in March 2013 proposed "the design and feasibility report to build Wuhan anti-cancer prevention and treatment of hospital" - to elaborate the necessity and feasibility of the establishment of the whole hospital,.

(See full text)

(4) how to overcome cancer? We must establish a "Institute of Innovative Molecular Cancer" to carry out multidisciplinary research related to cancer and set up a related specialist group. In order to overcome the cancer, improve the cure rate, reduce the mortality rate, improve the quality of life, improve the medical level, reduce the complications, the basic research must be carried out.

The study of oncology is the most complex and difficult problem in medical research. It involves multidisciplinary knowledge and theory, including pathology, cytology, immunology, virology, endocrinology, medical genetics, immunopharmacology, molecular Oncology; from the molecular level of the tumor pathogenesis to understand the causes of the disease it will be to provide effective intervention and the treatment measures for the prevention and treatment.

In view of the study of oncology involving multidisciplinary knowledge and theory, we must set up the relevant specialist group, further study, based on the knowledge and theory of the discipline, known medicine, to explore the unknown knowledge of the discipline, the future of medicine, Edge disciplines, interdisciplinary, in order to help overcome cancer.

It should be set up following the cancer and is closely related to the specialist group, special in-depth basis and clinical research.

① Immunology and Cancer Research Group

The study group of recent clinical research tasks should be: a, the assessment of the immune function of cancer patients; b, the efficacy of immunoregulatory treatment of cancer patients monitoring; c, put, chemotherapy in patients with immune function quantitative measurement.

② Virus and Cancer Research Group

Some of the cancer known to be closely related to the virus, the treatment should be considered the corresponding treatment, and the virus is closely related to human tumors are: Burkitt Muba; nasopharyngeal carcinoma; leukemia; breast cancer; cervical cancer; Gold lymphoma and so on.

The study of the etiology of human tumor has progressed rapidly in recent years. If you can prove that some of the human tumor virus causes, it is possible to use the vaccine to prevent the occurrence of cancer and control its popularity.

③ Endocrine hormone and cancer research group

Hormone is an important chemical substance that regulates the development and function of the body, and the hormones maintain a dynamic equilibrium relationship according to the law of unity of opposites. Endocrine disorders, due to the imbalance of hormones, so that some hormones continue to act on a tissue, this abnormal chronic stimulation may lead to cell proliferation and cancer.

A carcinogenic hormone can only promote the growth of tissue cells, such as ovarian estrogen, pituitary gonadotropin. Experimental studies have shown that hormonal imbalance caused by thyroid, pituitary, ovary, testis, adrenal cortex and the palace, cervix, vagina, breast and other organs of the tumor, estrogen has caused the role of breast cancer.

④ mycotoxin and cancer research group

it is necessary to have a further study on the carcinogenic factors of some known tumors closely related to mycotoxi. In the recent ten years, some mycotoxins are gradually observed to have carcinogenic or cancer-promoting action on animals.

Therefore, medical circle begin to pay more and more attention to studying the relation of fungus and its mycotoxin with human tumor.

Mouldy grains polluted by Aflatoxin in a liver cancer-prone area of China are mixed in feed to feed rats. After six moths, the inducing rate of liver cancer is up to 80%. This kind of feed can also cause monkeys' liver cirrhosis as well as other hepatic lesions and induce liver cancer. Most of the induced liver cancers are hepatocellular cancers. Furthermore, this kind of feed can lead to the adenocarcinoma of kidney, stomach and colon; intratracheal instillation can cause squamous cell carcinoma of lung.

Therefore, making a good job of mould proofing and ridding of oil and foodstuffs is important for exploring the prevention of some tumors and ensuring popular physical fitness.

In the esophageal cancer-prone area of China, Geotrichum candidum Link abstracted from edible pickled vegetable is proved to have the cancer-promoting action. Use the culture of Geotrichum candidum Link to feed rats for twenty months, and then papilloma in anterior stomach is induced. Some moldy food can cause precancerous lesion and early cancer in esophageal epithelium of animals

⑤ Environmental and Cancer Research Group

During the process of seeking for the cause of cancer and occurrence conditions, human have carried out an extensive research and accumulated rich knowledge, which have found that above 90% cancers are caused by or closely related to environment.

How to prove the relationship between environmental pollution and cancer? there are many examples of history; air pollution, water pollution, soil pollution, food pollution have the serious impact on human carcinogenesis.

The above study group composed of various schools

(5) how to overcome the cancer to attack the total attack? It must "set up the medical, teaching, research, science city to overcome the cancer and launch a total attack"

We strive for "to build Wuhan Science City to attack the cancer and launch a total attack"

The basic Envisage and design of XZ-C's launching the total attack

Xu Ze Professor proposed the following of the general idea of the total attack of conquering cancer and the basic design of science city

<u>Dawn spirit of scientific research</u>

<u>Hard work and struggle</u> ------18 years of cold window and

↓

hard work

<u>Review and reflection</u> -------------Follow-up, summed up the successful experience of treatment (In the second monograph there are the typical case); reflection failure treatment lessons (in the first monograph there are cases of failing to prevent from recurrence, failed to stop metastasis)

↓

<u>Open up and Innovation</u> ------------- 48 kinds of good tumor inhibition rate were screened out of 200 kinds of Chinese herbal medicine in the animal experiments ; 11 years of clinical validation of Z-C immunoregulation of traditional Chinese medicine series; it was realized to rise to theoretical knowledge, new concepts, new models.

↓

Facing future medicine --------- Recognizing the inadequacies and problems of traditional therapies in the twentieth century, recognizing the direction of the 21st century

↓

Look forward to look ----------- Suggest:

- Establishment of Innovative Molecular Tumor Hospital
  - Cultivating advanced cancer researchers for the country.
- Establishment of innovative molecular tumor hospital (at the molecular level of Western medicine combined) ------ benefit more cancer patients and serve more cancer patients.
- Establishment of Innovative Molecular Cancer Institute
  - Research cells begin to change
  - to the CT can be found between a long time, To achieve three early goals, "Target" metastasis, cancerous lesions, precancerous state.
- Build innovative molecular cancer pharmaceuticals
  - out of a new way to overcome the cancer with our characteristics

The science base of conquering cancer and launch the total attack(the science city)

The science city of medicine and teaching and research and development

The cancer animal experimental center

- The establishment of innovative molecular tumor hospital - for the national training of advanced oncology research talent.
- Establish an innovative molecular tumor hospital (combined with Western medicine at the molecular level) - to benefit more cancer patients and serve more cancer patients.
- The establishment of the Institute of Innovative Molecular Oncology - Research on cell initiation of malignancy - to CT can be found between a long period of time to achieve three early goals, "target" metastasis, cancer lesions, precancerous state.
- Build innovative molecular cancer drug factory - out of a new path with cancer of our country.

Sixth, while building a well-off society at the same time, it is suggested "ride research"- ------ the necessity and feasibility of cancer prevention and cancer control of medical research and cancer prevention and treatment

- Adhere to the anti – cancer and cancer prevention new path of the Chinese characteristics of well - off society

At present, the country is implementing the spirit of the 18th National Congress of the Communist Party of China to ensure the goal of achieving a well-off society in 2020. The country is building an innovative country, prosperity and technological innovation. National Science and Technology Innovation Conference to deepen the reform of the system, decided to enter the ranks of innovative countries in 2020.

Its goal for the key areas of scientific research is to achieve a major breakthrough in the original, a number of scientific results in the new areas come into the forefront of the world, the general scientific quality is increased generally and enters into the innovative country.

This great situation also creates a major opportunity for our capture of cancer for the direction of scientific research work and deeply encourage me to actively participate in, pioneering and innovative. I deeply appreciate that cancer should not only pay attention to treatment, but also pay attention to prevention, in order to stop at the source. The way-out of Cancer treatment is in the "three early" (early detection, early diagnosis, early treatment) and anti-cancer out of the way is in the prevention.

I deeply think that: this excellent situation and opportunity also creates a good opportunity for anti-cancer, anti-cancer research work. Therefore, I suggest: you can engage in "ride research", never missed, if it is missed, it will no longer come.

What is "riding research"? This is what I think that no one mentioned in the literature. At present, the construction of ecological civilization and the protection of the ecological environment and the construction of a well-off society and the construction of an innovative country are a historic great initiative and the power in the contemporary, in the future, for hundreds of millions of people for health benefits, for future generations to seek health and welfare of the great initiative.

I would like to take a "historical car" under the great historical wheel and put anti-cancer, anti-cancer and anti-cancer research work up and will certainly receive fruitful results and strive to China's medical care in the basis of cancer treatment and clinical research to achieve new results into the forefront of the world, and strive to capture cancer in this critical area of scientific research to achieve a major breakthrough in originality.

In the current energy-saving emission reduction and pollution prevention and pollution control of the excellent situation are conducive to carry out anti-cancer, cancer control of scientific research and prevention and control work. The environmental and cancer have a great relationship; the energy saving and the pollution abatement and building an environment-friendly society have the closely related to the prevention of environmental carcinogenesis. As early as the 20th century, 80 years of domestic and foreign experts, scholars believe that more than 90% of the cancer is caused by environmental factors; the protection and recovery of a good environment are an important part of the prevention of cancer.

I have been engaged in the experimental study of tumor surgery and clinical practice for half a century. Knowing that to achieve the purpose of cancer prevention and control must have the government-led, experts, scholars efforts and the masses to participate, mobilization of the whole people, thousands of households to participate in order to do. At present, China is building an innovative country, building a well-off society, it is the government-led, the masses involved, mobilization of the whole people, thousands of households involved in the work, so that it will be able to improve people's awareness of cancer, to prevent cancer and in our province, the city it significantly reduces the incidence of cancer effect.

I would like to suggest: in the building of a moderately prosperous society, rural urbanization work, the development of anti-cancer, anti-cancer outline, the development of anti-cancer, anti-cancer measures, the development of new towns, new rural cancer prevention and control planning and measures. Carry out anti-cancer, cancer control work. Adhere to the Chinese characteristics of anti-cancer, cancer control innovation path, to overcome cancer, built a well-off society, everyone healthy, away from cancer.

Therefore, I would like to put forward a proposal of "building a scientific research": building a well-off society, building an ecological civilization, protecting the ecological environment and building an innovation-oriented country. This work is in the contemporary, Great initiative, took the opportunity to the way "ride research" to carry out cancer control and prevention of research work and cancer control measures. The purpose is to the people healthy, away from cancer, reduce our country, our province, the incidence of cancer in our city.

First, building a moderately prosperous society is conducive to carry out the scientific research and prevention and control work of anti-cancer, cancer control

In order to build a well-off society, the construction of new socialist countryside, new towns should also carry out anti-cancer work, so that a well-off society, everyone to improve anti-cancer, anti-cancer knowledge, everyone's health, away from cancer. Well-off society, the new socialist countryside, the new town should be how to prevent cancer, anti-cancer? Should be from the clothing, food, shelter, anti-cancer, from improving the living environment, from improving the living habits of cancer, with this basic knowledge, the vast majority of cancer can be avoided, can be prevented.

In order to carry out anti-cancer, cancer control work, we should first understand, study the relationship between the environment and cancer:

(1) the relationship between environment and cancer

1, air pollution and cancer

Mankind has developed billions of tons of coal, oil and natural gas as fuel and energy, such as thermal power, smelting steel, cars and aircraft to circulate a lot of harmful gases such as tar, kerosene and dust into the atmosphere surroundings. Air pollution can cause many diseases to occur, the most serious is lung cancer.

2, water pollution and cancer

Water pollution, mainly industrial and agricultural production and urban sewage caused.

3, soil pollution, food chain and cancer

Human large-scale industrial and agricultural production activities, so that a large number of industrial waste water and pesticide fertilizer into the soil, so that the deterioration of soil quality, human health threat, is also carcinogenic factors.

China's industrial development has made great contributions to China's economic development. However, while industrial development has brought about environmental pollution problems, we must take active measures to strictly control pollution control.

Building a resource - saving and environment - friendly society on the industrialization, modernization of the development strategy of the prominent position, the implementation of each unit, each family. Building an environment-friendly society is an important action to highlight environmental protection and is a top priority in curbing environmental degradation.

At present, we are carrying out energy conservation and environment-friendly social construction comprehensive test for energy-saving emission reduction, sewage treatment. This policy has a great deal of relevance to work and cancer prevention work because:

1, human beings in the search for cancer etiology and factors in the process, carried out a wide range of exploration, accumulated a wealth of knowledge. One of the most prominent is the discovery of more than 90% of the cancer caused by environmental factors or closely related.

The current province, the city is ongoing energy-saving emission reduction, pollution abatement, environmental pollution control. It will greatly reduce the air, water, food contaminants and carcinogens. Therefore, and anti-cancer, cancer has a great relevance.

2, the United Nations Health Organization proposed: 1/3 of the cancer can be prevented; 1/3 of cancer can be cured by early treatment; 1/3 of cancer can be effective treatment and reduce symptoms and prolong life. Therefore, it can be considered that cancer can be prevented.

Must be fully aware of the importance of cancer prevention, environmental factors and improper social behavior is the most important pathogenic factors, these external or human factors can be avoided or intervene.

Through energy-saving emission reduction, pollution prevention, pollution control, people improve their health knowledge, environmental pollution and other carcinogenic factors for effective intervention, will reduce the incidence of related cancer.

3, environmental pollution can increase the incidence of cancer:

I deeply understand: why engage in energy-saving emission reduction, environment-friendly "two-oriented society"? Because with the development of modern industrialization, a large number of energy consumption, a large number of production and life during the day and night kept a lot of tar, soot, dust and other harmful gases into the atmosphere, atmospheric pollution, water pollution, soil pollution, Food pollution, occupational carcinogenic substances soared. In recent decades, the incidence and mortality of lung cancer in Western developed countries has increased rapidly. Such as the British lung cancer mortality in 1930 to 100 million, up to 1975 up to 120.3 / 10 million, 45 years, an increase of 12 times. The United States 1934 - 1974 male lung cancer mortality increased from 3.0 / 10 million to 54.5 / 10 million, an increase of 17 times. The above data is amazing. If not energy-saving emission reduction, it will be a lot of emissions of pollutants, greatly harming human health, to promote cancer incidence and mortality rate of rapid growth. Energy-saving emission reduction is for the healthy development of industrialization, continue to leap.

Because of environmental pollution, harmful to society, harmful to human life, to improve the environment and to prevent and control pollution and to defend health are conducive to building a healthy, happy, harmonious, environment-friendly society.

So, what is the risk of environmental pollution? The most frightening thing is that environmental pollutants contain many carcinogens that have led to an increase in the incidence of cancer, such as the destruction of nuclear power plants in Japan, resulting in a significant increase in the concentration of nuclear substances in the surrounding air, water, soil and food, and the promotion of leukemia, cancer, etc. Increased morbidity, not only to the contemporary and endanger future generations.

4, the harm of environmental pollution: As we all know, the harm of environmental pollution is:

① pollution of people's life and health, radiation, nuclear radiation, bacteria, viruses, harmful chemical poisoning, air pollution, water pollution, soil pollution, food pollution, not only harm people's life and health, and lead to an increasing incidence of human cancer;

② cause epidemic spread of infectious diseases;

③ a large number of pollution of chemical substances, harmful gases, harmful water, fertilizer, pesticides can lead to cancer, mutations, causing cancer high risk, high incidence.

Therefore, to reduce the incidence of cancer, we must improve the environment, prevention and control of pollution, building an environment-friendly society, a harmonious society.

Anti-cancer strategy should be anti-cancer, cancer control, the use of I-level prevention, II-level prevention, III-level prevention. I deeply think that the current pollution reduction, pollution control is I-level prevention, in fact, from the fundamental anti-cancer measures. In fact, under the auspices of the government, all the people mobilized to participate in the masses of anti-cancer measures.

Second, it is recommended that while creating a well-off society at the same time, it is put forward to have a "ride research" – to conduct the medical

research of cancer prevention and control work and cancer prevention and cancer control

1, I think the current energy-saving emission reduction, pollution prevention and treatment, in fact, are the I-level prevention of anti-cancer control . Its purpose and effect can reach the level of prevention of cancer I level. This is a golden opportunity and must seize this golden opportunity; if missed, no longer come. I have been engaged in the experimental study of tumor surgery and clinical practice for half a century, knowing that to achieve the purpose of cancer prevention and control must have the government-led, experts, scholars efforts and the participation of the masses and mobilization of all and thousands of households involved in the work. It will be able to improve the awareness of the whole people anti-cancer to achieve the role of preventing cancer and to receive the effects of reducing the incidence of cancer in the province and the city.

2, to carry out the prevention of cancer and cancer control, now there is no practical solution, only from the technical and tactical to proceed, but it should be from the strategic focus to implement people-oriented and fundamentally emphasize the harmony between man and the environment. It is necessary to carry out scientific research to explore innovation. Science is an endless frontier, and research is endless. With the development of the eyes, eyes forward, under the guidance of the scientific concept of development, energy conservation, pollution prevention, treatment and anti-cancer, cancer control, reduce the incidence of cancer related scientific research, will produce many now do not know The new knowledge, and even the original innovation of scientific research and produce new disciplines, new industries.

I deeply appreciate this policy and work: energy-saving emission reduction, pollution prevention, pollution control, which itself contains the significance and effects of the prevention of cancer and control cancer. But it did not really point out. I would like to make a proposal to suggest that our province, the city clearly pointed out that in building a moderately society at the same time, to carry out a number of cancer control and prevention research and the development of cancer control planning and measures. To improve people's awareness of cancer prevention is an innovation and also is the initiative for the benefits of a country and the people.

To improve people's awareness of cancer prevention and to do a good job of building well-off society are concerned about the vital health of the people's health and it will have the province's people's support and gratitude and it is to conduct the more serious and active energy-saving emission reduction and the prevention of - pollution and pollution control and the prevention of cancer and cancer control work.

The prevention of cancer and anti-cancer work are a hard nut to bite the bones, but it should also continue to bite down. Because cancer is human damage, the prevention of cancer and anti-cancer are mankind business. I know that to do this work will depend on the experts, scholars personal efforts; if it is never possible, it depends on the individuals only. It must be under the auspices of the government, mobilize the masses, the mobilization of the people which can be done and only socialism can do. It should walk out of our characteristics of the prevention of cancer and anti-cancer innovation path. I am convinced that in building a moderately prosperous society at the same time, "riding research" carries out anti-cancer and cancer prevention and control planning and the group prevention and the group control anti-cancer measures. In my province and my Wuhan city circle (8 +1) the cancer incidence and mortality rate will be significantly reduced.

Third, following the scientific concept of development and adhering to the road of innovation of the Chinese characteristics of anti-cancer, anti-transfer

Why do I put forward a well-off society at the same time when it is put forward a "ride research"? Why is it thought of that this is a good time to help "overcome cancer"?

This is gradually recognized from my study of conquering cancer over 30 years of scientific research and it is the journey that we have completed the application of the "eight five" research topics of scientific research, is a series of coherent research steps, scientific research, scientific research Exhibition times, before and after the phase together, step by step; in different stages there are different understandings.

Climbing Scientific research is like climbing the mountain, to a layer of peaks can see a layer of scenery, a mountain is more higher than a mountain, a mountain scencery is much better than a mountain scenery .

Follow the scientific concept of development, my research journey of ideological understanding and scientific thinking, all of these can be divided into three stages Introduction:

1, the first stage (1985 - 1999)

New discoveries, new acquaintances - finding problems - asking questions - innovating thinking and changing ideas.

In 1985, I made my own petition of more than 3,000 cases of thoracic and abdominal cancer patients, and it was found that most patients were relapsed or transferred after 2-3 years. Postoperative recurrence and metastasis are the key factors that affect the long-term efficacy of surgery. It must do the clinical basic research to prevent cancer recurrence and metastasis; if no basic research breakthrough, the clinical efficacy is difficult to improve. As experimental surgery is to a key to open the medical restricted area, so we established a tumor animal laboratory, set up a laboratory surgery laboratory, carried out a series of experimental tumor research: the implementation of cancer cell transplantation, the establishment of cancer animal model to find the mechanism and the regulation of the cancer metastasis and recurrence and to look for the regulation and the effective measures of cancer invasion, recurrence, transfer.

New discovery

From the experimental tumor study found that: ① resection of the thymus can make the animal model and the study was concluded: the occurrence and development of cancer and the thymus of the host have the positive relationship. ② our laboratory study of cancer metastasis and immune relationship, the experimental results suggest that the transfer has the relation with immune. ③ the experimental study found that with the progress of cancer, the host thymus showed progressive atrophy.

In order to further study, based on the experimental laboratory, Hubei Institute of Experimental Surgery was established in March 1991, Professor Xu Ze was as director and Qiu Fazu academician was as a consultant, the research objectives and tasks was "conquering cancer" as the main direction.

In 1994, we set up a cancer specialist outpatient department, through the review of clinical medical practice cases, postoperative adjuvant chemotherapy analysis, evaluation and reflection, it was found that the problems: ①some patients had recurrence and metastasis after the surgery because adjuvant chemotherapy failed to prevent recurrence; ②in some Patients the adjuvant chemotherapy failed to prevent the transfer; ③ in some patients chemotherapy promoted immune failure.

From the analysis and reflection of the clinical practice case, why did the patient fail to prevent recurrence and metastasis after surgery? From the chemotherapy drug in the cancer cell cycle to analyze the reflection, from the analysis and reflection of the chemical drugs to suppress the immune, from the chemical drug resistance to analyze, reflect, it was found that there are problems: ① In the current chemotherapy there are still some important errors; ②the current chemotherapy still exists Several major contradictions and it needs to be further studied and improved.

From the follow-up results it was found that postoperative recurrence and metastasis are the key to long-term efficacy of surgery. So we also raised an important question: clinicians must pay attention to and study the postoperative recurrence and metastasis prevention and control measures to improve postoperative long-term efficacy.

From 1985 to 1999, we conducted a series of animal experiments and clinical trials of cancer research and reviewed and analyzed and reflected and summed up the analysis of success and failure of both positive and negative experience and lessons learned, so finishing the above experimental study and Clinical practice review, reflection, analysis of scientific research materials, summary, collection, it was published the first monograph "new understanding of cancer treatment and new model" in January 2001 Hubei Science and Technology Publishing House, Xinhua Bookstore issued.

2, the second stage (after 2001)

The goal of the study and the "target" of cancer therapy is targeted at anti-metastasis, pointing out that the key to cancer treatment is anti-metastasis.

After 2001, our research work in-depth analysis of what is the key of the postoperative recurrence and transfer?

In view of the recurrence of cancer since the 1970s, the transfer rate is still high; in order to prevent postoperative recurrence and metastasis, it is the use of postoperative adjuvant chemotherapy and even before surgery it has begun chemotherapy, but the results are not Meaningful. Still in the postoperative shortly it had the recurrence and metastasis, or while it has the side chemotherapy, it has the side of the transfer; the more chemotherapy and the more metastasis. In some cases due to intensive chemotherapy, it was to promote immune failure. All of these are worthy for our clinicians to be serious and objective to think and analyze; cancer treatment should be how to prevent recurrence and anti-transfer in order to obtain a good long-term treatment effect.

Today, the most important problem of cancer treatment is how to stop the metastasis ; the transfer is the bottleneck of cancer treatment.

If you can not solve the problem of cancer metastasis after radical surgery, cancer treatment can no longer move forward.

Therefore, the key of the current cancer research is anti-transfer. The core issue of cancer treatment is to address the transfer and recurrence.

One of the keys to cancer treatment is anticancer metastasis. Transfer is just a phenomenon, how to clearly understand the cancer cell transfer process, steps and mechanisms? We should try to understand why cancer cells will be transferred? How is it transferred? What is the fate of the steps, routes, processes and transitions? What is the molecular mechanism of cancer cell metastasis? What is the weak link in the process of cancer cell metastasis? which link or part can be Hit or blocked in order to achieve the purpose of anti-transfer?

We spent more than three years on the cancerous animal model of the experiment, to observe and track the cancer in the regulation of the transfer, looking for interference and prevention of the transfer of cancer cells approach.

Through the review, analysis and evaluation of a large number of cases in clinical practice, we propose that the key of the current cancer research is anti-metastasis; (2) cancer is manifested in three forms in the human body, the third form is cancer cells that are being transferred; Cancer treatment goals should be aimed at these three forms; ④ cancer development process "two point and one line" cancer treatment, not only should pay attention to two points, should pay attention to cut off the line; ⑤ it was found that the specific measures of anti- Cancer cells were for surrounding, chasing, resistance, cutting . It was proposed the third field of anti-cancer metastasis therapy; the "main battlefield" which destroys the cancer cells on the way is in the blood circulation; it is important to improve immune regulation, immune monitoring.

By 2005, we have compiled a lot of information on the above experimental research and clinical acceptance, summed up, collected, and it was published the second monograph "new concept and new method of cancer metastasis therapy" in January 2006 published by the People's Medical Publishing House, Xinhua Bookstore, And in April 2007 by the People's Republic of China Press and Publication Administration issued the "three hundred" original book award.

3, the third stage (after 2006)

The focus of research for cancer was on the study of the prevention and treatment during the whole process of the cancer occurrence and development. Closely with the clinical reality and aimed for the problems and shortcomings of the current clinical traditional treatment, it was put forward reform and innovation, research and development.

Recognize the strategy of prevention and cure of cancer, the strategy must move forward, the way out of cancer treatment is in the "three early", anti-cancer out of the way is in the prevention.

The second monograph is the scientific research forward on the basis of the first monograph; the "target" of cancer treatment was located in the anti-transfer and it was pointed out that the key to cancer treatment is anti-transfer which is very correct.

But the transfer is only the final stage during the whole process of the occurrence and the development of cancer which is only a local problem, and can not reduce the incidence of cancer and may reduce the mortality rate.

After 2006, we realized that the goal of cancer treatment is necessary to treat severe patients with advanced metastases, but the effect is poor. The more treatment and the more the new patients; once diagnosed,that is the late, the effect is not good; in order to overcome cancer, it must do the "three early", it must be prevented in order to reduce the incidence of cancer and cancer mortality.

Cancer treatment of the way-out is in the "three early" and we must strengthen the "three early" research.

Cancer incidence and development experience the susceptible stage - precancerous lesions - invasive stage, in the tumor hospital of the province or the major hospitals of the tumor or cancer center cancer in the current China the treatment is mainly concentrated in the middle and late stages and the treatment effect is poor. In the late patients, if it can be surgery, it will have the surgical treatment; if it can not be done by surgery, it can only estimate the treatment.

Therefore, the path of cancer treatment should be in the "three early", early detection, early diagnosis, early treatment.

In the early patients the effects of the general treatment are better and it is to improve the treatment effect, it is necessary to reduce the mortality rate of cancer.

Therefore, we must pay attention to the study of early diagnosis methods and treatment methods, but also must pay attention to the treatment of precancerous lesions to reduce the invasion stage of the middle and late patients.

If we can treat cancer in the precancerous lesions or early stage, the cancer treatment is very good, then the progress into the invasion, metastasis, the late patients will be reduced, it can reduce the incidence of cancer.

Therefore, we believe that the current tumor hospital or oncology are mainly in the treatment of patients with advanced, even if the treatment results are good, can only reduce the mortality rate, while ignoring the susceptible stage and the precancerous lesions and the early patients, it is impossible to reduce cancer. So we think we must pay attention to the prevention and treatment of cancer during the whole process of the ccurrence and development of cancer and is a strategic concept of the overall, we must update thinking, change the concept.

I have been engaged in tumor surgery for 59 years, the more treatment and the more patients, the incidence of cancer is also rising, so I deeply appreciate that cancer should not only pay attention to treatment, but also to pay attention to prevention, in order to stop at the source. Therefore, I deeply appreciate the way out of cancer treatment in the "three early", we must strengthen the "three early" (early detection, early diagnosis, early treatment) research, anti-cancer approach lies in prevention, we must strengthen the preventive measures.

As mentioned above, the tumor prevention and treatment strategy center of gravity forward, its meaning has two aspects, one to change the way of life, improve environmental pollution and other preventive measures, the other for the treatment of precancerous lesions, to prevent its development to the invasion or Late.

The way out of cancer is to prevent the need to strengthen the preventive measures of the study.

Cancer has become the world's largest public health problem, compared with other chronic diseases, cancer prevention and control will face greater challenges.

Over the past 30 years, China's cancer mortality rate has risen significantly, has become the first cause of death of urban and rural residents, the average of every four deaths in one died of cancer.

Cancer is not only a serious threat to human health, but also an important factor in rising medical costs. China's annual direct use of cancer treatment costs nearly 100 billion yuan. So that patients and the whole society to bear a huge financial burden. Many patients spent tens of thousands or even hundreds of thousands, nor the corresponding effect, the results of human and two empty, cancer mortality rate is still the first, how should i do? Worthy of our clinician analysis, reflection, should be studied. How is the road to study? Be sure to understand the current problems in the treatment.

Although countries spend a lot of money on the treatment of cancer patients, but the past 20 years, some of the common 5-year survival of cancer has not improved significantly.

How to do? The way out of cancer is prevention, prevention and intervention is the most important in the field of public health.

In recent years recognized that more than 90% of the cancer is caused by environmental factors, the protection and recovery of a good environment, is an important part of the prevention of cancer. 1/3 of the cancer can be prevented.

The environment and the relationship between cancer, very close, environmental pollution, can cause a variety of carcinogenic substances into the human body or a variety of carcinogenic factors affect the human body. How to prove the relationship between environmental pollution and cancer, history, there are many examples confirmed.

Environmental pollution in the air pollution, can increase the incidence of lung cancer. Industrial developed countries, power generation, steel, automobile, aircraft, fuel, energy, a large number of soot and other harmful gases into the atmosphere, polluting the air, leading to lung cancer morbidity and mortality is increasing.

Environmental pollution in the water pollution and cancer, water pollution is mainly caused by industrial and agricultural production and urban sewage. Water pollution can induce or induce cancer.

Chemical pollution in environmental pollution, and the incidence of cancer is also closely related to human cancer more than 90% and environmental factors, which is mainly chemical factors.

Research on the source of environmental pollution carcinogens and how to eliminate this pollution is a very important issue in the prevention of cancer, the prevention of cancer must be pollution prevention and treatment.

I think the energy-saving emission reduction, pollution prevention and treatment of cancer is the I-level prevention, the occurrence of cancer resistance at the source. And that this is to help "overcome cancer" a good time, I am convinced that building a well-off society will be at the same time to achieve anti-cancer, cancer control and get a good effect, so that people are healthy, away from cancer.

In order to overcome the cancer for cancer prevention, cancer research, must carry out anti-cancer metastasis, recurrence of the basic and clinical research, multi-disciplinary collaboration joint research, it is necessary to set up Wuhan anti-cancer research.

After the approval of Qiu Fazu academician, Xu Ze, Li Huqiao and other professors declared preparation which was approved by the higher authorities of Wuhan City. In June 21, 2009 it had established a Wuhan anti-cancer research associate and then set up a cancer metastasis and relapse treatment professional Committee. It was formed a cancer transfer academic research team, academic research, academic research discussion, academic propaganda, academic workshops or academic seminars for our province, the city which have trained a number of young people in the anti-cancer metastasis and treatment to become the senior personnel.

Cancer research goal: foothold is "research", under the guidance of the scientific concept of development, with the development of the eyes, the spirit of innovation, eyes forward, facing the future, the development of medicine, anti-cancer, cancer control, the occurrence and development of cancer, the mechanism of cancer metastasis and recurrence and prevention and treatment. The research route is to find the problem → ask questions → research questions → solve the problem or explain the problem in order to help overcome cancer.

Wuhan Anti-Cancer Research Association combined with Wuhan city circle 8 + 1 hospitals set up Wuhan city circle 8 +1 anti-cancer alliance for cancer prevention and anticancer academic research meeting and academic exchange.

Wuhan Anti-Cancer Research Association in December 2009 visited the United States Houston Houston Stirling Cancer Institute for academic exchanges, and presented the second monograph "new concepts and new methods of cancer metastasis therapy" and "cancer metastasis experimental research book."

By 2010, we compiled a lot of research and clinical research data, summed up, brought together and it was published the third monograph "cancer treatment of new concepts and new methods", in October 2011 published by the People's Medical Publishing House, Xinhua Bookstore.

The third monograph "new concept and new method of cancer treatment" is a new concept, innovative content, both experimental research basis and clinically the proven "new concept of cancer therapies", it was put forward a series of cancer treatment Reform and innovation.

Fourth, adhere to the Chinese characteristics of building a moderately prosperous society, at the same time to carry out anti-cancer and cancer prevention new path

Through great efforts China's energy-saving emission reduction, pollution prevention and control, and building a moderately prosperous society will also be achieved to reduce the incidence of cancer great results at the same time. This is the characteristics of the socialism country of cancer prevention and control of cancer, which is building anti-cancer and cancer prevention new path of a well-off society in China; after 3-5 years of obtaining the experience of successful work, the prevention of cancer and cancer control innovation path with the Chinese characteristics of building a moderately prosperous society combined with prevention and control of cancer in the province and the city can be introduced and pushed to the country, to the world.

Why is it to prevent cancer and to control cancer in here? Because more than 90% of the cancer are related to environmental pollution; to improve the environmental pollution can have the role of preventing and controlling cancer. Control of pollution may prevent or control carcinogens into the human body. Both the improvement of the big environment and the small environment can reduce, prevent or control the environmental carcinogens into the human body or environmental carcinogens effects on the human body.

The current is to carry out energy-saving emission reduction of the excellent situation, it is engaged in "ride research" to carry out anti-cancer, cancer prevention research work a great opportunity, is a golden opportunity. In the past also recognized that anti-cancer is important, but only on paper, for popular science propaganda. Now in the construction of a well-off society under the specific practice, anti-cancer, cancer control can be a great time, can be achieved year by year to reduce the province, the city's cancer incidence. Anti-cancer, cancer control everyone is responsible, medical workers should be aware of their heavy responsibility. In this excellent situation, make the best use of the situation, do a good job of anti-cancer work, improve people's awareness of cancer, change some living habits, improve some living environment, environment-friendly, harmonious life, people will be healthy, happy, longevity, away from cancer.

In order to do this work, we have created the Wuhan Anti-Cancer Research Association, and the formation of the anti-cancer metastasis, relapse professional committee, organize more experts, scholars and people with lofty ideals for cancer prevention and control of medical science research work, Will make every effort to develop the work of the country and the people.

Therefore, in doing a good job of energy-saving emission reduction, pollution prevention and pollution, building a moderately society at the same time, I made the following recommendations: "ride research" to carry out "cancer prevention and control research, develop cancer planning and measures" (see Annex 2), To improve environmental pollution, eliminate or avoid some environmental carcinogenic risk factors, strengthen cancer prevention science publicity and education, popularize cancer prevention knowledge, establish a sound monitoring system, monitoring high-risk groups, government-led, experts, scholars, The whole people to raise awareness of cancer. I am convinced that will be environmentally friendly and reduce the incidence of cancer in Wuhan city of the double harvest of the great achievements.

Energy saving and emission reduction

pollution prevention and control

Well-off society, away from cancer

Anti-cancer and control cancer, conquer cancer

Power and work in the contemporary

Benefits in the future

How to build a well - off society, how to conduct the specific measures, principles, policies, procedures, and programs of building a well - off society in the fight against cancer? Government guidance is the key. The implementation of personnel training is also the key.

People must have modern life science knowledge; must have the modern scientific knowledge and technology of cancer occurrence and development of the whole process of prevention and treatment ; must have anti-cancer, the knowledge and technology of the cancer prevention ; must also have environmental science knowledge and technology. At present, universities have environmental colleges and life sciences, but we need modern high-tech and high-level talents with life science knowledge and skills, environmental science knowledge and skills to make anti-cancer, anti-cancer, anti-pollution, pollution control and science and technology Innovative experimental research into the colleges and universities laboratory, practical ability of experimental talents, so that China's tertiary institutions to establish a vigorous laboratory.

Therefore, in order to build a well-off society at the same time, "riding research" to overcome cancer, the modern high-tech talent training is the key, we must set up these modern high-tech secondary schools. Wuhan Anti-Cancer Research Association will apply for building the modern high-tech life science secondary school and modern high-tech environmental science secondary school, for the preparation talents for construction of well-off society and overcoming the cancer, and for the scientific innovation for the establishment of high-tech laboratories to develop high-tech experimental talents.

I deeply understand the building of a well-off society at the same time it is put forward a "ride research"; while building a new well-off society at the same time, anti-cancer and cancer prevention can be proceeded; it may become the new breakthrough of building the well-off society, but also for the construction of national central city added innovation Wuhan, innovation Hubei, Innovation of China's new content.

Seven, a number of suggestions of the construction of the personnel training, laboratory construction and the results transformation of the innovative countries on scientific and technological innovation

First, the construction of innovative countries should be thriving scientific and technological innovation

National Science and Technology Innovation Conference deepens the reform of science and technology system in 2020 to enter the ranks of an innovative country, its goal is for key areas of scientific research to achieve a major breakthrough; strategic high-tech areas to achieve leapfrog development; a number of areas of innovation into the world; Scientific quality generally improved, into the ranks of innovative countries.

How to build an innovative country? Innovative countries should not only prosper their own innovation, but also prosper the original innovation, it is not only catch the international advanced level, but also the international leading level.

What is independent innovation? Independent innovation is some people's products and we have to, do not rely on other people design, but our own design and a product. Independent innovation is their own design and is better than others, but also superior to competitive.

What is the original innovation? The original innovation is not someone else, or the world is not, is my unique invention of the plan, not to learn other people, but to others to come here to learn.

Innovation is not just product innovation, but should be the basis of theoretical innovation, theoretical innovation is the biggest achievement. Scientific development is based on the basic theory of innovation, this is the largest invention and creation, discover new theories, new laws, such as: Einstein's theory of relativity, Newton's law.

The establishment of scientific and technological innovation countries, we must prosper the achievements of scientific and technological innovation, not only the results of independent innovation, but also must have the original innovation results.

How can there be scientific and technological achievements?

Talent personnel is the key.

The standard of talent personnel must be genuine talent and practical, both ability and political integrity.

Whether it Is not really talented or not must be able to achieve scientific research results and technological innovation achievements.

How can there be innovative results?

Construction of the corresponding equipment laboratory is the key, with a good laboratory, there is the basic conditions for research, through experimental research, in order to produce the innovation achievement.

How can there be innovative results?

Cultivate talent is not the ultimate goal.

Construction of laboratories is not the ultimate goal.

The ultimate goal is to obtain innovative scientific research results and scientific research achievement, the ultimate goal of all scientific research is to obtain scientific research achievement.

It is to the results of the hero, to contribute to the results, to the academic level of achievement.

With the original innovation, it is more than the international level; the original innovation results must be confirmed by the new agency.

How can there be technology innovation?

First of all, it is to cultivate scientific thinking and scientific mind, to have academic atmosphere, and ask for some things why? At first, it is to ask questions, study the problem, and then solve the problem. It is to think more Why and to ask why? How to do? How to do it? What to do? In order to have a scientific and innovative atmosphere, it should be trained from young people.

Teachers at all levels should have scientific thinking, academic atmosphere, in order to train students to ask why? The teacher is the soul of the human engineer, to improve the quality of teaching, we must first improve the level and quality of teachers, we must first improve the academic team of academic atmosphere, scientific and technological innovation thinking and academic level. If the teacher did not have enough knowledge, he or she did not dare to ask students why.

Second, how can there be technology innovation? Talent personnel is the key.

How does talent come from, how to cultivate talent?

1, sent to study abroad, study abroad (students, visiting scholars) ; after the return students should participate in scientific and technological innovation, ; the person who is sent to other countries to learn should be brought back to the task of scientific and technological knowledge; after returning to the countries the person should have the results and contribution and produce out of talent.

2, to invite the talent personnel to come in, recruit domestic and foreign top scientific and technological personnel, to preside over scientific and technological innovation. How can the talent play my talents? How to apply?

① should have a better laboratory, to lead a group of people out of scientific and technological innovation. ② should be used to train personnel, cultivate a batch of China's own scientific and technological personnel, because please come in, when or will go, should be used for talent incubation, to help China to cultivate scientific and technological personnel. Even if it produces the talent, the results should be produced.

3, self-reliance, their own training. To be the original innovation of science and technology achievements, must their own country to develop their own scientific and technological personnel.

Now China is the world's second largest economy, how to continue to develop, how to continue forward, leap-forward development, catch up with the world's largest economy, you must self-reliance, their own training personnel.

The development of modern high-tech, should encourage the opening up of new research areas, can not always follow the people run behind People running inner circle, I ran the outer ring: people ran outside the outer ring, I ran in the circle, to go beyond the first. Otherwise run the same lap, people ran in front, blocked, and you can easily go beyond the front. So we can not run on the same lap followed by people running (I chose to study the subject of the past). Therefore, we have to catch up with the world's largest economy, personnel training can not rely on foreign study abroad, visiting scholars to train talent, should rely on our own training of personnel, we should rely on our own new technology, open up new areas of research, New industries, relying on our own talent training.

How to cultivate their own talent? The first of all it is to develop their own talent incubator.

To order to innovate the new technology, in order to leapfrog development, in order to go to the world's largest economy, to cultivate innovative talents is the key. To go beyond other countries, in order to open up new areas of research, and not to follow the study in other countries must rely on their own country to work hard, and to build up the ambition, self-reliance, self-cultivation of senior personnel, then it can keep sustainable development.

How to train talent? In the development zone a large number of talent are introduced. How to use and to play their talents? It Should be used for scientific and technological innovation, the development of science and technology, produce a result, innovate a new product, produce the amount of production, open up new business and new industries. On the other hand, the main task is to cultivate talents incubator, cultivate our high-tech talent, high-tech leading talent; not only the prosperity of China's scientific and technological innovation, but also high-tech talent.

How to train talent? I think of that traveling thousands of miles, starting from now on, from now on it should be self-reliance to cultivate modern high-tech talent plan on the agenda, organize self-reliance training modern high-tech talent institutions; the goal is to catch up with the international advanced level, toward the world's first economy body, it must be self-reliant and mainly depend on the self-cultivation of modern high-tech talent, sending to study abroad, visiting scholars supplement (because can not learn from foreign countries; because then our high-tech has gone beyond or keep pace).

Personnel training should walk on two legs:

1, one is to attract talent, recruit talent and send personnel to study abroad, visiting scholars, to be returned after participating in the construction and technological innovation, the current is an important way of personnel training, but this is only temporary, only Catch up, it is difficult to exceed.

2, the other is based on their own training personnel, the key is to build a good laboratory, in the long run, this is a permanent cure. Can not rely on foreign training and should rely on their own training. After the liberation of the early, China's medical talent are based on their own training. How to train themselves, is a large laboratory, through animal experiments, to carry out clinical research and work. To achieve scientific and technological innovation, so as to the original innovation, to go beyond.

After the liberation of the new China's medical development, from scratch, is to take this road self-reliance, by their own personnel training, pioneering work.

Such as cardiopulmonary bypass surgery

After the liberation of the early to not study abroad, visit, exchange, no foreign medical journals, publications, the late 50s of the last century, the early 60s, Xi'an, Tianjin, Shanghai, Wuhan, Nanjing, Anyang and other cities together Cardiopulmonary bypass and open heart surgery. Each group was done hundreds of dogs outside the cardiopulmonary bypass surgery in animal experiments, in animal experiments after surgery on the clinical success, Tianjin group also created a half cycle of extracorporeal circulation. I participated in the Wuhan animal experimental group, and group to Tianjin, Nanjing, Anyang to visit the study of animal experiments. China's cardiopulmonary bypass heart surgery is to rely on the dog through the animal experiments to explore their own experience to cultivate talent started.

Another example is liver transplantation

In the late 1970s, the United States has not established diplomatic relations, not to study, visit, exchange, no foreign medical journals, journals, Shanghai Ruijin Hospital Dong Fangzhong, Lin Yanzhen, Wuhan Tongji Hospital Qiu Fazu, Xia Suisheng established liver transplantation animal laboratory, Were carried out at the same time a few hundred dogs were liver transplanted animal experiments, both through the animal experiments after the clinical. Shanghai and Wuhan, the two groups of liver transplantation were carried out after the success of animal experiments carried out clinical liver transplantation. The In the 1980s, the animal experiments and clinical validation of Shanghai and Wuhan were all the same, and the survival rate of the patients was 3 days earlier than that of the Shanghai group., The Ministry of Health will focus on liver transplantation in Wuhan, the establishment of organ transplantation Institute, when I was the leader of liver transplantation identification experts, witnessed the liver transplantation in China is also through the dog's animal experiments to explore their own experience to cultivate talent started The

Based on their own training personnel, the key is to build a good equipment laboratory. I am deeply aware of the importance of the laboratory, I was the first batch of college students after the liberation of college students, I did not study, did not study, but I made a number of international level results, the key is that I have a good laboratory, I participated in the era of extracorporeal circulation animal laboratory, 80 years I established a cirrhosis of the liver laboratory, the early 90s I established the Institute of Experimental Surgery, to capture the main direction of cancer, my animal laboratory, equipment conditions are better Mice, rats, rabbits, rabbits, dogs, monkeys and other animal experiments, a better animal aseptic operating room, can be a dog's chest, abdomen, a variety of major surgery, and animal observation after the ward, Design, design, through the experimental operation, to achieve results or conclusions.

Therefore, the laboratory is a key condition, if there is no laboratory through the experiment, can only design, imagine, can not become a factual result.

Experimental surgery is extremely important in the development of medicine, it is a key to open the medical closed area, many disease prevention and control methods are after several animal experimental research, achieved a stable effect was applied to clinical and promote the development of medical career.

Therefore, the development of science, science and technology innovation, the laboratory is the key condition. Self-reliance, their own training of innovative talents, the laboratory is a key condition.

Third, how to train their own talent should establish a personnel training mechanism and personnel training institutions

It should meet the 21st century modern high-tech personnel training mechanism requirements and content:

1, should keep up with the development of modern high - tech;

2, should keep up with innovative countries and international metropolis needs of modern high-tech talent.

At present we have been in the 21st century, the first two years, how to understand and understand the concept of modern high-tech and content? Throughout the 20th century, human beings have recognized the discovery and application of thermonuclear reactions: the birth and popularization of computers; the establishment and development of molecular biology, is a major scientific research.

The scientific community predicts that the 21st century leadership science will be the life sciences with molecular biology as the core; computer-centric information science and environmental science.

Modern high technology will lead the new research field, new industry, new discipline. Modern high-tech innovation will lead the future, across the development.

Pedagogy should keep up with the development of the times. The specialties of running a school should serve the modern high-tech talents needed to build an innovation-oriented country and an international metropolis.

Since it is an innovative country, should strive to walk in the forefront of the world, the international competition should strive for the international advanced level or international advanced level. Since it is an international metropolis, it is necessary to strive to achieve international standards, including talent, technology, technological innovation, culture, humanistic quality, knowledge, construction, transportation and so on.

First clear a few concepts:

Science and technology refers to science and technology, from a more stringent sense, science and technology belong to two different categories, the original meaning of science refers to the human understanding of the natural law of the theoretical expression, and technology is the means of human transformation of the world. Scientific development has become the main foundation of technological development. Generally speaking, the majority of the people through scientific and technological achievements for the understanding of science, scientific development and technological progress through technological achievements and people's daily life contact.

The characteristics of modern scientific research:

"Theoretical science" refers to a comprehensive study of the basic concepts of science, basic principles and basic laws of science, and the application of science has a guiding role, and the application of scientific development, in turn, deepen and enrich the theoretical science. Sometimes also refers to the general basic science, "applied science" is the "theoretical science" relative to the concept, refers directly to the production or other social practice of science. It includes application theory and application technology. Applied science is sometimes referred to as technical science and engineering science, which is directly related to the speed of development of the national economy.

"Technology" includes two meanings: a variety of methods of operation developed in accordance with the principles of natural science, such as electrical technology, welding technology, laser technology, crop cultivation techniques, breeding techniques and production processes or operating procedures.

Building an innovative country, should be the prosperity of scientific and technological innovation, today are aware of the development of science and technology and basic research is sufficient to represent a country's comprehensive national strength, in other words, can also represent the national central city of comprehensive strength.

At present, some colleges and universities in our province and city have the College of Life Sciences. The School of Information Science of the School of Environmental Sciences focuses on theoretical science, applied science and basic science.

Technical level is more technical secondary schools and vocational schools, in fact, the technical level is very important, modern Hi-Tech technology is developing rapidly, with each passing day, but the current secondary school technical schools in China remained in the 20th century a single discipline, equipment obsolete, weak teachers, Should be taken seriously. The current teaching content can not keep up with the development of the times. The technical facilities and teaching contents of the technical college must keep up with the rapid development of modern high-tech technology. The technical colleges are mainly "applied science" and "technology", namely, technical science and engineering science and various kinds of scientific and technological principles developed according to these scientific principles. Operation methods and production process or operating procedures, it is directly related to the speed of development of the national economy, modern high-tech personnel level and quality level is also directly related to the sustainable development of China's science and technology product quality.

Such as aerospace industry, God nine off, the depth of the sail into the sea, high-speed rail … … are required modern high-tech skilled operation of the technology, workers, technicians, engineers, one by one, one minute, must be accurate.

The construction of innovative countries to become scientific and technological innovation center, we must attach importance to tertiary institutions, both ordinary secondary schools and secondary science colleges and universities, scientific and technological innovation thinking should be trained from young people, modern high-tech skilled skilled workers, technicians are the development of modern high One of the main technology. Therefore, the teaching content of Chinese intermediate science colleges and universities, teachers must learn to keep up with the development of modern science and technology innovation center, universities, scientific research institutions and large enterprises in the modern era (the 1920s) 21st century modern Gaoke technical personnel, laboratory personnel.

21st century modern high-tech knowledge, summarized as three aspects: life science and technology knowledge; environmental science and technology knowledge; information science and technology knowledge.

The current educational content can not keep up with the development of the times. For the development of modern high-tech disciplines, must have a good laboratory, but the current shortage of laboratory personnel, the status quo is a lot of doctors j nurse, will catch the mouse to do very little talent. Not the lack of college graduates, graduate students, but the lack of laboratory experiments of modern high-tech junior specialist talent. Construction of innovative countries to build science and technology innovation center, we must vigorously build a good laboratory, the construction of laboratories must first train the laboratory personnel. Scientific research personnel must be trained from young people, since ancient times heroes out of juvenile.

Therefore, the proposal: the establishment of the 21st century modern high profits. Technical experimental intermediate talent institutions, that the construction of laboratories to provide talent.

1, the founder of modern high-tech life science and technology college (secondary, three-year system)

Foster the establishment of laboratory personnel for tertiary institutions

Modern life science and technology is progressing rapidly, genetic engineering, molecular biology, cell inheritance, rapid development.

2, the founder of modern high-tech environmental science and technology school (secondary school, three years), environmental science has attracted global attention, it will be emerging disciplines, new industries, the current energy-saving emission reduction, pollution control, Two kinds of society ", must carry out a large number of research projects, to use modern high science and technology for pollution prevention and control, ecological balance, food hygiene supervision … … to cultivate a large number of environmental science and modern high-tech middle-level talent.

More than 90% of the cancer are caused by environmental factors or closely related, therefore, the current energy-saving emission reduction, pollution prevention and pollution, to create a "two-oriented society", in fact, anti-cancer, anti-cancer a preventive measures. Hoping to get government support for the construction of "two-oriented society" to cultivate a large number of environmental science intermediate professionals.

3, founded the modern high-tech information science and technology college (secondary, three-year system)

To enrich the construction of the corresponding university, college laboratory.

Information specialist technical quality and quantity, can represent a country's competitiveness and creativity.

Fourth, how can there be technology innovation? A good laboratory is the key

With talent, it does not mean that there is fruit. With talent, it does not mean you can prosper the scientific and technological innovation. Because, heroes have the places to use and to apply the skills; scientific research design and scientific research ideas must be through laboratory experiment research in order to draw conclusions and to produce the results.

Therefore, scientific and technological innovation must have a good laboratory, the laboratory is the key. If there is no good laboratory, although there are talent personnels, there are topics, there are projects, even if you get hundreds of thousands of dollars, if there is not the experiment, it can only be fantasy, empty talk, cannot have a result.

To turn scientific research design into scientific research results must have a good laboratory.

To compare China's universities with Europe and the United States, the gap between is not the size of the school and the number of teachers and students, the main gap is the lack of high-tech laboratories.

Although the universities in China are equipped with teaching and research group, that is, teaching and research, but many teaching and research groups do not have a laboratory, teachers can not carry out experimental research, it can not have a result and a master.

Science - is the endless frontier, the rapid development of modern high-tech, with each passing day, the quality of university teachers and teaching quality must also keep up with modern high-tech development, advancing with the times.

University teachers should have a dual task on the shoulders, one is to improve teaching; the second is the development of science.

University teachers should have a good laboratory for scientific research, follow the scientific concept of development, based on the known science, to explore the unknown science, for the future science, emerging disciplines, border disciplines, interdisciplinary, scientific frontier, innovation, Science hall, brick tiles.

Therefore, how can China's universities meet international standards? We should vigorously develop well - established laboratories.

How to fight for our university into the top 500, 200 strong? We should vigorously develop well - established laboratories.

How to build an innovative country? It should build a good laboratory.

How can scientific innovation out of the original innovation? It should build a good laboratory.

How can we open up new research areas? It should build a good laboratory.

How can basic research be carried out? It should establish a good laboratory.

How can we fight cancer? It should establish a good laboratory.

US technology booms, high-tech is developed, the main reason have the more laboratory and the equipment conditions are good; it is paid attention to the science and technology experiments, and attention to the laboratory. China sends a large number of students each year, visiting scholars to the United States to study abroad, graduate students, as visiting scholars, are basically working and studying in the laboratory. The main gap between China University and the United States and Britain and other countries of the University is universities modern high-tech laboratory in the United States and Britain and other with the excellent equipments, teaching and research groups are basically work, research, train graduate students, and guide students in the laboratory so that professors can be innovative results, open up new areas of research, produce a talent and produce a master of science.

Massachusetts Institute of Technology, the scale is small, the number of teachers and students only a few thousand people, but the school had 38 Nobel Prize winners, won a total of 39 Nobel Prize in Science, one of them won twice of Nobel Prize Award. It was ranking the highest in the world famous universities because the school has many modern high-tech high-level laboratories, laboratory talent, there are many academic masters, pioneered a number of cutting-edge research areas, strict style of study, rigorous and rigorous.

Therefore, it can be seen that the importance of modern high-tech laboratories in scientific and technological innovation; the importance of laboratories in achieving scientific research; the importance of laboratories in the development of science.

Laboratory is the incubator of scientific research results; laboratory is the training of personnel incubator.

In order to have scientific and technological achievements, it must has a good laboratory talent The talents can have a place to be useful and the heroes can play the skills, then the talent can be produced, therefore, the base of the development of science, prosperity and technological innovation, and the prosperity of scientific and technological achievements is the laboratory.

Many colleges and universities in our country, subordinates, provincial universities are equipped with many teaching and research group, but also cultivate a large number of graduate students, but some teaching and research group without a laboratory or laboratory. Strictly should only be called teaching group, teaching and not research. University teaching and research group without a laboratory or laboratory, how to study it? Recruit a large number of graduate students, how to train and guide graduate students for the experiment, for research? Teaching and research group without a laboratory or laboratory, professors can only prepare lessons, lectures, can not do experimental or research topics. University professors should not only talk about the knowledge of the textbooks, but also should talk about today's new progress, the development of new trends, new achievements and unknown knowledge. Teachers do not have a laboratory or laboratory, can not carry out research and research results. They have no place to do experiments, how to guide graduate students to do experiments?

Now a mentor, may recruit a few graduate students, to guide students how to choose topics, how to design, how to experiment, research process to obtain results or conclusions. But there are a lot of tutor of the teaching and research group without a laboratory, there is no research room, how to guide the experimental operation of graduate students? It is reasonable to say that a mentor should have a good laboratory, it may guide a good graduate students to conduct scientific research, writing papers, the development of science.

Development of science, scientific and technological innovation, the laboratory is the key condition.

It should vigorously build laboratories, and more training of high-tech talent, more innovative results.

It is therefore recommended that:

1, subordinate institutions of higher learning should have 1-3 state-level key laboratories

2, provincial institutions of higher learning should have 1-3 provincial key laboratories

3, municipal institutions of higher learning should have 1-3 municipal key laboratories

Laboratory rating, according to the talent, the level of results:

- State-level key laboratories, should be the leading international or international advanced level of results, scientific research leadership, scientific master, the results must be identified will be rated, the original results must be verified at the provincial level to verify the higher authorities acceptance.
- Three years can not be achieved at the international level, the level should be reduced, after the corresponding results to be restored.
- Provincial key laboratories, should be the leading domestic or domestic advanced level of scientific research, for the international advanced level of results, must identify the rating, higher authorities acceptance. Municipal laboratories are basically similar to provincial laboratories.

Since it is an innovative country, scientific and technological innovation, should be the leading international level, to be competitive and creative.

The establishment of high-tech laboratories, state-level key laboratories, should encourage the opening up of new research areas, innovative countries should establish a national high-tech laboratories, open up new areas of high-tech research center for the government to support and develop science.

Therefore, the construction of an innovative country, the construction of scientific and technological innovation center, must first vigorously build the laboratory, so that talent can make use of the product; scientific research and innovation of the land; so that people have to cultivate the land; so that graduate students have cultivated experimental areas; College professors have innovation, a result, a master of the land.

Should vigorously popularize the construction of laboratories, more scientific and technological achievements, so that the national central city into a national science and technology innovation center.

Fifth, the objectives of the scientific and technological innovation:

1, the innovative results

Should be the result, from the main innovation results, competitive, creative

And strive to out of the original innovation results, original results

Should be a product, a new industry, a new enterprise, production, learning, research combined

2, out of talent, a high-tech talent, science and technology leading talent, a master of science

Talent should be both ability and political integrity, medicine is benevolence, legislation for the first

Talent should be true to learn, should be fruitful, successful, innovative and superb technology

3, the importance of basic research, basic research leads to new knowledge, it provides scientific capital, it creates knowledge of the reserves, new products and new process is not a emergence is completely mature, they are built on the new Principles and new ideas, and these new principles and new ideas are in the scientific research work hard to develop.

The development of science is based on the basic theory of innovation, this is the greatest scientific achievement. Find new theories, new laws, new doctrines, new laws, is the greatest innovation.

Scientific progress depends on the emergence of new scientific knowledge, which can only be obtained through basic research.

Fundamental research in medical science is very important to progress in the fight against cancer. If there is no breakthrough in basic research, the clinical efficacy is difficult to improve.

The government should encourage the development of new areas of research, the fight against cancer, the development of new products, new industries, the realization of these tasks from the basic scientific research.

I deeply understand the importance of basic research: in 1985, I will do more than 3,000 cases of chest, general cancer patients after radical surgery to carry out a petition. The results showed that most of the patients were postoperative 2-3 years recurrence, metastasis, and some even after a few months after the transfer occurred. This makes me realize that although the operation is successful, but the long-term efficacy is not satisfactory, postoperative recurrence, metastasis is the key to long-term effect of postoperative. Therefore, we must carry out basic research, so we established the Institute of Experimental Surgery, and from the following three aspects spent 24 years to carry out a series of experimental research basic research and clinical validation work: ① explore the incidence of cancer, invasion and recurrence, The transfer mechanism, and the search for effective research and control of recurrence, transfer of effective research; ② from the natural medicine to find a new anti-cancer, anti-metastasis, pit recurrence of new drug research; ③ clinical validation work.

We conducted a four-year study in the laboratory for cancer incidence, invasion and recurrence, metastasis mechanism of the basic experimental study, and after 3 years from the natural drug screening experimental study to find a group of XZ-C1-10 immunoregulation resistance Cancer therapy, and then through 16 years in more than 12,000 cases of patients with advanced or postoperative metastatic cancer clinical validation; application of XZ-c immunomodulation anti-cancer traditional Chinese medicine, and achieved good results, can improve the quality of life of patients, improve patient symptoms, Patient survival.

After the above experimental study of basic research, from experimental to clinical, but also from clinical to experimental.

Experimental research and clinical validation data summary, and rise to theoretical sublimation, put forward new discoveries.

New understanding of the new theory: (1) the cause of cancer, one of the pathogenesis of thymus atrophy, thymic dysfunction, immune dysfunction; (2) proposed XZ-c immunomodulation therapy a chest lift The theoretical basis and experimental basis; (3) mention

(4) to promote cancer treatment of multidisciplinary comprehensive treatment of new models: the whole treatment to radical surgery, supplemented by biological immunity, traditional Chinese medicine, XZ-C immunoregulation, differentiation of cancer, treatment of cancer treatment should be updated ideas, change the concept, the establishment of a comprehensive treatment concept; Induced mainly. (5) the evaluation and challenge of systemic intravenous chemotherapy for solid cancer; (6) the initiative to reform, the physical cancer should be reformed as the target organ intravascular chemotherapy; (5) (9) 10 years has published three monographs: ① "new understanding of cancer treatment and new model" published in Hubei Science and Technology in 2001; ② "new concept of cancer metastasis therapy (1)

new concept of cancer treatment, new models, new methods; And the new method "published in 2006 by the People's Medical Publishing House, in April 2007 by the People's Republic of China Publishing Department" three hundred "original published engineering certificate; ⑨ "new concept of cancer treatment and new methods" in October 2011 people Military Medical Publishing House. Followed by American physician Dr. Bin Wu translated into English. The English version was published in Washington on March 26, 2013 and was issued internationally.

In summary, the experimental study, basic research is very important, if no experimental research, basic research breakthrough, the clinical efficacy is difficult to improve, it is difficult to put forward new ideas, new concepts, new theoretical insights. Which is the key laboratory, I have a good laboratory, I was director of the Institute of Experimental Surgery, but also clinical director of surgery, experimental research, basic research and clinical validation easy to take into account.

Sixth, the scientific and technological innovation, the results of timely development is the key. Scientific and technological innovation results should be timely transformation, development, and application so that people benefit from them.

One of the aims of scientific and technological innovation is to make innovative achievements, with the *results, should be identified acceptance, through the results of the appraisal or outcome of the Council* will be the results of identification, the results of the level of acceptance, the original innovation, should be verified.

Project is not equal to the results –

Currently, some of the university promotion, raising the duty, and graduate students recruit attach importance to the project. This is supposed to be, but this understanding is not enough because the project is not equal to the results. With the project it does not necessarily achieve results, only when the project has achieved results, only on behalf of academic level, scientific research. It should not be on the project on the hero, but should be the results of academic level, scientific research, scientific research contribution.

At present, some colleges and universities scientific research department only pay attention to scientific research projects, funding, do not attach importance to the acceptance of scientific research, there are many projects have not achieved scientific research results, hastily ended. The country put a lot of research funding each year in tertiary institutions, research institutes must be very cherished, be sure to obtain the corresponding results, should be strictly enforced, due to pay results, scientific research results identification, acceptance, So that the results of scientific research and acceptance of results, so that the work of scientific research work vigorously, every year innovation, fruitful.

Research Office should pay attention to the acceptance of scientific research, particle sweeping warehouse.

How to evaluate scientific research results? There should be scientific research results certificate or certificate; should have scientific research results or scientific and technological research results report; should have the above project scientific research or research papers at home and abroad academic exchange and academic influence at home and abroad; or research papers published in the magazine, Or published research monographs.

Scientific research results should be timely transformation and development

What about research results? It must be transformed and developed to be practical so that people can get benefit from it and the community can get benefit, should not be tied "high", should not be locked in the "purdah", should be timely transformation and development.

After identification or evaluation of scientific research, not the bundle of "high", or locked in the "purdah" should go down the cabinet, out of purdah, for transformation, development, application. Produce social and economic benefits, to serve the community.

How is the transformation of scientific and technological achievements? Over the years, this has been a big problem. In the country this is an unresolved big problem. But it is a problem that must be studied and discussed about the solution.

If not timely transformation, development, application, and people getting benefit, the scientific and technological innovation results are great waste.

To built an innovative country and to format a scientific and technological innovation center is bound to scientific and technological achievements, like springing up, thriving, scientific research will be numerous, harvest year after year.

How can these scientific and technological achievements be harvested? Is it "stacking" Is the bundle of "high"? Is locked in "purdah"? How to do? It should be timely transformation, development, application, so that the community gets benefit, the people gets benefit, the development of science, social progress, people's happiness.

Innovative countries, the prosperity of scientific and technological innovation, scientific research results, how to transform, how to develop, and how to apply, it becomes the key.

For the achievement transformation, development is the key. This issue must be put on the agenda in a timely manner, the establishment of the results of the transformation mechanism, the establishment of results transformation agencies, so that the results play a role in generating social and economic benefits.

The current status quo, many of our tertiary institutions have the hands of scientific research results or quasi-results, I have a series of results, no intermediaries, no brokers, no matchmaking, I do not know how to attract foreign investment, no scientific research, The development of mechanisms and institutions, I do not know what level of government to request guidance and support. Scientists, scientific research staff can not use the results, no one cares, the bundle of "high"; entrepreneurs want results, can not find, not. This is the current prominent of a pair of social contradictions.

How to do I would like to make a suggestion:

Government-led, matchmaking,

Government - led, investment

Talent market recruitment, scientific research should also be the results of the promotion, the results of the exhibition, the results introduced, investment.

Government-led, the establishment of scientific research achievements, the development of the working committee, under the results of the transformation of the work center and the transformation of the work of the Office, the establishment of the transformation mechanism and the transformation of work agencies, Chamber of Commerce for the promotion of products, the results will be the results of the promotion.

In short:

How to build an innovative country, national science and technology innovation center?

I think that the talent personnel and the laboratory are the key; with the results of innovation, the results of transformation and development are the key.

Talent ----a laboratory----a scientific and technological innovation results -----the transformation and development of the results

1, the talent personnel must be genuine talent, practical, and must be both ability and political integrity. How to evaluate and confirm the genuine talent? It must have access to scientific research, or have academic achievements. I am a senior doctor and have been a physician for 55 year and am a senior professor, so I think of medical ethics should be: medicine is benevolence, legislation is for the first.

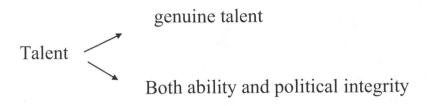

Scientific research leader must preside over the national research and international advanced level or the leading domestic level above the scientific research, and more mature scientific research experience.

2, the laboratory is the incubator of technological innovation results. Laboratory is the incubator of scientific research personnel training.

No laboratory can not be scientific and technological innovation fruit, no laboratory is difficult to science and technology talent. No equipment, excellent laboratory, it can not appear on behalf of high-tech innovation, scientific master Yang Zhenning, Ding Zhaozhong are through the equipment of excellent laboratory and won the Nobel Prize in Physics.

3, with the results of scientific and technological innovation, timely transformation, development and application is the key.

Innovative countries, built a scientific and technological innovation center, independent innovation or the original innovation of the results, how to timely transformation, development, application, so that people benefit. How to branch, industry, trade and production, learning, research pull line, bypass the combination of further development and prosperity and innovation. Must be put on the agenda, the establishment of the results of the transformation mechanism, the establishment of results transformation agencies.

Therefore, it is suggested that the government should lead the establishment of the transformation of the scientific research achievements, the development of the work committee, the establishment of the results of the transformation of the work center and the transformation of scientific research work office, the establishment of transformation mechanisms and transformation agencies.

We should vigorously build science and technology laboratories, the gap between China's universities and Europe and the United States is mainly their high-tech laboratory, China's high-tech laboratory less.

I think how to build an innovative country, talent, laboratory is the key, scientific and technological innovation is the purpose of innovation, innovation-oriented countries should be in key areas of scientific research original breakthrough, a number of areas of innovation into the forefront of the world. How to solve the problem of combining technology with economy and the transformation and development of scientific research achievements is the key. The problem must be put on the agenda in time. It must be government-led, establish the transformation mechanism of the results, establish the transformation mechanism, transform the work office, make the scientist and entrepreneur Combined with the results of the transformation and development, so that scientific research to play a role, resulting in economic and social benefits.

The benign relationship of the talent → laboratory → results → transformation and development is shown as the below:

Figure: The relationship of Talent → Labs → Results

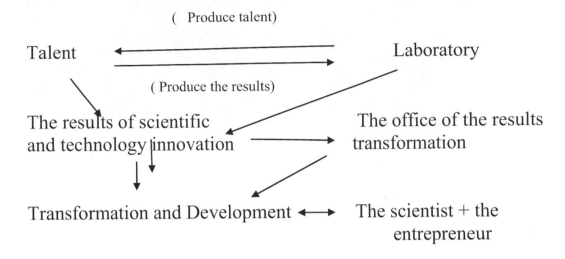

① **People Happiness**
② **The society progress**
③ **People benefit**
④ **The society benefit**

Eight, the strategic ideas and suggestions on the capture of cancer

The current cancer has become a major threat to human health, the incidence of the number of patients with an average annual rate of 3-5% increase in the incidence and death compared with 10 years ago, respectively, an increase of 24.7% and 19.2%. Three traditional treatment has been nearly a hundred years, the cancer patient mortality rate is still the first, what should be done or how do? How is the research road to go? It should be analyzed, reflected, and should be studied.

Victory over cancer, where is the road?

- Xu Ze (XU ZE) thinks of that the road is in the scientific research, the road is scientific research on the prevention and treatment of cancer; the road is the experimental basic research to explore the cause of cancer, pathogenesis, pathophysiology; road is in the study of cancer, the road is the reform and development in the traditional treatment; the road is in the multi-disciplinary research; the road is in the study of cancer metastasis and recurrence of prevention and control; the road is in the "three early" study.

Through the road in the prevention and treatment of cancer scientific research, human beings will overcome cancer, and ultimately will overcome cancer.

How to overcome the cancer I see one:

First, the road to scientific research is the experimental basic research to explore the cause of cancer, pathogenesis, pathophysiology

1, I believe that the development of cancer science research is the urgent need of the current status of tumor disciplines, we must recognize what the problems of the status of cancer disciplines are, how to do?

Although cancer treatment has been more than a century, has now entered the second decade of the 21st century, but "oncology" is still the most backward of the current medical disciplines, why? Because the etiology, pathogenesis, and pathophysiology of "oncology" are not clear. For the scientific research on ncology, it is still a virgin land, and it needs to be a lot of basic scientific research and clinical basic research. Although the application of the traditional three treatment (surgery, radiotherapy, chemotherapy) is for nearly a hundred years, tens of thousands of cancer patients undergo radiotherapy and chemotherapy, but how are the results? so far the mortality rate of cancer is still the first reason for the death of urban and rural residents in China . How should the road go? It should be in-depth reflection, in-depth analysis, in-depth study.

Why so? the main reasons are:

(1) the etiology of cancer is not clear, the pathogenesis is unclear, pathophysiology is not clear, there are a lot of basic theoretical problems which are not clear.

(2) the biological characteristics and biological behavior of cancer cells still lack sufficient understanding.

(3) the molecular mechanism of cancer cell metastasis still lacks sufficient understanding.

(4) the occurrence and development and cloning and proliferation, invasion, metastasis, planting, complex biological behavior of cancer are still lack of understanding which all are subject to conditional units for research.

The current cancer treatment program is still quite blind. Diagnosis means are behind and once the cancer is found, the cancer is already in the middle and late stage and the treatment effect is poor. Because the cause and the pathogenesis and the pathophysiology are still lack of adequate understanding and did not carry out the full experimental study of basic research, the current understanding of the tumor discipline seems still not clear enough fuzzy state or hazy state and the knowledge of the tumor is still in a very backward state.

Many large-scale tumor hospital or university affiliated hospital have not established cancer laboratory, can not carry out the basic research of cancer, nor the establishment of cancer animal laboratory, can not be carried out animal model test. Anti-cancer metastasis and recurrence must be carried out in the basic model of cancer animal model and it should be used in nude mice to establish a variety of cancer animal models to study the transfer of cancer cells and the mechanism. (My experimental surgery laboratory with the removal of mouse thymus to produce animal model 60 times, 7 years, with pure mice Kunming mice to replace the establishment of animal model of about 10,000 animals) Why pay attention to the basic research laboratory? Because, if there is no basic research breakthrough, the clinical efficacy is difficult to improve.

2, the experimental surgery is the key to open a closed area of medicine .

Experimental surgery plays a very important role in developing medical science, which is the key to open up the forbidden zone of medical science. The pathogenesis and control methods of many diseases have been achieved after countless animal experimental researches. The research results with stability can only be applied to the clinic, which promotes the progress of medicine, improves medical quality and develops new control methods.

The laboratory of experimental surgery in our college was set up in May 1980. Under the charge of Professor Xu Ze, researchers have carried out experimental researches of surgical therapy of refractory ascites caused by hepatic cirrhosis and the pathogenesis; have adopted the method of experimental surgery to explore the cause, pathogenesis and pathophysiology of pathological change of schistosomiasis japanica on lung; have studied the pathogenesis of hepatic portal vein hypertension caused by the hepatic cirrhosis of schistosomiasis japanica; have transplanted hepatic cells in the spleen to produce the second liver for treating hepatic failure. The above national-level and provincial-level scientific research items have laid a good foundation for experimental research.

In early 1987, this laboratory began to turn to the experimental tumor research. Researchers have carried out the transplantation of cancer cells, built experimental tumor animal models, explored the pathogenesis and pathophysiology of tumor, and investigated the law and mechanism of cancer cell metastases in cancer-bearing animal models and changes of the host's immune function. And then researchers have discussed Chinese herbal medicines with good anti-cancer effects, made a strict and scientific screening study of Chinese herbal medicines with anti-cancer and cancer inhibited effect in vivo of cancer-bearing animal models. In order to develop the career of cancer prevention and treatment, researchers commit themselves to the experimental researches of exploring the cause, pathogenesis and pathophysiology of cancer and further extracting Chinese herbal medicines with the effect of cancer prevention and cure.

With the practical requirement in our college's medical science situation, Institute of Experimental Surgery of Hubei College of Traditional Chinese Medicine was set up in March 1991 on the basis of experimental surgical laboratory. Professor

Xu Ze serves as director of the institute and Academician Qiu Fazu is invited as the mentor. Their research target and task are: Institute of Experimental Surgery is mainly to tackle key problems of cancer. The emphasis is to adopt the method of experimental surgery to carry out fundamental researches of experimental tumors and control researches of clinical patients. This research laboratory of experimental tumor adopts biological engineering technology and genetic engineering technology of cancer cells, exploits the fundamental research and clinical practice of tumor biological therapy and immunization therapy, develops and promotes the career of cancer prevention and treatment.

3. Our laboratory has found the following understandings from the experimental tumor research.

(1) Our laboratory has found that removal of mouse's thymus will not affect the buildup of cancer-bearing animal model and injecting immunosuppressant can also contribute to the buildup of cancer-bearing animal model. The research results indicate that there is an obvious link between the generation and growth of cancer and the host's immune organ- thymus and its function.

(2) The experiment, which explores tumor's effect on the host's immune organ, shows that with the gradual growth of cancer, thymus presents progressive atrophy. That is to say, the host's thymus presents acute progressive atrophy after inoculation of cancer cells.

(3) This experiment has also found that some experimental mice, which are inoculated unsuccessfully or have a very small tumor, do not have an obvious atrophic thymus. In order to know the relationship between tumor and atrophy of thymus, researchers resect the transplanted solid tumors in a set of experimental mice when the size of tumors equals to the size of thumb. The anatomy after one month shows that their thymus does not have a further progressive atrophy. Therefore, it can be speculated that the solid tumor may produce a kind of unknown factor to inhibit thymus. But accurate results still need the further experimental researches.

(4) The above experimental results prove that the growth of tumor can lead to the progressive atrophy of thymus. Then can we adopt some methods to prevent the host's thymus atrophy? Therefore, the writer starts to carry out animal studies to look for a way or drug to prevent the thymus atrophy of tumor-bearing mouse. He adopts cellular transplantation of immune organs to restore the function of immune organs, which is to explore a way to inhibit thymus atrophy of immune organs as the tumor grows and look for a method to restore the thymus function and reconstruct immunity. Then the writer conducts transplantations of fetal liver cells, fetal splenic cells and fetal thymocytes on mice, which is to reconstruct mice's immunologic function through adoptive immunity. The result indicates that after combined transplantation of three groups of cells (S, T and L), the completely regressive rate of short-term tumor is 40% and the rate of long-term tumor is 46.67%. The patient whose tumor has completely regressed can get the chance for long term survival.

4. The experimental study result reveals that one of cancer causes and pathogeneses may be the atrophy of thymus and the hypo-function of immune organs.

A series of animal experimental studies have been done for exploring the cause, pathogenesis and pathophysiology of cancer. The analysis and think of experimental results produce new discovery, new thinking and new revelation. That is, one of cancer causes may be the atrophy of thymus, the damage of thymus function and the hypo-function of immune organs. Therefore, Professor Xu Ze first proposes the idea in the world that one of cancer causes and pathogeneses may be the atrophy of thymus, the function damage of central immune organs, the hypo-function of immune organs, the reduction of immune surveillance function and immunologic escape. But what leads to the host's thymus atrophy? The writer ruminates over this question and speculates that the solid tumor might produce a kind of factor that can suppress thymus; nevertheless, the speculation needs further experimental researches. This kind of factor is temporarily called "thymus suppressor cancer-factor".

5. Subsequently, the writer raises the theoretical and experimental basis of "thymus protection for enhancing immunity; pulp protection for hemogenesis" in XZ-C immunologic mediation and control therapy.

Based on the inspiration from the above experimental results about the cause and pathogenesis of cancer, the new theory and new method of XZ-C immunologic mediation and control targeted therapy that first proposed by Professor Xu Ze have their theoretical and experimental basis. Our presented therapeutic principle and theory of "thymus protection for enhancing immunity; pulp protection for hemogenesis" are reasonable and scientific. Through sixteen years' clinical observation of over 12,000 patients with intermediate- or advanced-stage cancer in Twilight Specialist Out-patient Department, it can clearly show that this therapeutic principle with sixteen years' clinical application is correct and reasonable. The therapeutic effectiveness is satisfactory and trusted by patients.

As an old saying goes, "Once the headrope of fishing net is pulled up, all its meshes open." As long as the thymus atrophy might be one of cancer causes and pathogeneses, then theoretical basis of therapy must emerge at its proper moment.

6. Review the research history of cancer causes over the past one hundred years.

In the history of medicine, more than 2500 years ago, the scholar of ancient Greek-Hippocrates used a word "Cancer" to describe tumor. From then on people started the study and understanding of malignant tumor.

Until 1775, British doctor found that boys who sweep air flue for a long time are easy to suffer from carcinoma of scrotum. Then this doctor proposed the theory that the production of tumor is closely related to environmental factor.

In the late 19th, German doctor discovered that workers who touch dye have an impressively high proportion of suffering from bladder carcinoma. Afterwards some chemical substances successfully induce tumor in animals; tobacco components exert an influence on lung cancer; Aspergillus flavus has a definite relation with liver cancer. All these have provided direct evidences for the theory of cancer caused by chemical substances.

In 1908, Danish pathologist Ellerman and Bang found that chicken's leukemia can pass to healthy chickens through the filtered solution without cells. Two years later, American pathologist Rous proved that a kind of sarcoma in chicken is caused by virus, which establishes the theory of oncogenic virus.

The relation between human tumor and virus was established after EB virus was found in Burkitt lymphoma in 1964. The following researches show that EB virus and nasopharyngeal carcinoma, hepatitis b virus and primary carcinoma of liver, human papilloma virus and cervical carcinoma have an intimate relation. Those all lay a solid foundation for the theory of oncogenic virus.

People's knowledge of tumor causes continues to expand. Finding that sailors who often expose to the sun have a high risk of contracting skin carcinoma, people start to consider physical factors which may cause cancer. Until discovering that rate tumor can be induced after a large dosage of X-irradiation, people begin to confirm the theory of cancer caused by physical factors. In 1940s, after the explosion of atomic bombs in Japanese cities of Hiroshima and Nagasaki, various tumors and leukemias in survivors occur in high incidence. In the process of clinical cancer therapy, iatrogenic leukemia appears after the primary lesion is controlled. The two facts provide evidences for the theory of cancer caused by physical factors.

Although having had a preliminary knowledge of the tumor etiology, people still feel indefinite about the pathogenesis and pathophysiology of malignant tumor, and also lack effective preventive and therapeutic measures. Therefore, it is urgently necessary to have an extensive, in-depth and detailed study of tumor's pathogenesis and pathophysiology as well as prophylactic-therapeutic measures.

Reviewing the above research history of cancer over the past one hundred years, we can find that researches about cancer's cause, pathogeny, pathogenesis and pathophysiology are still quite rare. Until now whether or not cancer is a kind of disease can hardly be explained. That's because according to the definition, a disease must have the pathogeny, cause, pathogenesis, pathophysiology and pathology. But for one hundred years, people have always applied themselves to clinical and clinical fundamental researches of surgical operation, radiotherapy and chemotherapy. But in aspects of regular laboratory fundamental and clinical fundamental researches of cancer cell mutation, clone, proliferation, invasion, metastasis and implantation, people have done a little, such as invasion, metastasis, cancer embolus, immunization, endocrine and virus, etc. Exploring cancer's cause, pathogenesis, pathophysiology, metastasis and relapse must depend on the fundamental research of cancer-bearing animal models. All sorts of cancer animal models should be built with nude mice, in order to study the law and mechanism of cancer cells' invasions and metastases.

How to overcome the cancer I see two:

Second, the road of scientific research is to study the occurrence and the development of the whole process of prevention and treatment of cancer

1, Xu Ze (XU ZE) on the idea, strategy, planning diagram of conquering cancer

How to fight cancer

↓

Where is the road?

↓

Our ideas, strategies, experience should be divided into three parts

↓

Before the formation of cancer - for the prevention part - anti-mutation

↓

There may be malignant tendencies of precancerous lesions - for the intervention part

↓

Has been the treatment of primary cancer and the treatment of anti-metastatic part

2, the way-out of cancer treatment is in the "three early" and the way out of anti-cancer is to prevent

Cancer occurrence and development experience susceptibility stage, precancerous lesions and invasive stage; All the present tumor hospitals or tumor departments mainly focus on the cancer treatment in middle or advanced stage. The Therapeutic effects are poor. If patients in middle or advanced stage can accept surgical operation, then they will be treated surgically. But if not, they will only receive palliative treatment. Therefore, cancer treatment lies in "early detection, early diagnosis and early treatment". Generally, patients in the early stage will get a better therapeutic effect. The increase of therapeutic effect will certainly reduce the fatality rate of cancer. Consequently, we must put much emphasis on the study of early-stage diagnostic and therapeutic methods, and on the treatment of precancerous lesion for lessening medium-term or terminal patients in the invasive stage.

2 Occupying lesion can be seen through CT or MRI, middle or advanced stage

stage of susceptibility	precancerous lesion	early stage	no metastasis	have metastasized	
				local position	amphi position
①	②	③	④	⑤	⑥

① Cancer prevention

② Outpatient service of "three kinds of earliness"

③ Surgical operation

④ Place surgical operation first, radiotherapy, chemotherapy and biological TCM second

⑤ Possible to undergo surgical operation

⑥ To give treatment as carcinomatous metastasis

Figure 2: the whole process of cancer prevention and control

If patients have been treated well in the stage of precancerous lesion or early stage, then the number of patients in middle or advanced stage of invasion and metastasis will fall off. Thus, the cancer incidence rate will also decline. Therefore, we hold that the present tumor hospitals in various places mainly focus on the cancer treatment in middle or advanced stage. Even though the therapeutic result is effective, it can only bring the reduction of cancer mortality rate. But if ignoring the stage of susceptibility, precancerous lesion or early stage, it will be impossible to reduce the cancer incidence rate. Therefore, we must put much emphasis on the whole process of cancer production and growth. After all this is the real global change of strategic importance.

We have for many years of cancer surgery, the more treatment the more patients, the incidence of cancer is also rising, so I deeply appreciate that cancer should not only pay attention to treatment, but also to prevent prevention, to block the source. Cancer treatment was in the "three early" (early detection, early diagnosis, early treatment), anti-cancer out of the way is to prevent.

As stated above, the strategic center of gravity of tumor treatment and prevention moves forward. There are two aspects in its meaning. One is to prevent cancer by changing life style and improving environmental pollution; the other is to cure precancerous lesion for inhibiting cancer's development to the invasion stage, middle stage or advanced stage.

In 1990, our institute's specialist out-patient department of tumor surgery once opened the outpatient service of "three kinds of earliness" to carry out various endoscopies and biopsies, through which have found many atypical hyperplasia of stomach, intestinal metaplasia, atrophic gastritis and hyperplasia of mammary glands, etc. These "precancerous lesions" are difficult to treat. Then how to handle these precancerous lesions or precancerous conditions so as to prevent their cancerations urgently needs clinical researches to look for better treatment methods.

3, it should pay attention to the diagnosis and technology research of the basis and clinics of precancerous lesions.

The key to cancer treatment is in the "three early", and how to deal with precancerous lesions is a critical stage of cancer prevention and treatment.

The present cancer diagnosis mainly depends on image examinations of type-B ultrasonic, CT and MRI. But as soon as the cancer comes to light, it has reached the middle or advanced stage. Many patients have lost the chance of radical excision. Although the complex treatment has been done, the therapeutic effects are still poor. If the cancer is in the early stage or belongs to the carcinoma in situ, then the curative effect of operation will be better and the cancer can be cured. Therefore, the cancer treatment should strive for "three kinds of earliness", which refers to early detection, early diagnosis and early treatment.

Because cancer's pathogenic factors are not very clear, the primary prevention is still quite difficult.

Studies in recent years indicate that malignant tumor rarely has a direct carcinomatous change in normal tissues. Before the occurrence of tumor in clinical diagnosis, cancer often goes through quite a long evolution stage, which is the stage of precancerous lesion. Early identification and control of these precancerous lesions will bring positive significances for the secondary prevention of cancer.

What is precancerous lesion? The precancerous lesion is a histopathology concept, which refers to a kind of tissues with the dysplasia of cells. Precancerous lesion has the potential to become cancerous. If there is no cure in a long period, precancerous lesion will evolve into cancer. In other words, precancerous lesion just has the possibility of changing into cancer. But not all the precancerous lesions will eventually become cancer. Through proper treatments, precancerous lesions may return to their normal states or have a spontaneous regression.

Canceration is a developing process with several stages. There is a stage of precancerous lesion between normal cells and cancer. It is a slow process from precancerous lesion evolving into cancer, which needs many years or even more than ten years. The length of canceration course is closely related to the strength of carcinogenic factors, individual susceptibility and immunologic function. Therefore, the study of precancerous lesion is of great importance to cancer's prevention and control.

4, 1 / 3 above the cancer can be prevented

The tumor formation is a long process with several factors and stages. Precancerous lesion is of reversibility, so cancer is preventable.

The several factors, steps and stages of tumor formation have the following features.

The generation and growth of tumor can be roughly divided into several stages of initiation, promotion, metastasis and others. Cellular canceration induced by chemical carcinogen is a multistage process. The chemical carcinogenesis process of Experimental animals and the generating process of human tumors (such as colon cancer) have a series of changes, which are hyperplasia $\rightarrow$ pathological changes $\rightarrow$ benign tumor $\rightarrow$ malignant tumor $\rightarrow$ tumor metastasis, etc. The whole change process is complicated with multiple stages of initiation, promotion and evolution, etc. It often takes a long cytometaplasia time to change from normal cells to the tumor that can be detected clinically, which is a long cumulative process.

(1) Two-stage theory of tumor formation: In 1942, Beremblum carried out the experimental study of mouse's skin canceration induction, in which he used benzoapyrene to treat mice's skins for about one year, and only three out of one hundred and two mice suffered from skin tumors. If mice's skins were treated with benzoapyrene for several months and then treated with the tumor promoter-croton oil, thirty-six out of eighty-three mice suffered from skin cancers, whose incidence rate was ten times higher than that of using benzoapyrene alone. If mice's skins were first treated with croton oil for several months and then treated with a carcinogenic substance, there would be no induced tumor. If mice's skins were only treated with

croton oil for a long time, whose incidence rate of tumor would be lower than that of using benzoapyrene alone (1/106).

On the basis of this study results, Beremblum and Subik have proposed that cancerous process contains two different but intimate stages. One is a specific provocation stage. Small dosages of carcinogenic substance induce normal cells to become potential cancer cells. The other is nonspecific promoting stage. Potential cancer cells are further promoted to suffer from mutation and evolve into tumor under the action of tumor promoters, such as croton oil and others.

People hold that provocation process refers to the process that normal cells change into potential cancer cells under the action of carcinogenic substances. The time of promoting process is fairly short and generally irreversible. While promoting process is the process that potential cancer cells change into cancer cells under the action of tumor promoters. The early promoting stage is reversible but the late stage is irreversible.

Carcinogenic substance is a kind of mutagen, which plays a decisive role in canceration process. While cancer promoters do not have the mutagenicity, which can only promote potential cancer cells to have a further proliferation change and gradually evolve into cancer cells. During these two processes of provocation and promoting stages, induced cells grow out of control, escape from the host's immune surveillance, gradually form tumor cells with malignant phenotype and then evolve into tumor cells with infiltration and metastasis. This theory recognizes that tumor generation is quite a long process (months, years and even more than ten years) and will be impossible through a single factor or stage, which is very important to cancer prevention and control. It prompts that people have enough time to build up cancer-fighting ability, strengthen immunity, change life style and improve environmental pollution to prevent cancer. Intervention measures should be emphasized to tackle the reversible stage of cancer promoting.

(2) Multi-factor and multi-stage model of tumor formation: Vogelstein proposed the multi-stage model of genetics of colon cancer and histological change, which makes

people get a better idea of the formation of human colon tumor and molecular events happening in the process of development. It proves that the synergic action between cancer gene and cancer suppressor gene is the key factor for cellular canceration. The study conclusion is that canceration process of colon is a process with multiple involving genes and developing stages.

Carcinogenic action

Genetic change Variance of cancer suppressor gene

Genetic change Oncogene abnormality

Genetic change Oncogene abnormality Abnormality of cancer suppressor gene

Cloning expansion

Genetic change Oncogene abnormality Abnormality of cancer suppressor gene

Normal cells transformed cells precancerous lesion malignant cells clinical diagnosis of tumor metastatic tumor

Initiation stage promoting stage evolutional stage metastatic stage

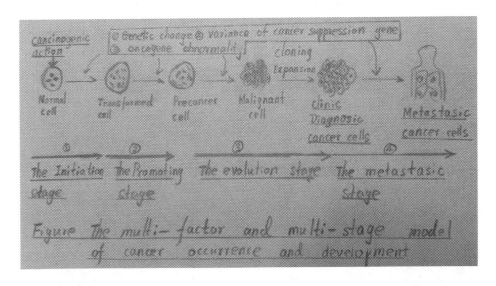

Figure 3 The Multi-factor and multi-stage model of Cancer occurrence and development

5, the way out of cancer is to prevent

For almost half a century, human spectrum of disease has undergone a drastic change. Most communicable diseases have been effectively controlled. Chronic diseases, such as cardiovascular diseases and malignant tumors have been the most serious diseases threatening human health.

Cancer has become the most serious public health problem in the world. Compared with other chronic diseases, cancer's prevention and control face a greater challenge.

Over the last thirty years, the fatality rate of cancer in China is on an obvious rise, which has occupied the number one in causes of death of urban and rural residents. On average, one out of every four deceased persons dies from cancer.

Cancer not only seriously threatens human health but also causes the rapid rise of hospitalization costs. The direct costs of cancer treatment in China are about one hundred billion RMB every year, which makes patients and the whole society bear a huge economic burden.

Although each country inputs a large number of funds to treat cancer patients, the five-year survival rate of some common cancers has no obvious improvement in the recent twenty years. For instance, during the years from 1974 to 1990 in USA, the five-year survival rate of esophagus cancer only rose from 7% to 9%, stomach cancer from 16% to 19%, liver cancer from 3% to 6%, lung cancer from 12% to 15% and that of pancreatic cancer remained the same as 3%.

What's to be done? Anti-cancer method lies in prevention. Prevention and intervention is the most important thing in the field of public health.

As for the malignant cancer, prevention outweighs therapy. Worldwide tumor researchers have reached a consensus of adjusting public health resources and policies, shifting strategic focus from therapy to prevention, and carrying out positive and effective studies of pre-warning, early diagnosis and intervention to lower tumor incidence rate and raise curative rate.

The evidence in *Cancer Report* provided by World Health Organization proves that up to one thirds of cancers can be prevented. As long as every national government, medical workers and the common people actively take actions and shift the research emphasis of tumor prevention and treatment to tumor prevention, they can prevent above one thirds or even about half of the cancers.

How to overcome the cancer I see the three:

Third, the road of scientific research is to carry out multidisciplinary research, special in-depth basis and clinical discipline research

1. Oncology study is the most complicated and difficult subject in the study of medical science. It ranges over multi-disciplinary knowledge and theories, which involves pathology, cytology, immunology, virology, molecular biology, medical genetics, immunopharmacology and molecular oncology. On the level of molecule, studying tumor pathogenesis and learning diseases causes can provide intervening and therapeutic measures for effective tumor prevention and treatment.

The present surgical operation is still the most important, frequently used, definite and effective therapeutic methods to treat malignant tumor. But relapse or metastasis often appears in the short or long term after surgical operation. Follow-up results of more than 3,000 patients who have accepted cancer surgeries of chest and abdomen discover that postoperative relapse and metastasis are key factors for long-term therapeutic effectiveness of surgical operation. Therefore, an issue is raised that the method and measure of preventing and treating postoperative relapse and metastasis are important for improving long-term therapeutic effectiveness. There is a must to carry out fundamental and clinical interdisciplinary study on resisting relapse and metastasis.

Since 1970s, in view of extremely high recurrence and metastatic rate after cancer operation, in order to prevent postoperative recurrence and metastasis, patients accept a series of adjuvant chemotherapies. Some patients have even started to accept preoperative chemotherapies, but the results are not fully up to expectations. Postoperative relapse and metastasis still come out in a short time. How to prevent recurrence and resist metastasis to get a good long-term effect is the matter that really deserves clinicians' serious and objective analysis, reflection, consider and study.

Now in the early 21st century, cancer recurrence and metastasis have become the "bottleneck" in cancer treatment. The main problem of cancer treatment still focuses on how to fight against metastasis. If not solving the metastasis after radical operation of cancer, cancer treatment cannot have a further improvement. We hold that tackling key cancer problem mainly depends on the resistance to metastasis. The key problem of cancer treatment is to tackle metastasis and recurrence.

2. Organize multi-disciplinary joint researches with large-scale cooperation among hospitals.

It is a must to carry out fundamental and clinical studies on resisting relapse and metastasis as well as multi-disciplinary joint researches with large-scale cooperation among hospitals. Organize professors, experts, scholars, doctors, master, and physicians in universities and colleges as well as their affiliated hospitals, independent hospitals and special hospitals on the level of Hubei province or Wuhan city and anti-cancer persons with lofty ideals to carry out research cooperation and walk the way of joint researches with large-scale cooperation. Advocate large-scale research cooperation, pay attention to organize scientific and technical force of each side and raise anti-cancer force on resisting cancer, metastasis and relapse.

Anti-cancer study needs to cover a wide range of subjects, which involve not only clinical medicine but also many borderline subjects, interdisciplinary subjects and basic subjects. The study of cancer metastasis and recurrence ranges over internal medicine, surgery, radiation, endocrine, drugs, immunity, molecular organism, virus, biological information, genetic engineering, life science, molecular chemistry, enzyme chemistry, environmental protection, traditional Chinese medicine and laboratory, etc. Wuhan city has talented persons in all of the above fields. Therefore, our city has a certain foundation to organize scientific and technical force of each side, pool the wisdom and efforts of everyone, walk the way of joint researches with large-scale cooperation, and raise the anti-metastasis and anti-relapse level together to benefit ten million of cancer patients.

Anti-cancer study, which is to overcome cancer, must involve fundamental and clinical studies on resisting relapse and metastasis, multi-disciplinary joint researches with large-scale cooperation among hospitals and the establishment of Wuhan anti-cancer institute.

With the energetic support of academician Qiu Fazu, through the declaration and preparation of Xu Ze, Li Huiqiao and other professors, upon the local tax authorities' approval, they finally set up Wuhan anti-cancer institute on June 21, 2009. Then they establish a special committee for treating cancer metastasis and relapse, also organize academic and research team of tackling cancer metastasis to carry out academic research, academic discuss and academic propaganda, and open academic workshop or seminar. Thu they have trained many batches of senior talented young and middle-aged people on the study and treatment of resisting cancer metastasis for our province and city.

The goal in anti-cancer study relies on "research". Under the guidance of scientific outlook on development, take the view angle of development and innovative spirit, focus on the front sight and look into the future to develop medical science, research into the cancer prevention and control, the generation and growth of cancer, the pathogenesis of cancer metastasis relapse as well as the prevention and treatment of cancer. The research line is to discover, raise, study, solve or explain the problem.

3. Assemble the following professional research groups which are closely related to cancer; deeply specialize in fundamental and clinical discipline researches.

In view of oncology study ranging over multi-disciplinary knowledge and theories, the related personnel must assemble relevant professional research groups to further specialize in and reply on the known knowledge and medical science in this subject, study and explore the unknown knowledge and future medical science in this subject, borderline subjects and interdisciplinary subjects to help conquer cancer. The following professional research groups should be set up. In the future, new subjects, interdisciplinary subjects or new industries may come out.

(1) Immunity and cancer research group: in the modern history of tumor treatment, surgical operation, chemotherapy and radiotherapy are basic treatment methods. They have made some progress, but the whole curative effects are still not fully up to expectations. Cancer still occupies the number one in human causes of death.

The modern immunological therapy of malignant tumor began in the early 1970s. Through decades of unremitting efforts, with the development of technology, different treatment methods and drugs, such as interferon, interleukin and LAK cells appear in succession and have also got certain curative effects. But the successful application of anti-CD20 monoclonal antibody (rituximab) in lymphoid tumor just truly realizes immunization therapy and also opens up a new tumor therapeutic area——immune targeted therapy.

The earlier chapters in this book have already made some introductions. After four-year experimental research history of exploring pathogenic factors, pathogenesis and pathophysiology with cancer-bearing animal models, our laboratory have found that removal of mouse's thymus will not affect the buildup of cancer-bearing animal model; injecting immunosuppressant can also contribute to the buildup of cancer-bearing animal model and with the gradual growth of cancer, thymus presents progressive atrophy. Therefore, Professor Xu Ze first proposes the idea in the world that one of cancer causes and pathogeneses may be the atrophy of thymus, the function damage of thymus and the reduction of immune function. He also raises theoretical basis and experimental evidence of new theory and method——XZ-C targeted therapy of immune regulation.

The latest clinical research task of immunity and cancer research group should be: ① to assess the condition of immunologic function in cancer patients; ② to monitor the curative effect of immune regulation therapy in cancer patients; ③ to quantitatively measure the condition of immunologic function in radiotherapy and chemotherapy patients.

2, virus and cancer research group

Some of the cancer is known to be closely related to the virus, the treatment should be considered the appropriate treatment measures.

(1) the etiology of certain cancerous tumors

As early as 1908 and 1911, people have found in succession that leukemia cells of chicken and filtering medium of chicken sarcoma can induce leukemia and sarcoma. In 1951, leukemia virus is found in mice. In the recent ten years, due to the rapid development of virology, immunology and molecular biochemistry, the study of tumor virus has also made fast progress. Thus it is confirmed one after the other that many viruses can induce tumor and even some human viruses (such as adenovirus and herpes simplex virus) can also induce the tumor of mouse. EB virus can induce the monkey's malignant tumor. Until now, only one quarter of over six hundred animal viruses are discovered to have the characteristic of causing tumor. Of special interest is chicken's Marek disease. It is a lymphoid tumor caused by chicken's simplex virus, which can lead to the mass mortality of chickens. Now this disease can be prevented with vaccine to get significant effect. Inspired by the important progress in the research of animal tumor virus, the research about virus pathogenesis of human tumor is also continuously developing. At present, it is discovered that some human tumors, such as Burkitt lymphoid tumor, nasopharyngeal cancer, leukaemia, sarcoma, breast cancer and cervical carcinoma, are relevant to virus.

3, hormone and cancer research group

it is necessary to have a further study on the carcinogenic factors of some known cancers related to hormone. Cancer treatment should lay stress on Hormone; while cancer prevention should pay attention to the further study of hormone based on the current knowledge.

Hormonal imbalance and tumor generation.

Hormone is an important chemical substance for neuron humor to adjust the body's development and function. Various hormones maintain a dynamic equilibrium according to the law of the unity of opposites. In the case of endocrine dyscrasia caused by diseases or some reasons, hormonal imbalance leads to some hormones' sustained action on sensitive tissues. This kind of abnormal chronic irritation may cause cell hyperplasia and canceration. Hormones with carcinogenic action refer to these that can promote histiocytes growth, such as estrogen of ovary, gonadotropic hormone of pituitary, thyrotrophic hormone and galactin, etc. To give the example of breast cancer, when lacking of pituitary and ovarian hormone promoting the growth of mammary gland, mammary gland will not grow. Undeveloped mammary tissue is hard to produce tumor. Therefore, hormone is a necessary factor to induce breast cancer. Experimental studies show that hormonal imbalance can induce tumors in thyroid gland, adenohypophysis, ovary, testicle, and adrenal cortex as well as accessory organs of uterine body, uterine neck, vagina and mammary gland. Hormone takes a long time to induce tumor; and the induction often needs a certain genetic background and environmental factors to be pathogenic conditions. Furthermore, hormone can also cooperate with other carcinogenic factors to cause canceration or act as the pathogenic condition of other factors. Some hormones, such as prostatic hormone, can promote cell differentiation and strengthen immune response. Whether the hyposecretion of prostatic hormone has an effect on canceration still needs a further study.

4, mycotoxin and cancer research group

: it is necessary to have a further study on the carcinogenic factors of some known tumors closely related to mycotoxin. Cancer treatment should lay stress on the study of relevant processing measures; while cancer prevention should pay attention to the further study of cancer prevention and treatment based on the current knowledge.

There are many metabolic products of fungus in nature, which can poison animal nervous, digestive, urinary or hematological system. These products are called Mycotoxin. Cases of human acute poisoning caused by mycotoxin have been reported a lot. In the recent ten years, some mycotoxins are gradually observed to have carcinogenic or cancer-promoting action on animals. Therefore, medical circle begin to pay more and more attention to studying the relation of fungus and its mycotoxin with human tumor.

① Experiment on cancerogenic mycotoxins: Experimental studies find that cancerogenic mycotoxins have lots of different kinds. At first feeding rates with ergot-infected grain can induce the neurofibroma of ear. Then the mouldy yellowed rice polluted by Penicillium islandicum Sopp are found in Japan; and the toxin extracted from rice can cause the hepatic cirrhosis, hepatic tumor and hepatic cancer of mice and rats. Only until 1960 when one hundred thousand turkeys were poisoned to death by groundnut flour polluted by Aspergillus flavus Liak in England and then Aflatoxin was found to have carcinogenic action on animals, cancerogenic problem of mycotoxin finally attracted wild attention. Repeated studies prove that Aspergillus flavus Liak and its derivatives have more than ten kinds, among which the best one with carcinogenic action is B_1. Mouldy grains polluted by Aflatoxin in a liver cancer-prone area of China are mixed in feed to feed rats. After six moths, the inducing rate of liver cancer is up to 80%, which also proves the carcinogenic action of mycotoxins. This kind of feed can also cause monkeys' liver cirrhosis as well as other hepatic lesions and induce liver cancer. Most of the induced liver cancers are hepatocellular cancers. Furthermore, this kind of feed can lead to the adenocarcinoma of kidney, stomach and colon; intratracheal instillation can cause squamous cell carcinoma of lung; subcutaneous injection can cause local sarcoma. There are relevant reports about causing tumors in other regions, such as lachrymal gland, mammary gland and ovary. Therefore, making a good job of mould proofing and ridding of oil and foodstuffs is important for exploring the prevention of some tumors and ensuring popular physical fitness.

In the esophageal cancer-prone area of China, Geotrichum candidum Link abstracted from edible pickled vegetable is proved to have the cancer-promoting action. Use 0.5ml fungus medium and 0.25mg / (kg · d) methyl benzyl nitrosamine to feed a series of A mice. During two to seven months, the incidence rate of proliferative lesion, papilloma and cancer in anterior stomach of A mice is obviously higher than that of other mice only fed with nitrosamine. Use the culture of Geotrichum candidum Link to feed rats for twenty months, and then papilloma in anterior stomach is induced. Some moldy food can cause precancerous lesion and early cancer in esophageal epithelium of animals. Some fungi abstracted from moldy food can increase the content of nitrite and secondary amine or produce nitrosamine in food. The above experiments expand the research field of the relation between fungus and tumor and also provide new clues for tumor pathogenesis.

So far some fungi and their toxins related to tumor generation have both carcinogenic action and cancer-promoting action. This kind of dualism deserves attention.

Victory over cancer, where is the road?

XU ZE thinks of that the road is in the scientific research —the road is the scientific research on the prevention and treatment of cancer, road under the guidance of the scientific concept of development, research and development. Through scientific research, human beings will overcome cancer, and ultimately will overcome cancer.

Why is the road in scientific research? Because it must be aware of the status of tumor disciplines exist what problems? How to do? "Oncology" is the most backward of a discipline in the current medical science, why? This is because the etiology, and pathogenesis and pathophysiology are not clear; the scientific research of the oncology is a scientific virgin land and it needs to have a lot of basic scientific research. Therefore, the basic and clinical scientific research is necessary.

How to carry out scientific research on cancer?

1, what is science?

Science - is the endless frontier. Our scientific research work, has been guided by the scientific concept of development, based on the known medicine, for the future of medicine, for the future science, emerging disciplines, edge disciplines, interdisciplinary, based on known science, known knowledge, to explore unknown science, Unknown knowledge. Longing hard work, practice the scientific concept of development, scientific research on the road, hard journey, step by step, step by step a scientific research footprint, for the forefront of science, for innovation, forward, to overcome the cancer research hall, By brick tian tile.

2, what is the study: research is to explore the truth of things, nature, law, medical research and theoretical research and clinical research, our dawn Cancer Institute specialist specialist research work, are following the following scientific research: A) that is, from the clinical work to find problems → ask questions → through experiments, research problems → through clinical validation, to solve the problem, and finally to solve the problem for the clinical or explain the problem. (B) our study is from the clinical → experimental → clinical → re-experimental → re-clinical, back to clinical to solve the problem. (C) our research are closely integrated with the theory and practice, our research topics are from the clinical, to find the focus of clinical problems and clinical breakthrough, after experimental and clinical validation, and then applied to clinical Clinical practical problems. Our research follows the evidence-based medicine, seeking truth from facts, talking with facts, using data to demonstrate that there are measurable experimental studies with clinical, validated data.

3, what should be studied? The object or target of the study is cancer, should study how to understand cancer, should study how cancer prevention and treatment. To study: ① to explore the truth of the cancer thing, nature, law; ② the occurrence of cancer, the etiology of development, pathogenesis; ③ cancer cell biological characteristics and biological behavior; ④ cancer cell transfer multi-step, multi-Cancer cells and the relationship between the host, who will determine the fate of cancer patients; ⑥ find a new method of prevention and treatment of cancer. Here refers to the occurrence of cancer, development, metastasis, recurrence and finally the whole process and its prevention and treatment.

The whole process of cancer occurrence and development is: susceptibility stage → precancerous stage → early → middle to late stage, ie, invasion stage and late stage of metastasis. So the cancer metastasis is not cancer all but only a stage of cancer. My second monograph is "new concept and new method of cancer metastasis therapy"; the third monograph is "new concept and new method of cancer treatment" is different, the former for the cancer stage of cancer, cancer Transfer therapy.

Cancer metastasis is only a stage of cancer occurrence and development - the stage of the invasion, the latter is the whole process of cancer development and the whole process of prevention and treatment, only the whole process of prevention and treatment, to overcome cancer.

4, how to study?

I made more than 60 years of tumor surgery, the more treatment and the more patients so that I deeply appreciate: cancer should not only pay attention to treatment, but also to pay attention to prevention, in order to stop at the source. The way-out of the treatment of cancer is in the "three early" (early detection, early diagnosis, early treatment). The way out of cancer is prevention. More than 90% of the cancer is caused by environmental factors and the protection and recovery of a good environment is an important part of the prevention of cancer. To Prevent cancer and to control cancer and to conquer cancer, why do I mention "control cancer"? Because energy-saving emission reduction, or /and pollution prevention or/and pollution control can effectively control the occurrence of cancer.

The prevention of cancer and cancer control should be used to prevent class I, II level prevention, III level prevention. The current emission reduction is a Class I prevention. Energy-saving emission reduction, pollution prevention, pollution abatement, is the scientific development and also is the great initiative of the prevention of cancer and cancer control for the benefit of the country and people. Scientific research must expand the horizon, the current forward, facing the future of science. Scientific research is mainly to study the unknown new scientific knowledge, so that science continues to move forward. All scientific research must be guided by the scientific concept of development. It should be under the guidance of the scientific concept of development, update thinking, change the concept of progress in the reform, innovation. Innovation must have the challenge of traditional ideas, cancer is a human disaster and the prevention of cancer and anti-cancer is the task of mankind.

Printed in the United States
By Bookmasters